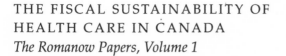

THE FISCAL SUSTAINABILITY OF HEALTH CARE IN CANADA
The Romanow Papers, Volume 1

Edited by Gregory P. Marchildon, Tom McIntosh, and Pierre-Gerlier Forest

The first of a three-volume set of selected papers from the Romanow Commission, this volume addresses the fiscal sustainability of health care in Canada from a variety of perspectives. The volume begins with an examination of cost factors, including those related to technology, ageing, and litigation, that directly affect the provision of health care. The next section deals with the financing and delivery of health services. The third set of essays looks at the intergovernmental dynamics of financing health care – one of the most contentious aspects of health-care policy in Canada. The final section discusses the influence of international trade regimes, particularly the World Trade Organization and the North American Free Trade Agreement, on the health-care system in Canada.

The contributors to the volume include well-known experts in the field, along with emerging scholars from Canada and abroad who bring fresh perspectives and insights to the topic. Presenting various diagnoses and policy prescriptions, the papers highlight the important issues that governments and health-care sector managers must confront to keep the Canadian health-care system viable in the twenty-first century.

GREGORY P. MARCHILDON holds a Canada research chair in public policy and economic history, and is professor of public administration at the University of Regina.

TOM MCINTOSH is assistant professor of political science and a member of the research faculty at the Saskatchewan Population Health and Evaluation Research Unit at the University of Regina.

PIERRE-GERLIER FOREST is professor of public policy and management in the department of political science at Université Laval. He currently holds the G.D.W. Cameron Chair with Health Canada.

The Fiscal Sustainability of Health Care in Canada

Edited by

Gregory P. Marchildon,

Tom McIntosh, and

Pierre-Gerlier Forest

UNIVERSITY OF TORONTO PRESS

Toronto Buffalo London

© University of Toronto Press Incorporated 2004
Toronto Buffalo London
Printed in Canada

ISBN 0-8020-8617-9

∞

Printed on acid-free paper

National Library of Canada Cataloguing in Publication

Romanow papers / edited by Gregory P. Marchildon,
Tom McIntosh, and Pierre-Gerlier Forest.

Contents: v. 1. The fiscal sustainability of health care in
Canada – v. 2. Changing health care in Canada – v. 3. The
governance of health care in Canada.
ISBN 0-8020-8626-8 (set).   ISBN 0-8020-8617-9 (v. 1).
ISBN 0-8020-8618-7 (v. 2.).   ISBN 0-8020-8619-5 (v. 3)

1. Medical care – Canada.   2. Medical policy – Canada.
3. Public health – Canada.   I. Marchildon, Gregory P., 1956–
II. McIntosh, Thomas A. (Thomas Allan), 1964–   III. Forest,
Pierre-Gerlier   IV. Title: The fiscal sustainability of health care
in Canada.   V. Title: Changing health care in Canada.   VI. Title:
The governance of health care in Canada.

RA449.R65 2004   362.1'0971   C2003-904073-9

University of Toronto Press acknowledges the financial assistance to its
publishing program of the Canada Council for the Arts and the Ontario
Arts Council.

University of Toronto Press acknowledges the financial support for its
publishing activities of the Government of Canada through the Book
Publishing Industry Development Program (BPIDP).

Contents

Acknowledgments

The papers in this volume, and its two companion volumes, were originally commissioned as part of the research activities of the Commission on the Future of Health Care in Canada headed by Roy J. Romanow and were first issued on the commission's web-site during the summer and autumn of 2002. From the outset of the commission's work, Mr Romanow made it clear to us that we had a mandate to ensure that the report's recommendations were based on the best available evidence and analysis. His support was unwavering for our contention that there were still important gaps in our knowledge about health care in Canada that needed to be filled. As the commission's executive director, director of research, and research coordinator, respectively, we were given an opportunity that few academics ever receive, and deeply appreciate the commissioner's trust in, and support of, our work on behalf of the commission.

We want also to acknowledge Steven Lewis's contribution to the development of the terms of reference for the authors and in helping us to match the right author with the right research assignment. Morris Barer, Rob Courchene, Donna Shilds-Poe, and Diane Watson of the Institute of Health Policy and Services Research of the Canadian Institutes of Health Research managed the often time-consuming independent peer review of the papers during the commission's work. The comments provided by the anonymous reviewers greatly improved the quality of the papers, and their efforts on behalf of the commission are appreciated. Louise Séguin-Guenette provided invaluable services in co-ordinating the tranlsation and publication of the papers on the commission's web-site and did so without ever losing her sense of humour. Don Moggridge, who reviewed the papers for the University of Toronto Press, was especially helpful in assisting us in turning a set of separate studies into three thematic volumes.

We also want to thank the staffs of the University of Toronto Press and the University of Ottawa Press, especially Virgil Duff (who acted as our experienced sherpa from the beginning), Bill Harnum, and Lynn Mackay, for their assistance in creating a more permanent legacy for these papers and for the work of the commission.

Finally, we want to thank our contributors, who approached their respective papers with enthusiasm and who so clearly shared our belief in the value of the overall project in which we were engaged.

GREGORY P. MARCHILDON
TOM McINTOSH
PIERRE-GERLIER FOREST

March 2003

Contributors

Gerard Boychuk is assistant professor of political science at the University of Waterloo.

Timothy Caulfield is associate professor in the Faculty of Law and the Faculty of Medicine at the University of Alberta.

Raisa B. Deber is professor of health policy, management, and evaluation in the Faculty of Medicine at the University of Toronto.

Robert G. Evans is professor of economics at the University of British Columbia.

Katherine Fierlbeck is associate professor of political science at Dalhousie University.

Pierre-Gerlier Forest is professor of public policy and management with the department of political science at Université Laval. He currently holds the G.D.W. Cameron Chair with Health Canada.

Sarah Hogan is a health economist working for the University of Otago School of Medicine in Dunedin, New Zealand.

Seamus Hogan is a senior lecturer in the Department of Economics at the University of Canterbury, Christchurch, New Zealand.

Jeremiah Hurley is professor of economics at McMaster University.

Martha Jackman is a professor in the Faculty of Law at the University of Ottawa.

Jon R. Johnson is a private lawyer specializing in international trade law and a partner in Goodmans LLP in Toronto.

Gregory P. Marchildon holds a Canada research chair in public policy and economic history, and is professor of public administration at the University of Regina.

Tom McIntosh is assistant professor of political science and a member of the research faculty at the Saskatchewan Population Health and Evaluation Research Unit at the University of Regina.

Steve Morgan is a professor at the University of British Columbia's Centre for Health Services and Policy Research.

Richard Ouellet is professor of law at Laval University.

Cynthia Ramsay is an independent health economist and business woman living in Vancouver.

Melissa Rode has an MSc from the London School of Economics and is currently an independent scholar and consultant living in Atlanta, Georgia.

Michael Rushton is associate professor at the Andrew Young School of Policy Studies at Georgia State University in Atlanta.

THE FISCAL SUSTAINABILITY OF
HEALTH CARE IN CANADA

The Many Worlds of Fiscal Sustainability

GREGORY P. MARCHILDON

At the core of the Romanow Commission's mandate was the expectation that its ultimate recommendations would 'ensure the long-term sustainability of a universally accessible, publicly funded health care system.' In April 2001, when the commission was established, the country was in the midst of a fierce debate about whether Canada's public system of health care was still sustainable or needed radical surgery to its funding and delivery. The debate then and now often generates more heat than light, largely because of participants differing and often-conflicting assumptions and definitions concerning sustainability.

The word 'sustain' originates from the Latin for hold or support. In contemporary environmentalism, 'sustainability' means achieving balance by avoiding the depletion or destruction of existing resources. In public finance, it means having a dependable revenue stream to finance ongoing government expenditures. Combining both usages, the Romanow Commission's final report (Commission 2002, 1) describes 'sustainability' as the sufficiency of resources 'over the long term to provide timely access to quality services that address Canadians' evolving health needs.' These resources extend beyond financial to human resources, including providers such as nurses, physicians, dentists and other direct providers as well as hospital, clinic, and health authority managers, and to physical resources, including hospital and clinic facilities; pieces of equipment, such as X-rays, magnetic resonance imaging (MRIs), and other advanced diagnostic imaging, as well as the information-technology infrastructure that supports the health system.

The word 'fiscal' generally refers to financial resources only. This in itself is not problematic, since all resources can theoretically be expressed in terms of the financial resources required to hire, purchase, maintain, and update human and physical resources over time. A problem, however, arises with the way in which the phrase 'fiscal sustainability' is then interpreted. Naturally, governments and public-finance economists focus on the state's ability to fund public health care with existing government revenues. Fiscal sustainability in this context involves not only revenues sufficient to fund line items in a government's health and health-care budget, but also the growth of those items relative to other expenditures and whether growing expenditures on health are 'crowding out' government's capacity to fund its other priorities.

Health-policy experts tend to look beyond existing government budgets to the effectiveness of health expenditures, whether funded through public, private, or mixed sources. If shifting resources from the public sector to the private increases total effectiveness, then societal welfare might be improved. More often than not, however, this type of cost shifting can actually reduce total welfare, even if it improves a governmental balance sheet in the short run. Moreover, citizens intuitively understand that they pay all the costs associated with health and health care, whether through taxes or through private user fees and insurance premiums. They therefore want to know the total cost for themselves and their families.

Public finance and health policy approaches are both useful – indeed essential – to any analysis of fiscal sustainability. But if their differing assumptions and definitions are not clearly articulated, they can and do hinder understanding. This has been the essential problem in the debate over fiscal sustainability in Canada. The commission's final report sets out total expenditures (public and private) in the first chapter, entitled 'Sustaining Medicare,' and evaluates the Canadian system in terms of both sets of costs. It is important not to limit assessments of fiscal sustainability to one or other approach and to examine spending on both total health care *and* public health care.

In terms of governance, financing, and delivery, Canada's health-care system can be categorized in four parts: hospital and physicians' services, governed by the federal Canada Health Act (CHA); specialized health goods and services financed and administered by the federal government; non-CHA portions of provincial plans; and private health goods and services. The first group, hospital and physicians' services, constituted about 42.4 per cent of total expenditures on health care in Canada in the fiscal year 2001–02. These services are administered through single-payer insurance systems by provinces and territories, but under a broad set of rules set by Ottawa through the CHA and enforced through federal cash transfers to the provinces. Funding comes from the provincial and federal tax systems and, in two provinces, from premiums that are also taxes by another name. Access is based strictly on medical need, and user fees are not permitted. Delivery is effected mainly through self-employed physicians, salaried nurses, and other health providers employed by regional health authorities (RHAs), hospitals, or other, mainly public or not-for-profit, non-governmental bodies.

The second category consists of federally administered health services and goods. These include public and preventive health initiatives, monitoring and regulation of drug and food safety, and health care services for members of the armed forces and the Royal Canadian Mounted Police and for First Nations and Inuit communities, which directly administer a number of programs and benefits. This category made up 5 per cent of total health expenditures in 2001–02.

The third group of services includes prescription drug plans, home care, and long-term programs, along with whatever else provincial health plans cover aside from hospital and physicians' services. Rules on access are set by the provinces. These services amounted to 25.2 per cent of health expenditures in Canada in 2001–02. Funding is provided through provincial tax systems, supplemented by user fees, including co-payments and insurance deductibles. Provincial plans coexist with (and are sometimes complementary to) private, often employment-based, insurance plans. Delivery takes many forms but tends to be non-governmental, generally involving the not-for-profit and for-profit sectors.

Finally, the fourth category – dental, vision, and other private health-care goods and services not covered by provincial plans – constituted 27.4 per cent of health expenditures in 2001–02. Consumers pay either directly or indirectly through third-party insurance policies, often employment-based. Health providers in this category, including dentists, dental hygienists, psychologists, pharmacists (outside hospitals), optometrists, and chiropractors and their support personnel, work predominantly within the private sector.

In its final report, *Building on Values*, the Romanow Commission (2002) relied heavily on a series of discussion papers prepared by authors who looked at fiscal sustainability from varying perspectives and assumptions. These scholars answered a spectrum of questions concerning fiscal sustainability, with some moving into new territory in order to provide clearer assumptions and definitions than are currently available in the literature. This volume begins with an examination of cost factors, including technology, ageing, and litigation, that directly affect the growth of health care. The next section deals with the financing and delivery of health services, especially with whether there are better alternatives to the way the Canadian system currently operates. The third set of essays grapples with the intergovernmental dynamics of financing health care, which has become one of the most contentious aspects of health-care policy in Canada. Going beyond domestic factors, the fourth and final section addresses the emerging influence of international trade regimes, particularly the World Trade Organization and the North American Free Trade Agreement, on the fiscal sustainability of health care in Canada.

Cost Factors

In broad terms, both private and public health expenditures have been on the rise in Canada since 1945. Approximately 7 per cent of gross domestic product (GDP) was devoted to health care in 1970, compared to 9.1 per cent thirty years later. The figures for public health care are 5 per cent of GDP in 1970, compared to 6.5 per cent in 2000 (Commission 2002, Appendix E). This trend holds whether as a percentage of GDP or in inflation-adjusted per-capita expenditures.

The same upward trend has been observed in every OECD country. Health is a superior good – as incomes rise, people and societies spend progressively more on health care, on leisure activities, and on luxury goods, relative to other goods and services. Indeed, growing income is the most robust variable associated with higher levels of health spending in all countries (Gerdtham and Jönsson 2000).

Canada does differ from other OECD countries in experiencing a sharper decline in public health-care expenditures in the early to mid-1990s. This was a consequence of the recession of the early 1990s, combined with aggressive fiscal 'belt tightening' by the provinces after years – in some cases, decades – of deficit financing. Virtually every province made a major attempt to contain health costs, often restructuring delivery of health care. 'Health reform' became inextricably linked with cost cutting, making such efforts more difficult in subsequent years. Then, beginning in 1997, provincial health-care costs began to bounce back up, despite implementation of the Canada Health and Social Transfer (CHST) and, with it, sizeable cuts in Ottawa's cash transfers to the provinces. For the next five fiscal years, real (1997 constant-dollar) public-sector health expenditures grew by an average of close to 5 per cent per year (Commission 2002, Appendix E). The sudden switch to spending after cost reduction was the product of a number of factors – pent-up demand for health care after years of cost containment; the cost of educating, training, and hiring new health professionals after years of restricting supply; and government and public fatigue with cost cutting and reform.

According to the Canadian Institute for Health Information (CIHI 2002), this rapid growth is beginning to slow, but the pressure of health-care spending on provincial budgets has been intense since 1997. By the fiscal year 1999–2000, health spending was accounting for more than 35 per cent of total provincial and territorial program spending, compared to 28 per cent 25 years earlier. 'Cost-drivers' within health budgets – the individual sectors that are growing much more rapidly than others – have been crucial here. A short list of the more commonly identified cost-drivers would include prescription drugs, technology, ageing, genetic testing, and medical-malpractice litigation.

There is little argument concerning prescription drugs. In 1975, they made up about 6 per cent of health-care spending in Canada – a share that remained stable until the mid-1980s, when drug costs began to soar. By 2001, they accounted for 12 per cent of total spending on health care. Combined with over-the-counter drugs, they cost more in total than physicians' services. Clearly, provincial governments have been much affected by rising costs for prescription drugs given their drug plans.

Other cost-drivers are less well understood, however, and the Romanow Commission asked various experts to explore them in greater detail. Steve Morgan and Jeremiah Hurley (chapter 1) analyse the health-technology cost-driver. They distinguish between change caused by the introduction of new products and new technologies and by major changes in the way existing technologies are used. The introduction of new prescription drugs, for example, would fall within the former category, while new uses for positron-emission tomography (PET) scanners – a technology that has been around for over 30 years – would be an example of the latter. Both types of change can be significant cost-drivers.

Morgan and Hurley identify three major present and future technological cost-drivers: increases in the use and cost of certain classes of
prescription drugs; the expanded use of advanced diagnostic imaging;
and the cost of genetic testing and associated goods and services. All
are directly affected by broader societal and scientific factors, including
an ageing population, the influence of consumer-directed marketing of
health technologies, and advances in the genetic sciences.

The average family in Canada today consumes just over $1,200 a
year in prescription drugs and receives about 30 prescriptions for a
family of three, at about $40 per prescription. This statistical average
obscures the fact that drug consumption is unevenly distributed, with
a majority of Canadians using far less than the average, but a sizeable
minority, far more. At least one-half of these drugs now fall into five
classes: lipid-reducing agents, psychotropic, gastrointestinal, anti-
hypertensives (analgesics), and anti-infectives. In Québec alone,
spending on these five classes of drugs amounted to almost $1.8 billion
in 2000 (Quebec 2001). Most of these drugs are patented products, with
20 years of protection from competition. As Morgan and Hurley point
out, the policy role of governments should be to ensure that the price
that Canadians collectively pay for these prescription drugs is equal to
their benefit relative to all other alternatives. This means going beyond
testing the clinical effectiveness of drugs to a full pharmaco-economic
evaluation. This is essential, given that drugs will probably remain the
fastest growing component of health-care expenditures for at least the
next decade.

Diagnostic imaging has been a major cost factor in all OECD countries, but in Canada efforts at cost containment in the early to mid-
1990s reduced capital expenditures, including purchases of diagnostic
equipment, just as new techniques were being introduced or old ones
were being adapted for new purposes. Canada found itself well below
the OECD average in availability of computed-tomography (CT) scanners and magnetic resonance imaging (MRIs). This has created bottle-
necks in access and a market for private, advanced diagnostic clinics to
allow people to jump queues in the public system. Advanced diagnostic imaging is a valuable tool, and only significant investments can
improve the quality of diagnosis and shorten waiting times.

In contrast, genetic testing is just beginning to affect health-care
costs. It is too early to tell how it will influence expenditure patterns,
but some observers believe that it will become the fastest-growing sector of health care within the decade. Moreover, government policy will

shape the trajectory of costs, given the patent protection built into the extremely high selling price of genetic tests and their associated products and services.

Recently, the impact of ageing on health-care costs has become a major issue. Debate has polarized around two starkly conflicting scenarios – a pessimistic view, in which a swelling number of ageing 'baby boomers' will swamp public health care, and an optimistic view in which ageing will have little or no appreciable impact, in the light of the experience of countries currently facing a similar demographic challenge.

It is estimated that the population bubble created by the baby boom will peak in 2030. Seamus Hogan and Sarah Hogan (chapter 2) attribute 0.9 per cent of the forecast 2.9 per cent real annual growth in Canadian health expenditures per capita to demographic factors. Of this amount, they assign two-thirds to the 'baby boom' bubble (i.e., fertility) and one-third to people living longer (i.e., mortality). They see neither the pessimistic nor the optimistic perspective as correct. The age structure of Canadian society will have a modest but noticeable impact on health-care costs. While the Hogans argue that it would be foolhardy to redesign health care solely to meet this challenge, they urge governments to plan ahead in order to meet a growing demand for certain types of medical care, including cardiovascular and orthopaedic surgical procedures. They also suggest that governments consider redesigning funding mechanisms, by introducing some pre-funding mechanism or by building a demographic factor into future federal health transfers to assist the provinces under greatest pressure from an ageing population.

Pre-funding would make sense probably only at the provincial level, which control the majority of revenues used for funding health care and almost all service delivery. While the Romanow Commission rejected major change in funding mechanisms, it did agree to some experimentation with a 'population-based' federal formula for transfer funding. As a consequence, it recommended two short-term funds – one for diagnostic services, the other for rural and remote health – to be distributed on a population-health basis that takes into account demographic ageing. Although the larger and wealthier provinces resist anything other than a per-capita formula for transfers, a well-designed population-based formula would alleviate some of the pressure on the provinces hardest hit by the demands of an ageing baby boom.

In U.S. health care, litigation, particularly medical-malpractice actions against physicians, is increasing health costs. While the volume of lawsuits per capita is far less in Canada, and the damage settlements and court awards for malpractice are far lower, this activity may become more prevalent and costlier. For this reason, the commission asked Timothy Caulfield (chapter 3) to examine the current legal framework and see whether it will aid or hinder health reform. The purpose of tort law is to ensure that the victims of medical malpractice receive compensation from the health providers at fault and thereby to discourage similar mistakes in the future. Given the time and cost involved in launching and sustaining a lawsuit, however, only a fraction of those people harmed ever actually receive compensation.

More important, as Caulfield points out, the current malpractice system may pose a significant barrier to systematic reform intended to reduce the incidence of medical error, improve overall quality, and introduce a team approach to primary care. Fearing litigation, health providers are reluctant to admit errors and may even hide them to avoid lawsuits, whereas quality improvement requires greater 'transparency.' The common law of fiduciary responsibility makes *individual* health providers responsible for a standard of care appropriate to provider's professional qualifications and experience. If a given physician is the most highly trained and experienced member of a primary-care team, then he or she will probably be held relatively more responsible for the treatment of a patient, thereby discouraging the physician from sharing responsibility.

For all these reasons, Caulfield argues that tort reform may be an essential complement to quality improvement, such as the quality-council approach recommended by the Fyke Commission (Saskatchewan 2001) and the 'shared-care' method of primary care recommended in all recent reports on health reform in Canada. He suggests replacing the common-law tort system with provincially legislated medical no-fault insurance, similar to the central-government schemes in New Zealand and Sweden.

Although it has not influenced Canada's approach to medical malpractice, the introduction of the Charter of Rights and Freedoms in 1982 has changed many other aspects of Canadian law. The question is whether the Charter has yet created, or could potentially create, a legal right to essential medical care enforceable by the courts and thereby increase pressure on public health-care spending. Martha Jackman (chapter 4) suggests that the cost implications of the Charter are modest. Its Section 7 establishes the 'right to life, liberty and security of the person and the right not to be deprived thereof except in accordance with the principles of fundamental justice.' So far, the 'right to life' does not confer an unqualified right to receive or to provide (or even to refuse) health care, but 'fundamental justice' does 'raise the bar' in terms of the standard that is, and will be, imposed by the courts for decision making in health care by requiring more input from patients. The requirement to offer meaningful patient participation in decision making, as well as more inclusive decision making at the broader policy and regulatory levels, may increase short-term costs but should result in more effective decisions in the medium or long term.

Although the Romanow Commission was sympathetic to the logic of Timothy Caulfield's essay, provincial tort reform lay a little beyond its mandate and expertise. However, legal reform needs to be considered by provincial governments that are serious about improving quality and reforming primary care. The commission was also influenced by Martha Jackman's view concerning the impact of the Charter and hoped that its recommendation concerning some public representation in its proposed Health Council of Canada would help increase patients' participation in decision making.

The Financing and Delivery of Health Care

Given the long-term trend of rising costs in health care, recent attention to the financing of these expenditures is hardly surprising. Naturally, the exact form of financing varies, at times quite considerably, from country to country, and in a federation such as Canada, even from province to province. And while issues of service delivery can be viewed as analytically separate from financing, there are important links between them, as the mode of financing can influence the type of delivery, while the nature of delivery can also have an impact on funding.

There are three basic sources of funding for all health-care systems (Mossialos and Dixon 2002). First, taxation comes in many forms, including direct taxes, such as personal income tax, and indirect taxes, such as consumption taxes on goods and services. In Canada, personal income and consumption taxes provide most funding for major social programs such as public health care. The federal government levies the Goods and Services Tax (GST), and the provinces, sales tax. Unlike other OECD countries such as France, Germany, and Japan, Canada does not rely on a social-insurance form of taxation – generally payroll taxes on employment income – to pay for health care.

Second, user fees are costs imposed directly on people as they consume health and health-care goods or services. They include co-payments made by individuals to share the cost of a particular health good or service, as well as deductibles under any insurance plan (public or private) whose payment is triggered by the use of health care. The key element is the direct linkage between use and payment. Canada, unlike most Western european countries, prohibits user fees under the terms of the Canada Health Act, for publicly insured hospital and physicians' services. But, unlike many citizens of wealthier European countries, Canadians often pay very large user fees for non-covered goods and services, including prescription drugs and dental care. In terms of public insurance coverage, the Canadian system is considered to be narrow but deep relative to European public plans that include prescription drugs, home care, and (in some cases) dental care, but with co-payments for hospital and physicians' services.

Health economist Robert Evans (chapter 5) describes the nature of health funding in Canada and presents a revenue-expenditure-income model that is the health equivalent of a national income model. Any shift in the existing federal–provincial financing mix will generate distributional gains and losses to individual citizens, as well as to regions. As a consequence, the controversy over financing is essentially a debate over 'who pays' and is by definition heavily value-laden.

According to the evidence presented by Evans, single-payer systems funded through general taxation are both more effective in terms of cost control and more equitable, in distributing benefits to those with the greatest health needs, than the alternatives. Moreover, public health care in Canada is highly redistributional, to the point that there is an inverse relationship between tax contributions and actual usage of services (Mustard et al. 1998). In other words, wealth and health are strongly correlated, as are poverty and illness. This means, according to Evans, that any move to a system based more on user fees, whether through medical savings accounts (MSAs), co-payments, or making health care a taxable benefit, will result in an additional burden on those least able to pay. Even if those individuals are exempted from paying, the additional burden inevitably falls on the middle class. And if individuals are allowed to purchase private insurance to cover such user fees, then the tax-expenditure subsidies generally used to support such multi-payer insurance schemes increase the regressiveness of the system.

Cynthia Ramsay (chapter 6) argues that while single-payer systems appear efficient, the cost-saving methods actually imposed by governments may be as destructive of equity as partial insurance coverage in a multi-payer system as in the United States. In her view, the goal of universal coverage can be achieved through the market, and she suggests that there is no direct causal link between the degree of public financing and positive system outcomes in terms of access, quality, and cost.

Ramsay points out that waiting lists are now a common feature of the Canadian system and are a product of public-sector rationing that blocks access for everyone. The inference is that some market-determined access based on user fees might actually produce a better outcome for the majority of Canadians. Ramsay argues that governments are more effective in containing costs than private systems, but they do so through the application of 'brute force – capping physicians' fees, closing hospitals, and delisting services' and without the quality features of some private systems. She points to the quality (and efficiency) outcomes of California's Kaiser Permanente – a non-profit health management organization (HMO) – as an example of what could be achieved through a private, competitive health system. Citing the RAND study used by David Gratzer (1999), Ramsay supports the introduction of user fees to reconnect cost with use. In particular, she recommends MSAs, with exemptions for the poorest members of society and a cap once a certain level of catastrophic cost is reached.

Both the RAND study and the imputed impact and incentive effects of user fees are highly contested. Nonetheless, it is difficult to argue with the evidence presented by Robert Evans that user fees, however imposed, will have a regressive impact on those who need and use the system most. Nor has the administrative efficiency of a single-payer system of public health insurance ever been disproven. On the contrary, the Romanow Commission relied on a series of studies led by Stephanie Woolhandler and David Himmelstein (1991; 2002) demonstrating that U.S. administrative costs – related to billing, contracting, reviewing utilization, and marketing involved in multi-payer insurance – are triple Canada's. In the end, relying in part on the evidence adduced in a comparative study of European co-payment schemes on its behalf (CES 2001), the Romanow Commission recommended against user fees for hospital and physicians' services, concluding that any potentially beneficial incentive effects in curbing unnecessary medical use were more than outweighed by their negative impact on necessary medical use.

Finally, the commission rejected policy options involving replacing parts of the current provincial single-payer insurance systems with multi-payer private insurance, recommending instead the gradual expansion of the single-payer system beyond hospitals and physicians, in part because of its proven administrative efficiency. The commission also endorsed the evidence presented by Robert Evans that the tax system remains the most efficient and equitable system in which to raise revenue for public health care. That said, rationing through the public system can create other barriers to access that are as unacceptable as those generated by user fees, and these must be reduced or eliminated on an ongoing basis for any public system to remain viable.

Cynthia Ramsay's use of the Kaiser Permanente illustration also shows that, while questions concerning financing and delivery are separate in theory, they are often linked in practice. The example also highlights the confusion surrounding the debate over public versus private modes of financing and delivery that is currently raging in virtually all OECD countries – a debate that Raisa Deber (chapter 7) attempts to clarify by dissecting the different modes of delivery and the characteristics associated with each. As she points out, the key reason for the argument has been the perceived inability of organizations associated with public systems to meet patients' needs. These problems may include the growing length of waiting lists, the low morale of health providers, the lack of service orientation towards the users of the system, and inflexible labour and budgetary arrangements. In contrast, private organizations are often seen as free from restrictive collective labour agreements and inflexible job descriptions and more efficient in managerial and administrative terms because of market disciplines. Critics respond by pointing out that private organizations achieve this efficiency by hiring non-union personnel, evading government cost controls, and 'cream skimming' healthier patients, leaving the difficult and costly cases for the public system.

The debate is much confused by the polar views of the 'public' and 'private' sectors in health-care delivery. As Deber explains, most of the organizations actually delivering health care in Canada are not-for-profit (NFP) organizations rather than public bodies directly controlled and operated by government, although they are sometimes lumped in the private-for-profit category because of their 'private' character and at other times classified as 'public' because of their non-profit, public purpose. Deber proposes four categories, rather than the usual bipolar 'public–private' classification – public delivery, private NFP delivery, private for-profit small business delivery, and private corporate delivery. This scheme is more analytically powerful than bipolar classifications. The only organization that remains difficult to pigeon-hole is the regional health authority (RHA), a body that has delegated powers from the province for health administration and delivery but is more connected to, and acts less at arm's length from, government than the typical private NFP organization.

Deber summarizes the literature concerning the performance of these various organizational forms and concludes that there are 'some systematic differences' at least in terms of 'incentives and values inherent.' For example, public and NFP organizations have few incentives to increase efficiency or improve client services, but for-profit firms have few incentives to minimize the amount that they bill payers, to invest more in the quality of care (unless not doing so will harm their businesses), or to spend on non-profitable activities, including research and community services. These 'tendencies can only be controlled through effective performance monitoring and measuring measures that are costly and difficult to implement for public, NFP, and for-profit organizations.'

Deber concludes that the type of competition introduced through private delivery can often set up providers as rivals. Naturally, they will behave accordingly, treating information as proprietal and keeping their distance from other providers. Such behaviour can run counter to the integration and co-ordination of services that has been called for by most patients, providers, and recent reports on health care. The Romanow Commission concluded on the basis of Deber's review, as well as other studies, that the private-for-profit sector is no more efficient than the public or NFP sectors. At the same time, however, it saw monitoring and measurement performance as necessary spurs to existing public and NFP organizations to improve service delivery.

Federal–Provincial Fiscal Dynamics

These questions of financing and delivery are further complicated by the nature of a federal state and the fact that public health care in Canada is governed and funded by two orders of government. Provinces have primary, but not sole, jurisdiction over the organization and delivery of health-care services, largely because the constitutional division of powers does not address health and health care directly. While the provinces are responsible for most aspects of administration and delivery, the federal government has major responsibilities in health protection and regulation, including the regulation and approval of prescription drugs, and for providing health services to specific groups, most notably First Nations and Inuit peoples. On the fiscal side, Ottawa exercises a spending power through transferring to the provinces funds notionally earmarked for health care, in return for which provincial governments are expected to comply with the principles of the Canada Health Act.

The 'federal spending power' is the focus of much of the dynamic tension between the two orders of government. The convoluted history of these fiscal transfers is almost incomprehensible to the uninitiated and further complicated by shifts in the actual transfer regimes over time. For the first twenty years of public health care, federal cash transfers for provincial hospital and physician plans were based on the principle of the federal government's sharing expenses with the provinces on a 50–50 basis. This changed in 1977 with the introduction of Established Programs Financing (EPF), in which Ottawa 'split' the transfer into two, with roughly half going eventually to the provinces in the form of a permanent tax transfer and the other half flowing annually in the form of a cash amount calculated in relation to growth in the economy rather than to health-care expenditures. This capped the growth of transfers for Ottawa and gave greater flexibility to the provinces for spending. It also shifted fiscal risk to the provinces, gave Ottawa less say on the overall direction of the system, and mixed policy objectives by including postsecondary education with health. In 1996, the new CHST regime added transfers for social assistance and social services to health and education. It also removed the escalator based on economic growth. The actual amount of cash transfers fell significantly, in return for which provinces were to receive even more flexibility in their programmatic use of the transfers.

No matter how calculated, federal cash transfers to the provinces for health care (and for other major provincial social programs, including postsecondary education and social assistance) have declined over the past two decades (Commission 2002, Appendix E). This has suggested to many observers that only a federal reinvestment in social spending can ensure that provinces will not, as time goes on, be forced to 'buy' health care at the expense of education and social welfare. This complements political arguments concerning what is 'fair,' based on the original medicare deal between the provinces. In fact, in their paper, public-finance economists Melissa Rode and Michael Rushton (chapter 8) conclude that no new taxes or user fees are required to make up the public funding shortage, as long as the federal government returns to its 'historic' share of funding.

Indeed, few argue against the need for an additional federal contribution. The real debate focuses on the nature and form of that contribution. Concerned about the federal government's past behaviour in unilaterally reducing transfers for health and the resulting damage to the predictability of health funding, Rode and Rushton argue that a transfer of additional tax room to the provinces would be more effective at 'locking in' the federal government for the long term while giving the provinces the flexibility that they need in administering and delivering health care. This policy recommendation contrasts sharply with the view, expressed by Tom Kent (2002) and others (Maslove 1998), that only an increase in the cash portion of the transfer can guarantee a continuing federal role in order to preserve the national dimensions of health care.

Of the three major research projects initiated by the commission, one dealt with the federal–provincial dimensions of health care, including the transfer regime. Led by the Institute of Intergovernmental Relations (2002) at Queen's University, the study also endorsed the view that only a federal cash transfer could achieve the broader policy objective of a health system with significant pan-Canadian features. This was the view ultimately endorsed by the Romanow Commission, which rejected a tax transfer in favour of a pure cash transfer for three reasons: first, tax transfers may encourage rather than reduce the likelihood of future intergovernmental warfare if provinces ignore or discount them shortly after obtaining them; second, the public has no guarantee that the revenue generated from tax points will go to health care; and, third, Ottawa's ability to exercise leverage in setting and upholding the national dimensions of public health care is directly proportional to its cash contribution.

Despite the long-term decline in federal cash transfers, as well as the rapid growth in provincial health spending since the late 1990s, Gerard Boychuk (chapter 9) argues that there is little evidence of a fiscal crisis in health funding. The provinces are playing 'catch-up' after historically low levels of investment in the early to mid-1990s – an argument recently detailed by Carolyn Tuohy (2002). Boychuk points out that while provinces' health expenditures have been rising as a proportion of their total program expenditures, they make up the same proportion of total provincial revenues as they did in 1991, and he argues that the latter comparison is a superior measure of fiscal sustainability, as it compares spending to resources actually available. With the decline in federal transfers, an increasing proportion of provincial own-source revenues has been flowing to health care rather than to other provincial programs and debt retirement. Add to this a relatively shrinking revenue base through tax cuts (where this has occurred), and a real 'health squeeze' emerges in provincial budget setting. Boychuk argues that this has created the impression of 'crowding out.' A permanent increase in federal transfers will make provincial health expenditures 'sustainable,' assuming that provincial governments are willing and able to control costs and do not slash taxes.

The issue of tax cutting is an important one and is linked to the challenge of debt repayment. Since at least the early 1970s, both orders of government have engaged in systematic deficit financing. By the 1990s, provincial and federal debt levels were dangerously high and threatened the fiscal sustainability of the entire public sector. Taxes, including sales and income tax, were increased to reduce deficits, even while public services were cut back. As a consequence, the general public was paying more yet getting less service in return, and governments responded by beginning to reduce taxes as the debt began to be tamed by the late 1990s. According to Armine Yalnizyan's (2002) estimate, federal and provincial tax cuts since that time now amount to approximately $40 billion worth of forgone revenues on an annual basis, and the debate over the choice between tax cuts and increased investment in public programs such as health care continues.

Boychuk also makes the important point that the structural features of federal–provincial relations themselves create much of the current instability and dysfunctionality in health care, as does the lack of transparency in funding and responsibilities. On the one hand, Ottawa wants to minimize its fiscal liability while maximizing its visibility as the defender of health care through enforcing the Canada Health Act. On the other hand, the provinces want to minimize any constraints on their health-care spending and program design while maximizing federal funding. Since it is almost impossible for the general public to evaluate the relative contributions of each order of government,

Ottawa can allow its contribution to slide, even as it continues to hold itself out as the defender of national medicare. The provinces, in contrast, have much incentive to encourage the perception of a health-care crisis in order to lever more money out of the federal government, thereby relieving the pressure on their overall provincial budgets. The end result is a loss of confidence by the general public in both Ottawa and the provinces and a decline in the ability of government generally to manage, much less improve, public health care.

Consistent with this analysis, Katherine Fierlbeck (chapter 10) argues that any policy solution for health care in Canada also requires a new intergovernmental arrangement, one that both respects and makes more transparent the roles and responsibilities of both orders of government. The need for additional federal cash as a result of the long-term decline in transfers provides a 'window of opportunity' for real change in the relationship between Ottawa and the provinces. As a starting point for this new compact on health care, Fierlbeck recommends the approach adopted in the Social Union Framework Agreement (SUFA), agreed to by all governments (save Quebec) on 4 February 1999. This would include public accountability and transparency, joint planning and collaboration, predictability in transfer funding, and some type of arrangement for opting out in agreed-on program areas if the accountability framework and defined Canada-wide objectives are accepted.

International Trade Regimes and Canadian Medicare

In analysing the fiscal sustainability of public health care in Canada, it is not enough to understand domestic policy. International factors now affect the manoeuvrability of both orders of government – particularly international agreements that set the rules for trade, investment, and intellectual property. Jon Johnson (chapter 11) and Richard Ouellet (chapter 12) have carefully reviewed the impact of both trade regimes on the future of public health care in Canada. Both focus on the North American Free Trade Agreement (NAFTA) and the World Trade Organization (WTO) agreements, given the marginal impact of bilateral trade agreements (of which there are 30) on health care. Because of the many points of overlap, their analyses of NAFTA and the WTO arrangements are summarized together, followed by a brief review of their principal policy suggestions.

Enacted in 1994, NAFTA is a single agreement between Canada,

Mexico, and the United States covering trade in goods and services, investment, and intellectual property. Reservations protecting public health care and other social programms appear in lengthy appendices to the main agreement. The most important, Annex II, states that Canada 'reserves the right to adopt or maintain any measure' for health services 'to the extent they are social services established or maintained for a public purpose.' As Jon Johnson points out, this reservation applies as much to provincial public health-care services as to federal measures.

Although much debate has ensued concerning the type and degree of protection afforded by this reservation, Richard Ouellet notes that public health care in Canada has been entirely protected from NAFTA thus far. Johnson agrees with this analysis but sounds the cautionary note that the social-services reservation has not yet been tested and questions whether it would be effective where for-profit organizations deliver public health services. He also raises this concern in terms of one or another province's experimenting with multi-payer insurance replacing the single-payer system and whether American (or Mexican) firms would have a right to compete for health-care business under the NAFTA national-treatment obligations. These concerns were amplified in the major research study on globalization led by the Canadian Centre for Policy Alternatives (2002) on behalf of the commission. But Johnson also points out that there is further (albeit limited) protection under the so-called Annex I general reservation. All provincial measures, including provincial health plans, existing as of 1 January 1994 that do not conform with NAFTA are deemed to be protected. However, any new health programs or measures enacted after that time must come under the social-service (Annex II) reservation to be protected.

Unlike the situation with NAFTA, Canada's obligations under the WTO come under separate agreements negotiated under the aegis of the WTO, including the General Agreement on Trade in Services (GATS), the General Agreement on Tariffs and Trade (GATT), and the Agreement on Trade-related Aspects of Intellectual Property Rights (TRIPS). More important, as Ouellet points out, the WTO takes a 'piecemeal commitments approach,' in which liberalization of trade in goods and services and the protection of property continue incrementally through separate subject agreements *without* reservations and exceptions. While such provisions are generally interpreted narrowly (and therein lies the risk), much more attention must be paid to how provisions in the actual agreements will affect public health care, given that the sector cannot be exempted as a whole.

To deal with this problem, Ouellet recommends that the government of Canada argue that public health care be taken off the table in future WTO negotiations, including the current Doha round. Johnson goes one step further in suggesting that the federal government seize the opportunity presented by a heightened concern with social issues, including population health and health care, that developing countries have recently put on the WTO negotiating table. Both arguments support the Romanow Commission's recommendations to ensure that health care remains a protected social space in future trade negotiations and that the federal government should build alliances with other members of the WTO so that publicly insured, financed, and delivered health care can be maintained and even expanded over time.

Conclusion

The influence of these essays can readily be seen in the Romanow Commission's final report (Commission 2002), particularly in the first two chapters, on sustainability and governance. Current and future 'cost-drivers' in health care are manageable if governments and delegated health organizations exercise a degree of foresight and planning. At the same time, some leading-edge sectors of health care will grow faster than the economy, and this historically has produced a growth rate for health costs that is somewhat higher than that in the economy. This creates its own challenges in terms of public finance, but a simple response that amounts to little more than shifting costs from the public to the private sector can actually lead to higher total health-care expenditures.

The weight of evidence favours a tax-based, single-payer system for both efficiency and equity. Some debate continues concerning the narrow but deep character of the Canadian model as it relates to the prohibition on user fees for hospital and physicians' services. Here again, the comparative experience of other countries points to the high administrative costs (and low net revenue-generating nature of) user fees, as well as their undesirable impact on equitable access to necessary health care. However, less than 50 per cent of health care in Canada conforms to this model. Elsewhere, user fees and multi-payer insurance are the norm. And at this time, it is provincial drug plans and non-CHA services such as home care and mental health care that are often under the most fiscal pressure. However, they often directly affect the cost of hospital and physicians' services, since they offer a superior and/or lower-cost substitute for such services. If reform efforts do not include these critical areas, this lacuna will indeed undermine the fiscal sustainability of the Canadian model of health care.

An important part of retaining a system that has Canada-wide objectives is federal health transfers that are adequate, stable, and predictable. Ideally, this funding should be transparent, so that the public understands the relative contributions of both orders of government to the system as a whole and to provincial programs in particular. This would go some distance towards establishing a clearer regime, which would reduce the more dysfunctional intergovernmental wrangling of the last few years. It would also help restore Canadians' confidence in the ability of government to manage public health care in their interest.

REFERENCES

Canadian Centre for Policy Alternatives. 2002. *Putting Health First: Canadian Health Care Reform, Trade Treaties and Foreign Policy.* Summary Report of Consortium Research Project on Globalization and Health Prepared for the Commission on the Future of Health Care. Ottawa, Oct. 1992.

CES (Collège des Économistes de la Santé). 2001. *Utilization Fees Imposed on Public Health Care System Users in Europe. Proceedings of the Workshop on November 29, 2001.* Organized for the Commission on the Future of Health Care in Canada. Paris: CES.

CIHI (Canadian Institute for Heatlh Information). 2002. *National Health Expenditure Trends, 1975–2002.* Ottawa: CIHI, Dec.

Commission. 2002. *Building on Values: The Future of Health Care in Canada.* Final Report of the Commission on the Future of Health Care in Canada. Saskatoon, Nov.

Gerdtham, U.G., and B. Jönsson. 2000. 'International Comparisons of Health Expenditure: Theory, Data and Econometric Analysis.' In A.J. Culyer and J.P. Newhouse, eds., *Handbook of Health Economics*, vol. 1A. New York: Elsevier, 11–53.

Gratzer, D. 1999. *Code Blue: Reviving Canada's Health Care System.* Toronto: ECW Press.

Institute of Intergovernmental Relations. 2002. *Federal–Provincial Relations and Health Care: Reconstructing the Partnership.* Summary Report of Consortium Research Project on Fiscal Federalism and Health. Nov.

Kent, Tom. 2002. *Medicare: It's Decision Time*. Ottawa: Caledon Institute.

Maslove, A.M. 1998. 'National Goals and the Federal Role in Health Care.' In *Striking a Balance: Health Care Systems in Canada and Elsewhere. Volume 4*. Ottawa: National Forum on Health, 367–99.

Mossialos, E., and A. Dixon. 2002. 'Funding Health Care: An Introduction.' In E. Mossialos, A. Dixon, J. Fugueros, and J. Kutzin, eds., *Funding Health Care: Options for Europe*. Buckingham: Open University Press.

Mustard, C.A., et al. 1998. Use of Insured Health Care Services in Relation to Income in a Canadian Province. In M.L. Barer, T.E. Getzen, and G.L. Stoddard, eds., *Health, Health Care and Health Economics: Perspectives on Distribution*. Chichester: John Wiley.

Quebec. 2001. *Pour un régime d'assurance medicaments equitable et viable. Rapport prepare par le Comité sur la pertinence et la faisabilité d'un régime universel public d'assurance medicaments au Québec*. C. Montmarquette, Président. Quebec: Ministère de la Santé et des Services Sociaux.

Saskatchewan. 2001. *Caring for Medicare: Sustaining a Quality System* (Final Report of the Commission on Medicare). Regina: Saskatchewan Health.

Tuohy, C.H. 2002. The Costs of Constraint and Prospects for Health Care Reform in Canada. '*Health Affairs*' 21, no. 3: 32–46.

Woolhandler, S., and D.U. Himmelstein. 1991. 'The Deteriorating Administrative Efficiency of the U.S. Health Care System.' *New England Journal of Medicine* 324, no. 18: 1253–8.

– 2002. Paying for National Health Insurance – and Not Getting It.' *Health Affairs* 21, no. 4: 88–98.

Yalnizyan, A. 2002. Paying for Keeps: How the Feds Can Save Medicare. Unpublished monograph.

PART ONE

COST FACTORS

1 Technological Change as a Cost-Driver in Health Care

STEVE MORGAN AND JEREMIAH HURLEY

'Prediction is very difficult, especially if it's about the future.'

– Nils Bohr

When asked about the importance of technological change to the future of the health-care sector, economists might turn to the markets for answers. The message found there is clear, summarized in a recent headline from the business section of the the *New York Times*: 'This decade belongs to health care' (Munger Kahn 2002). Average price–earnings ratios in high-tech health sectors are currently about twice as high as those in other industries, indicating that investors assume that health technologies are poised to pay big dividends in the near future. These beliefs are no doubt fuelled by the highly publicized enthusiasm over the prospects for medical technology in the twenty-first century. 'Health Technology' is a regular feature in the daily news, particularly in the financial press, where a steady stream of featured breakthroughs promises to change the medical landscape, the health of the population, the financial fortunes of one firm or another, and the future cost of health care.

The recent burst of the e-commerce 'bubble' should give one pause when considering economic forecasts based on stock-market activity. There is, however, good reason to anticipate that 'technological change' will significantly influence health expenditures in the coming decades. This shift will consist of innovation and utilization. Innovation is the arrival of new products and techniques – the flow of new ideas into the stock of available technology. 'Utilization' concerns use of both new and old technologies in health care – what is done with the stock of available technology. In this paper, we argue that both techno-logical innovation and utilization will be driven by three influences in the coming ten to twenty years: demographic change, the genetic sciences, and consumer-directed marketing. We consider probable tech-nological change in health care and review expert opinions regarding likely innovation in selected fields of health care – genetic testing, pharmaceuticals, surgery, and imaging – and relate these trends to age-ing, genetics, and marketing. We next discuss the 'pricing' of health-care technologies, emphasizing apparent tensions between the incen-tives created by patents and the desire to regulate health care prices. We then examine issues in the evaluation and allocation of health tech-nologies that are central to efficient use of both new and old technolo-gies, offering as well a case study of pharmaceuticals. We conclude with recommendations on how various levels of government can work to create institutional structures to achieve that end.

Future Technological Change in Health Care

'I have seen the future and it is very much like the present, only longer.'

– Kehlog Albran

In past eras of profound change in basic scientific understanding, revo-lutions in the health of populations and the practice of medicine have not materialized as rapidly as experts predicted (Porter 2000). Conse-quently, the safest prediction for health-care technology in the coming decade is that progress will also be incremental – important, but none the less incremental, if we measure progress in terms of improvements in population health. This is because technological progress generally moves in a logical sequence. Most new ideas, products, and techniques tend to build incrementally and somewhat predictably on existing ones. Breakthroughs will occur, but their nature and magnitude are virtually impossible to forecast. Indeed, anyone who could foretell a specific technology that would dramatically improve population health in the near future would be very rich.

While dramatic shocks are almost impossible to predict, changes in the tides of technological progress may be foreseen if forces that influ-ence the direction of scientific inquiry are known to be shifting. More-over, changes in the rate of use of existing technologies or adoption of new ones may also be predicted if related and identifiable trends could also be foreseen. Health-care planning can (and should) adapt to these reasonably predicable influences of demographic change, genetic sciences, and consumer-directed marketing of health technologies while remaining prepared for unexpected shocks in health-care technology.

Technology and the Baby Boomers

Born between 1946 and 1965 in North America (and other developed countries), members of the 'baby boomer' generation are just now entering their years of high health-care use. The impact that these baby boomers will have on health-care costs will not be independent of the availability, cost, and utilization of health-care technology which will in turn affect the availability, cost, and use of that very technology.

The total cost of population ageing is a function of both changes in average health-care needs as the population ages and changes in the quantity, type, and cost of technologies used to meet those requirements. When the latter factors are held constant, the needs-related effect of population ageing has been a modest 'cost-driver' in recent decades (Fuchs 1984; Barer, Evans, et al. 1987; Barer, Evans, et al. 1995; Evans, McGrail, et al. 2001). It is likely to remain so in the coming decades. However, historical experience suggests that changes in the availability, use, and price of technologies to meet the needs of the elderly population will be important determinants of the cost of population ageing (Evans, McGrail, et al. 2001).

Innovation in health technology are related to demographic change these days because the health-care 'market' is shifting as the baby boom ages. Age-related needs of baby boomers increase the financial incentives for development and promotion of health-care technologies. Bringing to market products that ageing baby boomers will probably need is good business: 'That's where the money is.' Baby boomers are not only more numerous than other generations, they are also more affluent and independent than previous cohorts of elderly health-care consumers, and they have relatively high expectations about healthy ageing and consumer-oriented health care (Clark 1998; Dychtwald 1999).

Significant investment is already in place to develop forms of technology likely to be in high demand by the baby-boomer generation. Almost two-thirds of drugs currently in U.S. development are intended to 'lengthen and improve the quality of life for seniors' (PhRMA 2001b).

Therapeutic 'markets' currently experiencing rapid growth due to the boomer generation include treatments for hypertension, type II diabetes, high cholesterol, and arthritis pain (Scott-Levin 2001).

Treating Patients as Consumers

Some observers believe that increases in the consumer-orientation of health care may be one of the most significant challenges of health care in the coming years (Porter 2000). This shift results partly from the advent of new health technologies that go beyond the conventional definitions of health care and disease (Moynihan, Heath, et al. 2002; Smith 2002) and partly from a combination of growing affluence and increased access to information that has engendered higher expectations among consumers of health care. As well, new health-care marketing practices aim at capitalizing on notions of 'consumer empowerment' and 'patient-centred' health care (Mintzes 2002; Mintzes, Barer, et al. 2002).

Health-care technologies have traditionally been promoted through marketing activities aimed at health professionals who make decisions about allocation on behalf of, and in consultation with, patients. However, recent changes in the marketplace have caused companies – pharmaceutical manufacturers, in particular – to seek new means of promoting sales by marketing directly to consumers, in addition to conventional marketing aimed at professionals. Perhaps most notably, increased emphasis on expenditure controls by managed care organizations (in the United States) and governments (elsewhere) appears to have forced manufacturers to target patients directly in order to promote particular brands (Pinto, Pinto, et al. 1998; Morgan 2002a). A recent paper commissioned by Pfizer Inc. promotes consumer-directed advertising as a way to counter unduly restrictive policies imposed by insurance providers (Rubin and Schrag 1999).

While most forms of direct-to-consumer advertising for prescription drugs are illegal in all but two countries – the United States and New Zealand – the trend towards consumer-oriented marketing is unmistakable (Mintzes 2002; Morgan 2002a; Rosenthal, Berndt, et al. 2002). A watershed in this trend came in 1997, when the U.S. Food and Drug Administration relaxed restrictions on television and radio advertisements. Promotional activities aimed at U.S. consumers expanded explosively and now approach $3 billion per year. Canadians see much of this product, although such marketing practices remain illegal in

Canada (Mintzes, Barer, et al. 2002). U.S. pharmaceutical manufacturers are lobbying for the opportunity to advertise to consumers in other countries, including Canada. Companies holding patents on predictive genetic tests will not be far behind.

The consumer orientation of health-care marketing will be a determining factor in the utilization of health-care technologies in the coming decades. Technologies most heavily promoted directly to consumers will expand dramatically: if this were not likely to be the case, firms would not engage in such marketing practices.

Health Technology in the Genomic Era

While human genetics has been studied for some time, the complete mapping of the human genome is said to have launched 'the era of post-genomic science,' in which many commentators claim that virtually all aspects of medicine will change (Baltimore 2001; Collins and Guttmacher 2001; Collins and McKusick 2001). The promise of this new era is far reaching. When leading scientists were recently asked to report on the prospects of medical research in the twenty-first century, they cited genetics as central to developments in the treatment of most diseases – autoimmune diseases (Koopman 2001), cancer (Livingston and Shivdasani 2001), cardiovascular illnesses (Lefkowitz and Willerson 2001), adult onset (Type 2) diabetes (Olefsky 2001), and neurological and psychiatric illnesses (Cowan and Kandel 2001). The scientists also cited genetic information as a spur to diagnostic imaging (Tempany and McNeil 2001) and to pharmacological and biological therapy (Bumol and Watanabe 2001; Kaji and Leiden 2001).

The holy grail in the genetic era of health care consists of products that will allow 'physicians ... not only to use therapies to help patients live better with their genetic constitutions, but also [to] use novel therapies to alter the genetic makeup of the patient' (Kaji and Leiden 2001). Despite the high expectations of many people involved (or investing) in the race for such discoveries, radical genomic therapies will not appear on the Canadian market or in the health-care system within the next decade.

Innovations will occur, but they are likely to emerge gradually. As the genes and proteins related to more illnesses are identified, the amount of genetic 'data' is increasing dramatically; the task of turning that data into useful information, and ultimately helpful treatments, will take decades. For example, the list of potential targets for drug therapy is expected to balloon from the 500 biological receptors currently targeted by conventional pharmacological therapy to as many as 30,000 targets for bio-pharmaceuticals and genetic therapies (Drews 2000; Horrobin 2000; Bumol and Watanabe 2001; Lemonick 2001). Some observers question whether this impressive gain in 'data' has uncovered more needles or bigger haystacks (Horrobin 2000).

Even when the genetic origins of illnesses are known, 'cures' are hard to find. The genes that cause single-gene disorders such as sickle cell disease, cystic fibrosis, and muscular dystrophy have long been known; yet no cures have been found for them (Baird 2002). As we look to detect the genetic causes of and find cures for common illnesses, the complexity of the problem increases substantially. Most common diseases result from such a complex combination of environmental and multiple genetic factors that few (if any) are really 'genetic disorders' (Baird 2002). The number of genes with links to illness, combined with the complexity of biological systems, creates analytical challenges so immense that 'bio-informatics' has emerged as a new sub-discipline of computer science to help analyse related data (Pennisi 2001). In January 2000, for example, IBM launched a five-year, $100-million project to develop supercomputers dedicated to bimolecular simulation (IBM 1999). These developments portend the kind of obstacles that must be overcome to convert the massive amounts of data being generated into useful information and, ultimately, 'gene therapies.'

Although correcting genetic disorders remains science fiction, the information elucidated from genomic research has led to productive pharmaceutical research. Scientists are using genetic information about diseased and cancerous cells to find biotechnological 'magic bullets' – products that attack target cells without harming healthy tissues (Drews 2000; Horrobin 2000; Bumol and Watanabe 2001). While few such bio-tech products are currently on the market, there are an impressive number in clinical testing, and they now account for approximately one third of drugs currently in clinical testing (PhRMA 2001a). Some therapeutic breakthroughs are expected there, particularly in cancer treatment – which accounts for half of such products under development today.

Genetic Testing

Among genetic technologies, genetic testing will probably have the greatest influence on health care in the next few decades. While it has long been used to predict the health of future generations (through prenatal genetic testing and carrier screening), the tests that now capture the imagination of patients, providers, and investors are those that can predict the living generation's future health status (Miller, Hurley, et al. 2002) – 'medicines new gold mine.' Firms search massive databases of genetic information to discover and patent tests for genotypes that are correlated (however strongly) with illness (Herper 2001).

Although the genetic origins of common diseases are not currently well understood today (Baird 2000; Evans, Skrzynia, et al. 2001), some leading genetic researchers predict that risk-factor tests for as many as a dozen common illnesses – such as diabetes, cancer, and heart disease – will be available within a decade (Collins and McKusick 2001). Such developments could increase use of genetic testing because of the increased breadth of its applicability. Their total impact on health-care costs may, however, far exceed the cost of the tests themselves and will depend on changes in health behaviour induced by the testing process and its results (Miller, Hurley, et al. 2002).

Several cost components come into play here, including the cost of the tests and the effect of test results on the use of disease surveillance, prevention, and treatment services. Because of the complexity of gene–environment interactions and the profundity of certain test results, some experts argue strongly that genetic testing should be available only under supervision and only following counseling about the strengths and weaknesses of a given test (Caulfield 1999; Emery and Hayflick 2001; Baird 2002). Both positive and negative test results may change individuals' approaches to seeking health care. Some of these changes may reduce health-care costs; others may raise them. With the benefit of hindsight, analysts may find some of these changes useful and others wasteful; the balance depends on the ultimate predictive power of the test (Miller, Hurley, et al. 2002).

Pharmaceuticals

Pharmaceuticals will be one of the biggest cost-drivers in health care in the next ten years. Drugs have been one of the fastest-growing components of health expenditures in recent decades, and current predictions are for continued double-digit growth in expenditures on prescription drugs for North America until at least 2005 (IMS 2002b). At these rates of growth, such expenditures should double in five to seven years.

Recent growth in pharmaceutical expenditures has not followed a dramatic increase in drug discovery (Drews 1998). It has been driven largely by increases in both the cost of and the exposure to treatments in established therapeutic classes (Dubois, Chawla, et al. 2000; CIHI 2001; Morgan 2002b). Both expansion of and cost escalation within therapeutic categories are long-standing trends and have often resulted from the intensive promotion of new products that offer (at best) incremental improvements over existing therapies (Canada and Canada 1963; Temin 1980; Morgan 2001). This pattern is likely to continue, as utilization of direct-to-consumer advertising increasingly drives newer, patented products (Rizzo 1999; Mintzes, Barer, et al. 2002; Morgan 2002a).

As we saw above, ageing baby boomers will boost demand in several drug segments – including arthritis, certain cancers, depression, diabetes, heart disease, hypertension, and eventually Alzheimer's and other dementias. Investment in pharmaceuticals responded to this trend long ago, and now many products are about to be launched in major therapeutic classes for adult-onset diseases, including anti-hypertensives, anti-ulcer drugs, drugs for arthritis pain relief, insulins (diabetes) and, statins (lipid-lowering drugs) (CCOHTA 2001; PhRMA 2001a; PhRMA 2001b). Most of these products will offer some improvement – often for particular types of patient – over current therapies (CCOHTA 2001). If history is a guide, these entrants will probably achieve wide application through intense promotion (Canada and Canada 1963; Temin 1980; Morgan 1998).

Pharmacogenomics to Tailor Drug Therapy
'Pharmacogenomics' – the screening of patients for genes that predict the capacity to benefit from or be harmed by pharmaceuticals – is expected to become more common in the next decade (Phillips, Veenstra, et al. 2001; IMS 2002a). Because certain genotypes metabolize drugs differently from others, it may be possible to screen patients to avoid adverse reactions or to select a customized therapy. In the near term, genetic information will most probably be used to reduce adverse reactions among populations taking costly and potent medicines, such as those for the treatment of HIV/AIDS and cancer (Phillips, Veenstra, et al. 2001). Manufacturers of products with known relationships between genes and adverse reactions may find commercial advantage in advocating screening of patient candidates before administration of premium-priced drugs (IMS 2002a).

Genetic information is now being employed to screen patients in the early stages of clinical testing, so that only suitable patients receive a product during clinical trials, as a means of reducing the cost of taking products to market (Wallace 2000). When pharmaceutical products are marketed for the treatment of diseases and risk factors identified by specific genotypes, individual treatment will be substantially dearer than conventional therapies, partly because the value of treatments will increase if customization leads to more certain outcomes. As well, to the extent that genotype specificity reduces the potential market size for each customized treatment brought to market, each user must bear a greater share of the research costs (Drews 1998; Danzon and Towse 2000; Bumol and Watanabe 2001; IMS 2002a).

Pharmacogenomics to Expand Markets
Genetic testing can be used to expand markets for new and existing products, and manufacturers of some products in testing today are expected to seek approval to use them to treat genetically identified risk factors (Herper 2002). In particular, genetic testing for common, late-onset diseases has the potential to add substantially to the demand for existing and evolving models of pharmacological disease management. It is known that the uptake of genetic testing services depends on the test, the context, and patients' perceptions of the value of resulting interventions (Marteau and Croyle 1998). Much of the perceived benefit from testing will depend on sources of information regarding the value of tests and complementary preventive care or treatment. Consumer-directed advertising will play a major role in this regard. Both testing-service operators – potentially dominated by multinational patent-holding firms – and providers of preventive therapies will seek to reach not just clinicians and genetic counsellors, but also patients.

In the near future, new generations of established pharmacological models will probably help manage genetically indentified risks. Treatment modalities for non–genetically identified hypertension and high cholesterol, for example, may find expanded markets in populations identified as being at risk for elevated blood pressure or cholesterol. Evaluation of the clinical utility and economic benefit of treatments for genetic risks of late-onset disorders will require years, in some cases decades, because of the delay between treatment and expected health benefits. Treatments to manage biological factors associated with the risk of later illness – such as blood pressure or cholesterol levels – have historically received approval based on changes in the biological marker as a surrogate (albeit imperfect) of their impact on long-term health. It is yet unknown whether such surrogates will apply to risks of a genetic origin. This may force radical changes in evaluation methods, clinical trials, or even patent length in order not to waste time, money, and lives while the world experiments with unproven therapies. If treatments are approved only on the conjecture of long-term benefits (a possibility made real by limited patent length), the health-care system may bear substantial costs while waiting for evidence of benefits.

Surgical Procedures

Commentators appear to be relatively modest in predicting the scale of change in the surgical theatre (Mack 2001). Trends in surgery are towards less and less invasive procedures, with robotic assistance and other techniques building on progress made in laparoscopic procedures over the past twenty years (Darzi and Mackay 2002). These changes will result in faster recovery times, fewer complications, and therefore a broader pool of candidate patients. The fixed cost of machinery for such procedures is just one of two major cost considerations for health-care systems, along with – more important – the scale and scope of procedures conducted when infrastructure is in place. Baby boomers are creating growing demand for technologies related to cardiovascular and orthopaedic surgery (Boskey 2001; Lefkowitz and Willerson 2001; Hench and Polak 2002; Marshall 2002).

Diagnostic Imaging

Technological advances in diagnostic imaging are expected to come from refinements to and newer applications of existing imaging formats such as computed tomography (CT) scanning, magnetic resonance imaging (MRI), and positron emission tomography (PET) (Tempany and McNeil 2001). The biggest financial consequences of such change will come from increased use of imaging-based screening technologies. Diagnostic imaging will increasingly monitor individuals at high risk of illnesses for which ongoing diagnostic and surveillance costs might be justified. The largest potential growth in candidates will stem from the identification of people at risk of cancers and other illnesses by means of their genetic makeup – for example, women diagnosed with the BRAC1–2 gene associated with early-onset breast cancer (Tempany and McNeil 2001). Like genetic testing itself, diagnostic imaging must be rationalized by validity of the information that it generates and by the clinical utility of interventions that follow. The need for assessment is formidable: for example, despite the use of PET for over thirty years, evaluations of PET scanning are scarce, making it difficult for analysts to draw many conclusions about the cost-effectiveness of its use in Canada (ICES 2001).

Summary

The cost-impact of health-care technology in the coming decade will be driven not solely by the discovery of new products, devices, or procedures, but also by changes in the use of both new and old technologies. These shifts in utilization will be driven only partially by natural increases in needs as the population ages. Major determinants of the use of health-care technologies – pharmaceuticals and diagnostic imaging, in particular – will be increases in the demand for services induced by testing for genetic risk factors associated with common illnesses and demand for new technologies that are promoted directly to patients.

Pricing Health-Care Goods and Services

Internationally, a great deal of attention has been paid to the pricing of health-care technologies, particularly of pharmaceuticals (Andersson 1993; Monaghan and Monaghan 1996; Danzon and Kim 1998; Towse 1998; Berndt 2000; Calfee 2000; Danzon and Chao 2000). Purchasers of health care bemoan the high price of new products, while providers lament the cost of product development. What is the right price for medical technology?

From an economic perspective, the appropriate price is typically that which is equal to the marginal cost of production. This is the price that prevails in a perfectly competitive market, wherein free entry ensures that producers earn no more than a fair profit. A market outcome is said to 'fail' when the prevailing price does not equal the marginal cost of production. Such failures often provoke calls for price regulation.

Price regulation cannot always mimic what would happen in a competitive market – i.e., pricing at marginal costs – nor would we necessarily want it to. Marginal cost pricing cannot be sustained in industries with high fixed costs of production, including research and development. In such cases, the regulated firm would operate at a loss if it could not charge a price that exceeded the marginal cost of production. The loss would be equal to the fixed costs associated with setting up operations. Price regulations typically attempt to keep prices as near as possible to the average cost of production, including fixed costs.

Should the prices of patented health-care technologies be regulated such that they equal the average cost of production, including the fixed costs of research and development? No. They should be equal to the benefit that the product creates for the health-care system relative to all alternative technologies, including those competitively supplied at marginal cost. This price may bear little or no relationship to costs of production or of research and development. Nor should it.

The purpose of a patent is to provide incentive to innovate. A patent creates a temporary monopoly over the sale of an innovative product or process by prohibiting the unlicensed entry of competitors. If an innovator was not protected from competition, other firms could enter the market and bid prices down to marginal cost. To the extent that potential innovators could expect this to happen, they would have no incentive to pay for the research necessary to innovate in the first place. Allowing prices above marginal cost – during the period of the patent – is the purpose of patents.

But markets do not guarantee that a patent holder will recoup the research investment, nor do they limit the return to such investment. The market mechanism regulates the value of the monopoly conferred on patent holders such that the reward for innovation is proportionate to consumers' willingness to pay for the patented product or service. If a patented product is of little value to consumers, the market may not support sufficient sales at a sufficient markup for patentees to recoup investment. This should be of no concern to consumers or governments. Firms that gamble sometimes lose. And firms that gamble sometimes win.

There is no requirement that a patent holder charge a price that reflects average costs if the market will support much more. Patentees may charge much higher prices and earn large profits. This, too, should not be a concern to consumers or governments. If prices were held equal to that which covers the cost of production and research, there would be no more incentive for innovations of high value than for ones of little or no value. Moreover, if allowable prices were related to the research expenses on a company's books, there would be incentive for inefficiencies in the research process or for 'creative accounting' about what constitutes the cost of developing a product – we already observe much of the latter for the purposes of public relations and political lobbying (Young and Surrusco 2001).

The important question to ask is whether patented health-care technologies are being rewarded in a manner that provides incentives for research of the greatest value to society as a whole. This would require that their price when they are protected by patent should reflect their therapeutic value relative to the existing arsenal of health technologies – both new and old. Unlike ordinary goods and services, for which consumers' willingness to pay might reasonably approximate its social value, determining the value of health technologies will require expert evaluation and critical assessment (Evans 1984; Rice 1998). The 'purchaser' of health technologies – typically the health-care funder – must therefore engage in clinical evaluation and economic assessment when determining a reasonable price – its willingness to pay, so to speak. This we discuss further below.

The opportunity to set prices according to domestic goals and evaluations of technologies is decreasing with the internationalization of the price of health technologies, especially pharmaceuticals (Towse 1998; Jacobzone 2000; Willison, Wiktorowicz, et al. 2001). While price discrimination does occur on the international market, reduced prices are increasingly attained through hidden discounts or disguised through price-volume agreements. Canada, via continued, if not more rigorous, assessment and evaluation of technology, may be able to negotiate prices to some extent, but the agreed-on prices will probably have to fall within a narrow 'price corridor' established by international pricing precedents. Once prices are set, the appropriate and cost-effective allocation of technologies will depend in part on how technologies are chosen for individual patients.

For society, creating efficient incentives for future innovation in health care also requires an environment in which firms expect to be able to sell their technologies only to those for whom the technology is appropriate and cost-effective. The system for allocating such technologies must thus ensure appropriate utilization. It is nonsensical to overuse health technologies or to rely too much on newer, more costly ones, in the name of promoting innovation for tomorrow. Doing so provides all the wrong incentives. Once again, health care is unlike ordinary goods and services, for which consumers' willingness to pay for a product might serve as a reasonable rationing mechanism. Allocating health technologies may require other forms of rationing. This we also discuss further below.

Technology Assessment and Economic Evaluation

Technology assessment and economic evaluation are tools that may be used to inform decisions about use of new and existing technologies in clinical settings, to help with priority setting at local and regional levels, and to ration technologies at provincial or national levels. Each form of assessment involves a systematic attempt to collect and analyse data on the use of a technology. Assessment concerns evaluation of the consequences stemming from use of a medical device, product, or technique and measures consequences by various standards, including clinical safety and efficacy – established in the controlled setting of a clinical trial – as well as 'real-world' safety and effectiveness. Economic evaluations are systematic and comparative evaluations of both costs and consequences (Drummond, O'Brien, et al. 1997).

If either method informs priority setting, it is essential to separate evidence from anecdote and to minimize bias from assessments conducted at the behest of the health-technology industry (Morgan, Barer, et al. 2000). Given that at best half of health-care technologies have been evaluated for effectiveness, and even fewer for efficiency, such processes play limited roles in priority setting (Hurley, Birch, et al. 1997; Robinson 1999; Ham and Coulter 2001). While they can play an important role in price negotiations and in certain 'gate-keeping' functions, such as formulary decisions, but they have less effect in day-to-day allocation decisions.

Allocation Decisions

Allocation decisions in health care generally come in two broad forms. Whether based on formal assessment or on other processes, decisions on approval of the use of a technology often relate to a given setting – and take the form of a discrete interpretation, either yes or no. After this, decisions are then made about how and under what conditions a technology is used. Much has been written on the use of formal technology assessment in the related area of deciding about coverage – 'covered' or 'not covered.' In practice, however, decisions made by, or on behalf of, particular patients are more important in the allocation of health technologies.

In Canada, assessment issues have typically tended to be framed in terms of coverage vis-à-vis provincial fee schedules or drug formularies. This framing invites a discrete yes/no decision for technologies with potentially broad application. Indeed, this is exactly how 'delisting' (de-insurance) exercises are framed – as a problem of items being in the fee schedule/formulary that should not be. This situation has led to calls for explicit definitions of medical necessity to facilitate such determinations.

The challenge for coverage is to make a one-time decision wherein 'good things' are covered and 'bad things are not.' Many technology-assessment frameworks set out an algorithm for making such decisions (Deber, Ross, et al. 1994; Evans, Barer, et al. 1994; Deber, Narine, et al. 1997). The most thorough aim to rate standards of explicitness, rationality, relevance, and accountability. Theoretically, after such processes have been used to eliminate items from coverage, the system may go about operations as usual within the range of covered items.

There are a number of problems with framing priority setting in this discrete way. First, very few health-care technologies are effective/ efficient or ineffective/inefficient in all circumstances. Thus discrete, yes–no decision criteria for coverage are too blunt. They often result in broad use of technologies appropriate only under defined circumstances or in blanket denial of access to technologies that are effective in limited circumstances. Therefore, although coverage decisions and the related processes help determine ultimate access, traditional applications of broad coverage decisions are too blunt to result in efficient use of available technologies.

This has led to the notion of conditional coverage/access – access to and coverage of technologies only under conditions that render them effective and efficient. Health systems do not necessarily need to be strictly 'managed' (as in the practices employed by 'managed' U.S. care organizations), or regulated in a top–down fashion, to make coverage of and access to technologies conditional on appropriateness. However, when adequate information, opportunities, and incentives are given to those taking part in micro-level decision making, technological adoption may be efficiently rationed from the bottom up.

The information to make judgments on effectiveness and efficiency of a health-care service or technology often emerges only during a clinical encounter. It is at this point of exchange that information about signs, symptoms, and personal circumstances (including attitudes towards risks and outcomes related to treatments) is revealed. While additional information essential to appropriate rationing – including medical history and evidence about costs and benefits of alternative treatments – may be made available at the point of the clinical encounter, information uniquely accessible to the clinician cannot always be centralized. This lack explains in part the failure of top–down strategies for managing health technologies.

Attempts to centralize the approval process and use of inflexible, blunt rules are precisely the aspects of formal managed care that most rile physicians and patients and that have created the backlash against managed care in the United States. To ensure prudent adoption/use of services/technologies, policy might aim to influence the decisions of thousands of providers in millions of clinical encounters. Framing the issue in this way (as is done in Canada) shifts the focus for resource allocation (decision making about coverage priority setting, and so on) from a formal, defined process (whether or not based on technology assessment) to ensuring that providers/patients make good choices that reflect system goals. In this case, the mechanisms expand to consider financial and non-financial incentives, professional norms and socialization, the regulation of technology developers and marketers, and so on.

Notwithstanding the benefits of decentralizing incentives and opportunities to ration specific health-care services, formal decision-making processes about coverage will remain important. Indeed, with technology blurring the boundaries between medical treatment and cosmetic or 'lifestyle' therapy, maintaining a formal boundary around the 'medical' nature of public health care will only grow more important. The point of the preceding discussion is that too often the proposed solution to the problem of resource allocation is simply an explicit process for making discrete coverage decisions.

International Experiences: Containing Costs for Pharmaceuticals

Prescription drugs are probably the most studied form of 'health-care technology cost-driver.' Despite diversity of approaches, virtually no country has controlled expenditure inflation for a sustained period (Morgan 1998; Jacobzone 2000; Willison, Wiktorowicz, et al. 2001). Failure to control drug costs on an ongoing basis is largely a function of politics. Those policies that are, or would be, successful in achieving real cost control meet with strong opposition in the political economy of the pharmaceutical industry. The strongest opposition comes from the concentrated interest of pharmaceutical manufacturers. Manufacturers have overturned effective cost-control policies on numerous occasions – including the global drug-budget system in Germany and the independent product-evaluation system in Australia (Busse and

Wismar 1997; Henry and Birkett 2001). Sustained control over expenditures requires the political will to confront opposition to effective policy. It also requires the management of both the cost and the use of technologies. Managing each of these factors is a difficult task.

Price is a common target for policy intervention. In most developed countries, prices are either negotiated between manufacturers and national purchasing or priority-setting bodies or regulated directly (Jacobzone 2000; Willison, Wiktorowicz, et al. 2001). Many countries use pharmaco-economic evaluation in their centralized decision-making and price negotiations. In Australia, where it has been applied most rigorously and (until recently) independently, such evaluation has reduced the national price of top-selling medicines (Henry and Birkett 2001; Willison, Wiktorowicz, et al. 2001). Some countries – and provinces such as Ontario – negotiate expenditure caps or price-volume agreements with the manufacturers of new products to restrict financial risk for the public payer when demand is uncertain (Braae, McNee, et al. 1999; Willison, Wiktorowicz, et al. 2001). These negotiations reduce the unit price of a new product if its sales volume exceeds certain limits. Finally, some countries, such as the United Kingdom, regulate profits, sacrificing price regulation for the sake of negotiated research investment (Towse 1996; Jacobzone 2000).

Price regulations are not sufficient to control expenditures. As we saw above, negotiations that result in discrete, yes–no decisions at the aggregate level fail to account for decisions on use. No drug will be cost effective for all patients at given prices; typically, it will be so in some cases and not in others. Consequently, decisions at the clinical encounter are critical to determining the cost-effectiveness of drug use.

Strategies to address utilization have generally focused on blunt policy tools such as co-payments and prescription limits. Most countries resort to user charges of one sort or another as a means of containing costs (Jacobzone 2000; Willison, Wiktorowicz, et al. 2001). These policies have the effect of restricting public liability, but there is no sign that they produce sustained control of total expenditures. Indeed, untargeted co-payments and co-insurance have been shown to increase overall costs of health systems, since patients reduce both essential and non-essential drug use in the face of such charges (Soumerai, Ross-Degnan, et al. 1993; Adams, Soumerai, et al. 2001; Tamblyn 2001).

More advanced strategies for controlling use incorporate information and incentives targeted at the two major parties – patients and physicians. Through the dissemination of unbiased, comparative information about alternative drug treatments, public agencies have been able temporarily to make prescribing more appropriate. Tailored incentives, such as reference-based pricing (for consumers) and the integration of primary care and pharmaceutical budgets (for physicians), have shown promise at 'steering' use towards more cost-effective choices – as opposed to simply curbing utilization altogether – but limited implementation or complex changes surrounding such policies have made evaluation of these systems complicated (Braae, McNee, et al. 1999; Mays, Mulligan, et al. 2000; Willison, Wiktorowicz, et al. 2001).

Recommendations

Institutional structures will be necessary to deal with the inflationary pressures caused by, among other factors, health technologies in the coming years. If not managed carefully, these pressures may gradually erode the principles underlying the Canadian health-care system. This does not have to be the case. By ensuring the most appropriate and cost-effective use of technologies – both new and old – Canadian policy makers can achieve a health-care system for tomorrow that is both more equitable and more efficient than today's.

Through the regulation of safety and efficacy, the federal government should continue to play a rationing role by allowing access only to products that can do more good than harm. Through public funding of organizations such as the Canadian Coordinating Office of Health Technology Assessment, Ottawa can foster rigorous technology assessment and economic evaluation. And by disseminating guidelines (or 'guidances,' as Britain's National Institute for Clinical Excellence does), it can help 'inform' decision makers at the provincial, regional, and clinical levels (Ham and Coulter 2001). Furthermore, it can foster the innovation in health-care policy necessary to adapt to new health technologies by increasing its investment in health services and policy research. It can do so through institutions such as the Canadian Health Services Research Foundation and the Canadian Institutes of Health Research.

Provinces too support research for policy innovation, but they also have to implement policy. Whether acting by themselves or through regional authorities, they allocate health-care technologies. Provinces and their representatives allocate capital budgets, developing priorities with communities and becoming increasingly involved in the monitoring and evaluation of health outcomes and patients' satisfaction. Furthermore, their establishment of budgets and operating capacity – for example, hospital beds or MRIs – engenders rationing by practitioners within those constraints. The incentive for considering cost decreases for services around which no limits are placed. Consequently, how provinces structure and reimburse health care at the clinical level is a crucial decision.

Controls over health technology will not work if they do not relate to broader reform of primary care. Ultimately, efficient allocation of health technologies will depend on the dissemination of independent, balanced, and unbiased information to physicians and patients and on the financial incentives for them in the clinical encounter. Consequently, if Canadian policy makers wish better to control the inflationary pressures created by health-care technologies, they must substantially reform the organization and funding of health-care services.

REFERENCES

Adams, A.S., S.B. Soumerai, et al. 2001. 'The Case for a Medicare Drug Coverage Benefit: A Critical Review of the Empirical Evidence.' *Annual Review of Public Health* 22: 49–61.

Andersson, F. 1993. 'Methodological Aspects of International Drug Price Comparisons.' *Pharmacoeconomics* 4, no. 4: 247–56.

Baird, P.A. 2000. 'Genetic Technologies and Achieving Health for Populations.' *International Journal of Health Services* 30, no. 2: 407–24.

– 2002. 'Genetic Testing for Susceptibility to Common Diseases: Is Regulation Needed?' *Perspectives in Biology and Medicine* in press.

Baltimore, D. 2001. 'Our Genome Unveiled.' *Science* 409: 814–16.

Barer, M.L., R.G. Evans, et al. 1987. 'Aging and Health Care Utilization: New Evidence on Old Fallacies.' *Social Science and Medicine* 24, no. 10: 851–62.

– 1995. 'Avalanche or Glacier? Health Care and the Demographic Rhetoric.' *Canadian Journal on Ageing* 14, no. 2 (summer): 193–224.

Berndt, E.R. 2000. 'International Comparisons of Pharmaceutical Prices: What Do We Know, and What Does It Mean?' *Journal of Health Economics* 19: 283–7.

Boskey, A.L. 2001. 'Musculoskeletal Disorders and Orthopedic Conditions.' *JAMA* 285, no. 5: 619–23.

Braae, R., W. McNee, et al. 1999. 'Managing Pharmaceutical Expenditure While Increasing Access. The Pharmaceutical Management Agency (PHARMAC) Experience.' *PharmacoEconomics* 16, no. 6: 649–60.

Bumol, T.F., and A.M. Watanabe. 2001. 'Genetic Information, Genomic Technologies, and the Future of Drug Discovery.' *JAMA* 285, no. 5: 551–5.

Busse, R., and M. Wismar. 1997. 'Health Care Reform in Germany: The End of Cost Containment?' *Eurohealth* 3, no. 2: 32.

Calfee, J.E. 2000. 'The Increasing Necessity for Market-based Pharmaceutical Prices.' *Pharmacoeconomics* 18 Suppl 1: 47–57.

Canada, 1963. *Report Concerning the Manufacture, Distribution and Sale of Drugs. Combines Investigation Act.* Ottawa: Department of Justice, Restrictive Trade Practices Commission.

Caulfield, T. 1999. 'Gene Testing in the Biotech Century: Are Physicians Ready?' *CMAJ* 161, no. 9: 1122–4.

CCOHTA. 2001. *Emerging Technologies Bulletin.* Canadian Coordinating Office for Health Technology Assessment.

CIHI. 2001. *Drug Expenditures in Canada, 1985–2000.* Ottawa: Canadian Institute for Health Information.

Clark, B. 1998. 'Older, Sicker, Smarter and Redefining Quality: The Older Consumer's Quest for Patient-Driven Service.' *Healthcare Forum Journal* 41, no. 1 (Jan.–Feb.).

Collins, F.S., and A.E. Guttmacher. 2001. 'Genetics Moves Into the Medical Mainstream.' *JAMA* 286, no. 8: 2322–4.

Collins, F.S., and V.A. McKusick. 2001. 'Implications of the Human Genome Project for Medical Science.' *JAMA* 285, no. 5: 540–4.

Cowan, W.M., and E.R. Kandel. 2001. 'Prospects for Neurology and Psychiatry.' *JAMA* 285, no. 5: 594–600.

Danzon, P.M., and L.W. Chao. 2000. 'Cross-National Price Differences for Pharmaceuticals: How Large, and Why?' *Journal of Health Economics* 19, no. 2: 159–95.

Danzon, P.M., and J.D. Kim. 1998. 'International Price Comparisons for Pharmaceuticals. Measurement and Policy Issues.' *Pharmacoeconomics* 14 Suppl 1: 115–28.

Danzon, P., and A. Towse. 2000. 'The Genomic Revolution: Is the Real Risk Under-investment Rather than Bankrupt Health Care Systems?' *Journal of Health Services Research and Policy* 5, no. 4: 253–5.

Darzi, A., and S. Mackay. 2002. 'Recent Advances in Minimal Access Surgery.' *BMJ* 324, no. 7328: 31–4.

Deber, R., L. Narine, et al. 1997. *The Public–Private Mix in Health Care.* Toronto: University of Toronto, Department of Health Administration.

Deber, R., E. Ross, et al. 1994. *Comprehensiveness in Health Care*. Toronto: Ontario, University of Toronto, Department of Health Administration.

Drews, J. 1998. 'Innovation Deficit Revisited: Reflections on the Productivity of Pharmaceutical R&D.' *Drug Development Technology* 3, no. 11: 491–4.

– 2000. 'Drug Discovery: A Historical Perspective.' *Science* 287, no. 5460: 1960–4.

Drummond, M.F., B. O'Brien, et al. 1997. *Methods for the Economic Evaluation of Health Care Programmes*. Oxford: New York, Oxford University Press.

Dubois, R.W., A.J. Chawla, et al. 2000. 'Explaining Drug Spending Trends: Does Perception Match Reality?' 19, no. 2: 231–9.

Dychtwald, K. 1999. '"Age Power": How the New-Old Will Transform Medicine in the 21st Century. Interview by Alice V. Luddington.' *Geriatrics* 54, no. 12: 22–7; quiz 28.

Emery, J., and S. Hayflick. 2001. 'The Challenge of Integrating Genetic Medicine into Primary Care.' *BMJ* 322, no. 7293: 1027–30.

Evans, J.P., C. Skrzynia, et al. 2001. 'The Complexities of Predictive Genetic Testing.' *BMJ* 322, no. 7293: 1052–6.

Evans, R.G. 1984. *Strained Mercy: The Economics of Canadian Health Care*. Toronto: Butterworths.

Evans, R.G., M. Barer, et al. 1994. *It's Not the Money, It's the Principle: Why User Charges for Some Services and Not Others?* Toronto: Ontario Premier's Council on Health, Well-being and Social Justice.

Evans, R.G., K.M. McGrail, et al. 2001. 'APOCALYPSE NO: Population Aging and the Future of Health Care Systems.' *Canadian Journal on Aging* 20 Suppl 1 (summer): 160–91.

Fuchs, V.R. 1984. '"Though Much Is Taken": Reflections on Aging, Health, and Medical Care.' *Milbank Memorial Fund Quarterly Health and Society* 62, no. 2: 143–66.

Ham, C., and A. Coulter. 2001. 'Explicit and Implicit Rationing: Taking Responsibility and Avoiding Blame for Health Care Choices.' *Journal of Health Serv Res Policy* 6, no. 3: 163–9.

Hench, L.L., and J.M. Polak. 2002. 'Third-Generation Biomedical Materials.' *Science* 295: 1014–17.

Henry, D., and D.J. Birkett. 2001. 'Changes to the Pharmaceutical Benefits Advisory Committee.' *MJA* 174: 209–10.

Herper, M. 2001. 'Genet Tests: Medicine's New Gold Mine.' *Forbes*.

– 2002. 'Pharmacia's Next Trick: Gene Tests.' *Forbes*.

Horrobin, D.F. 2000. 'Innovation in the Pharmaceutical Industry.' *J R Soc Med* 93, no. 7: 341–5.

Hurley, J., S. Birch, et al. 1997. 'Medical Necessity, Benefit and Resource Allocation in Health Care.' *Journal of Health Services Res Policy* 2, no. 4: 223–30.

IBM. 1999. IBM Announces US$100 Million Research Initiative to Build
World's Fastest Supercomputer. IBM.

ICES. 2001. *Health Technology Assessment of Positron Emission Tomography.* Institute for Clinical Evaluative Sciences.

IMS. 2002a. *Leading the Personalized Medicine Revolution.* IMS Health.

– 2002b. *US Innovation Will Drive Domination.* IMS Global.

Jacobzone, S. 2000. *Pharmaceutical Policies in OECD Countries: Reconciling Social and Industrial Goals.* Paris, France, Organisation for Economic Co-operation and Development.

Kaji, E.H., and J.M. Leiden. 2001. 'Gene and Stem Cell Therapies.' *JAMA* 285, no. 5: 545–50.

Koopman, W.J. 2001. 'Prospects for Autoimmune Disease: Research Advances in Rheumatoid Arthritis.' *JAMA* 285, no. 5: 648–50.

Lefkowitz, R.J., and J.T. Willerson. 2001. 'Prospects for Cardiovascular Research.' *JAMA* 285, no. 5: 581–7.

Lemonick, M.D. 2001. 'Brave New Pharmacy: Using High-speed Robots and the Secrets of the Human Genome, Scientists are Changing Forever the Way They Discover New Medicines [The future of drugs].' *Time* 157, no. 2: 32–7.

Livingston, D.M., and R. Shivdasani. 2001. 'Toward Mechanism-based Cancer Care.' *JAMA* 285, no. 5: 588–93.

Mack, M.J. 2001. 'Minimally Invasive and Robotic Surgery.' *JAMA* 285, no. 5: 568–72.

Marshall, E. 2002. 'A Space Age Vision Advances in the Clinic.' *Science* 295: 1000–1.

Marteau, T.M., and R.T. Croyle. 1998. 'Psychological Responses to Genetic Testing.' *BMJ* 316: 693–6.

Mays, N., J.A. Mulligan, et al. 2000. 'The British Quasi-market in Health Care: A Balance Sheet of the Evidence.' *Journal of Health Serv Res Policy* 5, no. 1: 49–58.

Miller, F., J. Hurley, et al. 2002. *Predictive Genetic Tests and Health Care Costs: Final Report Prepared for the Ontario Ministry of Health and Long Term Care.* Hamilton, ON, Centre for Health Economics and Policy Analysis, McMaster University.

Mintzes, B. 2002. 'Direct to Consumer Advertising is Medicalising Normal Human Experience.' *BMJ* 324: 908–9.

Mintzes, B., M.L. Barer, et al. 2002. 'Influence of Direct to Consumer Pharmaceutical Advertising and Patients' Requests on Prescribing Decisions: Two-Site Cross-Sectional Survey.' *BMJ* 324, no. 7332: 278–9.

Monaghan, M.J., and M.S. Monaghan. 1996. 'Do Market Components Account for Higher US Prescription Prices?' *Ann Pharmacother* 30, no. 12: 1489–94.

Morgan, S. 1998. Issues for Pharmaceutical Policy. In *Canada Health Action: Building on the Legacy. Papers Commissioned by the National Forum on Health. Volume 4: Striking a Balance, Health Care Systems in Canada and Elsewhere.* Sainte-Foy, Que: Éditions MultiMondes.

Morgan, S.G. 2001. *Price and Productivity Measurement in a Pharmaceutical Sector Sub-market: The Real Cost of Treating Hypertension.* Vancouver: UBC Centre for Health Services and Policy Research.

– 2002a. 'An Assessment of the Health System: Impacts of Direct-to-Consumer Advertising of Prescription Medicines (DTCA).' In *Volume V: Predicting the Welfare and Cost Consequences of Direct-to-Consumer Prescription Drug Advertising.* Vancouver: CHSPR, UBC.

– 2002b. 'Quantifying Components of Drug Expenditure Inflation: The British Columbia Seniors' Drug Benefit Plan.' *Health Services Research (HSR):* forthcoming.

Morgan, S.G., M. Barer, et al. 2000. 'Health Economists Meet the Fourth Tempter: Drug Dependency and Scientific Discourse.' *Health Econ* 9, no. 8: 659–67.

Moynihan, R., I. Heath, et al. 2002. 'Selling Sickness: The Pharmaceutical Industry and Disease Mongering.' *BMJ* 324: 886–91.

Munger Kahn, V. 2002. Managers Say this Decade Belongs to Health Care. *New York Times.* New York: http://www.nytimes.com/2002/01/06/business/yourmoney/

Olefsky, J.M. 2001. 'Prospects for Research in Diabetes Mellitus.' *JAMA* 285, no. 5: 628–32.

Pennisi, E. 2001. 'So Many Choices, So Little Money.' *Science* 294: 82–5.

Phillips, K.A., D.L. Veenstra, et al. 2001. 'Potential Role of Pharmacogenomics in Reducing Adverse Drug Reactions: A Systematic Review.' *JAMA* 286, no. 18: 2270–9.

PhRMA. 2001a. *New Medicines in Development: Biotechnology. Washington.* Washington, DC: Pharmaceutical Research and Manufacturers of America.

– 2001b. *New Medicines in Development for Older Americans.* Washington, DC: Pharmaceutical Research and Manufacturers of America.

Pinto, M.B., J.K. Pinto, et al. 1998. 'The Impact of Pharmaceutical Direct Advertising: Opportunities and Obstructions.' *Health Mark Q* 15, no. 4: 89–101.

Porter, R. 2000. 'Millennial Musings.' *BMJ* 321, no. 7269: 1092–3.

Rice, T. 1998. *The Economics of Health Reconsidered.* Chicago: Health Administration Press.

Rizzo, J.A. 1999. 'Advertising and Competition in the Ethical Pharmaceutical Industry: The Case of Antihypertensive Drugs.' *Journal of Law and Economics* 42: 89–116.

Robinson, R. 1999. 'Limits to Rationality: Economics, Economists and Priority Setting.' *Health Policy* 49, nos. 1–2: 13–26.

Rosenthal, M.B., E.R. Berndt, et al. 2002. 'Promotion of Prescription Drugs to Consumers.' *New England Journal of Medicine* 346, no. 7: 498–505.

Rubin, P.H., and J.L. Schrag. 1999. 'Mitigating Agency Problems by Advertising, with Special Reference to Managed Health Care.' *Southern Economic Journal* 66: 39–60.

Scott-Levin Inc. 2001. *The Pharmaceutical Industry: 10 Trends to Watch*. Quintiles Transnational Corp. press releae, 7 Nov. 2001.

Smith, R. 2002. 'In Search of "Non-disease."' *BMJ* 324: 883–5.

Soumerai, S.B., D. Ross-Degnan, et al. 1993. 'A Critical Analysis of Studies of State Drug Reimbursement Policies: Research in Need of Discipline.' *Milbank Quarterly* 71, no. 2: 217–52.

Tamblyn, R. 2001. 'The Impact of Pharmacotherapy Policy: A Case Study.' *Canadian Journal of Clinical Pharmacology* 8 Suppl A: 39A–44A.

Temin, P. 1980. *Taking Your Medicine: Drug Regulation in the United States*. Cambridge, Mass.: Harvard University Press.

Tempany, C.M., and B.J. McNeil. 2001. 'Advances in Biomedical Imaging.' *JAMA* 285, no. 5: 562–7.

Towse, A. 1996. 'The UK Pharmaceutical Market. An Overview.' *PharmacoEconomics* 10 Suppl 2: 14–25.

– 1998 'The Pros and Cons of a Single "Euro-price" for Drugs.' *Pharmacoeconomics* 13, no. 3: 271–6.

Wallace, M. 2000. 'Genotype Screening: The Impact on Clinical Trial Costs [Abstract].' *Annual Meeting of International Society of Technology Assessment in Health Care* 15: 79.

Willison, D., M. Wiktorowicz, et al. 2001. *International Experience with Pharmaceutical Policy: Common Challenges and Lessons for Canada*. Hamilton: Centre for Health Economics and Policy Analysis.

Young, B., and M. Surrusco. 2001. *Rx R&D Myths: The Case Against the Drug Industry's R&D 'Scare Card.'* Washington, DC: Public Citizen.

2 How an Ageing Population Will Affect Health Care

SEAMUS HOGAN AND SARAH HOGAN

Concern over ageing is not exclusive to discussions of the future of health care, nor are Canadians alone in dealing with this issue. Many countries are facing the prospect of an increase in the percentage of the population aged 65 or older because of the ageing of the baby-boom generation, as in Western nations, and/or increasing life expectancy, as in a number of countries, most notably Japan. An older population tends to increase the need for public spending – on pensions, health care, and other services – while reducing the proportion of the population paying substantial income tax.

Forecasts of the impact that ageing will have on the Canadian health system vary widely. Some commentators predict a dire future and use the spectre of ageing to justify major structural changes to the public-health system or alteration of federal transfers to the provinces; others see the problems as overstated and argue that no special action is needed. The former view is expressed mostly in the media or in political debates, as in the well-publicized provincial report of 2000 on 'cost-drivers.'[1] The academic literature has tended to take the latter view (see, for instance, Evans et al. 2001a, and references there), although some papers find ageing, while not a dire threat, a serious concern that does require some policy action now (for example, Robson 2001).

The starting point for all such analyses is deriving a projection of current trends into the future, taking into account demographic change, but there are many uncertainties about the continuation of current trends. The diversity of policy conclusions concerning the impact of ageing on the health system stems partly from differences of opinion about assumptions to make when projecting current trends and about how to interpret the projections and derive policy conclusions from them. The first section of this paper shows how we derive our projection. After presenting the basic facts on demographics, ageing, and expenditures, we offer a simple baseline projection and a sensitivity analysis of six factors that could make the future deviate from that baseline. The second section discusses four policy proposals that arise from this analysis, focusing on financing Canadian public-health systems, rather than on issues of delivery, such as service levels and delivery mechanisms. A brief look at federal implications completes the second section.

The main message of this paper is that there is sufficient uncertainty as to the effect of ageing on health care to sustain either pessimistic or optimistic conclusions, depending on what assumptions one chooses from a wide menu of reasonable alternatives. Our policy analysis is therefore based on asking what a prudent course of action would be, given the inherent uncertainty. Our conclusion is that the ageing issue is serious and cannot be ignored, but there is no need for drastic measures like significantly reforming the health system. What is needed is an immediate decision to save for the specific purpose of meeting increased needs for the future, rather than spending now in the naïve expectation that an ageing strategy designed today will turn out to have been perfectly clairvoyant in the future. Finally, the one area for increasing current spending is the remuneration of health sector human resources, a shortage of which must be avoided in the years to come.

Deriving a Projection

Basic Facts

This subsection briefly presents the basic facts about the ageing of the Canadian population, the relationship between age and use of health care, and the relationship between age and health-care expenditures. This information will lay the groundwork for the projection made in the next section and the policy implications discussed in the remainder of the paper.

Basic Demographics

Over the past 70 years, the age structure of the Canadian population has changed significantly, with the fraction aged over 65 increasing from 5 per cent to 12 per cent, and the fraction aged over 85, from 0.2

Figure 2.1
Population age structure, 1997

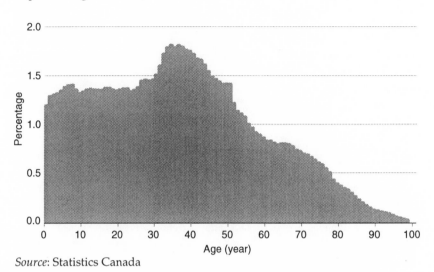

Source: Statistics Canada

per cent to 0.8 per cent. As a result, the average age of Canadians has risen by almost 10 years. Changes in mortality and migration patterns, and a fluctuating fertility rate, have all contributed to this increase.

The main focus for the current concern over ageing is the baby-boom generation, which arose from the big increase in fertility immediately after the Second World War, followed by a steady decline in fertility from the 1960s on. The post-baby-boom decrease in fertility helps explain the effect of the baby boom: initially the boom reduced Canadians' average age, simply because of the large and sudden increase in the number of children; but once the fertility rate fell back, the population steadily aged along with the baby boom, since that cohort represents a very large proportion of the whole. Currently, however, because baby boomers are only in their forties and fifties, the fraction of the population over 65 is lower than would be the case if the fertility rate had remained constant. Consequently, in fifty years or so, when most of the boomers will have died, the elderly fraction will be larger than it is now. These trends are illustrated in Figure 2.1, which shows the age distribution of the Canadian population in 1997, and in Figure 2.2, which shows both historical and projected changes in the fraction of the population over 65.

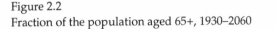

Figure 2.2
Fraction of the population aged 65+, 1930–2060

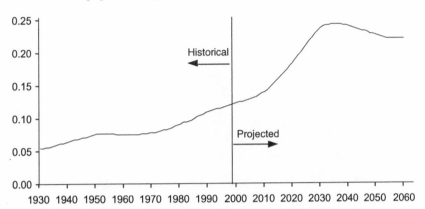

Source: Historical Data, Statistics Canada; Population Projections, Health
Canada (2002).

While the ageing of the baby-boom generation is the main reason
why ageing figures prominently in policy discussions, fertility cycles
have not been the main determinant of ageing over the past century.
Rather, the steady decline in mortality rates at all ages has led to a con-
tinual increase in the fraction of successive cohorts reaching old age.
Since shifts in mortality rates depend heavily on long-term factors
such as changes in nutrition, medicine, health care, and behaviour,
they usually follow long-term trends rather than displaying cyclical
behaviour. One can thus expect mortality rates to continue to decline
(though more slowly than in the past) and therefore add to the pressures of ageing brought about by the baby boom.

The Relationship between Ageing and Expenditure
The fact that a person's health tends to deteriorate with age is self-
evident and clearly backed up by the available data, and one would
expect a corresponding increase in health expenditures with age. This
relationship is confirmed by Figure 2.3, which breaks down total (public and private) health expenditures by age group and sex and shows
that per-capita health expenditures increase very rapidly after age 65.[2]
Although age-specific figures for health expenditures are not always
reliable, it is clear that the data reflect an underlying truth.

Figure 2.3
Health expenditures, 1980–1

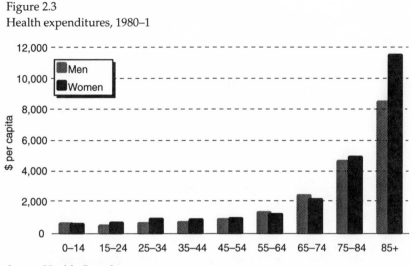

Source: Health Canada.

The fact that expenditures seem to start to rise rapidly soon after people reach 65 is the reason why the fraction of the population over 65 is the most common summary measure of the age of the population. The behaviour of expenditures after citizens turn 65 also highlights why ageing is very much a current concern. The baby-boom generation is still under 65 but rapidly approaching that point, with the first members of the generation reaching 65 in 2011. The choice of 65 as the cut-off between young and old is, however, somewhat arbitrary, but none of the projections presented in this paper depends on this particular cut-off.

The combination of an ageing population with a positive relationship between age and expenditures is the starting point for concerns over the future of the health system, as these elements form the basis for projections showing escalating expenditures.

Baseline Projection

This subsection briefly describes a baseline projection of the contribution of ageing to future growth in health expenditures. This projection then forms the organizing framework for the rest of the paper. The policy implications discussed in the remainder of the paper centre on

Figure 2.4
Ageing and health expenditures, 1980–2060

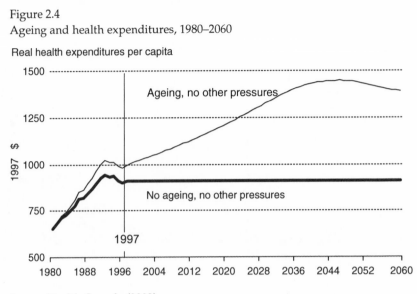

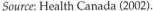

Source: Health Canada (2002).

whether the projected increase in expenditures would have serious implications for policy, whether the projection is reasonable, and how to address the underlying sources of uncertainty.[3]

There has been significant growth in health expenditures over the last twenty years. But ageing is not the only factor behind this increase: Some of it may result from other factors, including wage pressures in the health sector and the development of new technologies. The effect of ageing on health expenditures can be determined by decomposing expenditure data into different effects (Figure 2.4). For the period prior to 1997, the top line shows total health expenditure, and the lower line, likely expenditures if the population had remained constant at its 1980 level while per-capita expenditures for each age group and sex had changed in the way observed over the period 1980–97. Thus this line represents the change not attributable to ageing and thus caused by other factors. The effect of ageing is the difference between this figure and the total. The first bar in Figure 2.5 shows the average annual growth in expenditure attributed to ageing and other factors, respectively, over this period. Ageing is estimated to have had a small effect relative to other factors – only 0.5 per cent out of an average annual growth rate of 2.5 per cent.

Figure 2.5
Health cost drivers, 1980–2030

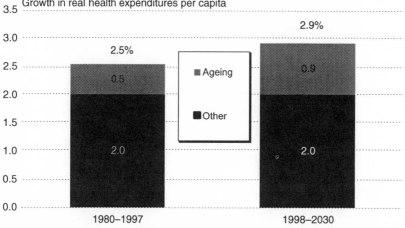

Source: Health Canada (2002).

The picture looks different when we project expenditure pressures into the future (Figures 2.4 and 2.5). If we assume that the relationship between real per-capita health expenditures and age will stay at its 1997 level (the last year in the data used in this paper) while the population ages according to a simple demographic projection, ageing alone would create pressure for an average annual growth in health expenditures of about 0.9 per cent over the next 30 years. The cumulative effect would be an increase of more than 30 per cent in health expenditures by the year 2030 purely as a result of population ageing. In Figure 2.4, in order to isolate the projected effect of ageing, we assume that ageing is the only source of real per-capita growth in expenditure. In Figure 2.5, however, to keep the numbers in perspective, we assume that other factors will continue to contribute an average of 2 percentage points to growth each year. Relative to this figure, the projected average annual growth in health expenditures of 0.9 per cent caused by ageing is still relatively small.

It is also interesting to decompose the historical and projected effects of ageing into the effect of an increasing life expectancy (decreasing mortality) and the effect of fluctuations in fertility. The policy implications of expenditure growth and the sensitivity of the projection to

Figure 2.6
Fertility and mortality effects, 1980–2030

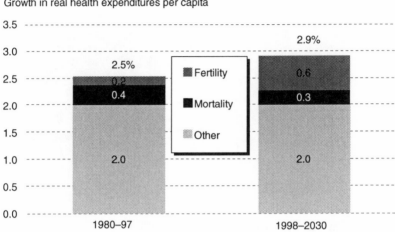

Source: Health Canada (2002).

demographic assumptions may differ depending on which effect is the
principal cause of population ageing. Figure 2.6 reveals that 70 per cent
of the 0.5 per cent average annual historical growth attributable to ageing comes from reductions in mortality, and only 30 per cent from fertility fluctuations, highlighting the point that the ageing of the baby-
boom generation has yet to have a major impact on health expenditures. The relative weight of the two effects reverses almost exactly in
the projection to 2030, with 71 per cent of projected growth due to ageing coming from the fertility effect and only 29 per cent from reductions in mortality.

Whereas the debate on ageing generally focuses on the idea that an
ageing baby boom is causing an increase in the number of older people, the baby-boom generation is currently younger than 65. Therefore
there is currently a disproportionately large fraction of the population
in ages with low health-care costs. As a result, costs for health care are
much lower than they would have been in the absence of the post-war
baby boom. As that generation ages, a greater fraction of the population will move into older and more expensive ages, causing a temporary, yet significant, increase in per-capita health expenditures.

Nonetheless, the results also suggest that, although the contribution of ageing to average annual expenditure growth will rise to about 0.9 per cent over the next 30 years as the baby boom reaches its high health-expenditure years, ageing will continue to represent only a secondary source of pressure on health-care costs, while other factors cause most of the pressure.

Sensitivity Analysis of Variables

The expenditure projection made in the previous subsection is just a projection, not a forecast. It is a statement of what would happen if certain conditions applied – namely, assumed changes in fertility, migration, and mortality rates, and no change in the relationship between health expenditures and age. The reality could differ for each of the following seven reasons, examined in this subsection:

- changes in demographic trends
- trends in population health
- a cost-of-dying effect
- baby-boom-specific capital investments, which push up the relative cost of older age groups
- technological change
- policy-induced changes
- ageing-related changes in the overall cost of health services delivery.

This subsection considers each of these possibilities in turn and then assesses their importance for policy.

Uncertainties over Demographics

It is difficult to argue with demographic projections because there is really very little meaningful uncertainty in demographic projections over 60 years or less. Most of the projected effect of ageing on expenditures arises from the baby-boom effect, which, because it is predetermined, is not subject to uncertainty. Furthermore, most of the effect of falling mortality rates is also predetermined: that is to say, the fraction of people aged over 65 who will survive each year will be much higher than in the past, not because of falls in mortality in the future, but because of those that have already occurred. Finally, while future birth rates may affect the fraction of the population that is old, they cannot seriously change the ratio of the elderly to the working-age population over the 30-year horizon that we are looking at here.

Future immigration patterns may, however, also make demographic projections inaccurate. Significant immigration can dampen the speed at which the population ages, but it does not change the main conclusion that the baby boom will lead to significant increases in the fraction of the population aged 65 and over. Similarly, emigration can affect projections, but because emigrants tend to be relatively young it may actually speed up population ageing.

Trends in Population Health
Changes in the health status of Canadians, particularly older people, could dampen or amplify the health-expenditure effects of an ageing population. Unfortunately, it is very difficult to answer definitively whether older Canadians' health status has been improving or declining, let alone project what might happen in the future.

Using data from the Canada Health Survey (1978–9) and the National Population Health Survey (1998–9), Hogan (2002) has shown that by at least one measure – the age-adjusted prevalence of chronic conditions, a particular problem for the aged – Canadians are not becoming healthier; so it seems unreasonable to expect any savings from reduced health-care needs. For some of these conditions – notably hypertension and arthritis – this increase in age-adjusted prevalence arises from the current cohort of elderly Canadians. Chen and Millar (2000) show that baby boomers, however, have a lower prevalence of these conditions and so can expect to reach the 65+ age groups in better health than the current elderly.

Changes in the prevalence of conditions are, however, only one way of measuring alterations in health status, and other measures of morbidity such as health-adjusted life expectancy (HALE) take the duration of ill health into account, since expenditures are affected by not only how many people require care but for how long they require it.

HALE figures were calculated by Martel and Bélanger (1999) for activity limitations and by Hogan (2002) for a number of chronic conditions, including activity limitations. They found that in 1998–9 Canadians could generally expect to live more years free of chronic conditions than they would have in 1978–9, indicating that the onset of chronic conditions is generally later than in the late 1970s. The fraction of life that an individual can expect to live free of a given chronic condition, however, has decreased for seven conditions among both males and females because of the proportionately greater increase in life expectancy at age 12 than in HALE at age 12. Although Canadians can expect to be healthy for longer than previously, a greater proportion of the increase in life expectancy will be unhealthy. These results suggest a significant positive survival effect for most chronic conditions – an increase in the number of years a person can expect to live *with* a given condition rather than dying. When the increase in survival is proportionately larger than the increase in healthy years, there is, by definition, an expansion of morbidity. This has been the case for most chronic conditions. None the less, there has been some compression of morbidity – a proportionately greater increase in the number of healthy years – for several serious conditions: heart disease, arthritis, emphysema, and activity limitation.

Perhaps most significantly, the compression of morbidity for activity limitation, achieved through a simultaneous increase in the number of years expected to be free of limitations and a decrease in the number of years expected to be spent with limitations, suggests that Canadians are generally living a greater percentage of their lives with a reasonable quality of life. Since this has occurred at the same time as an expansion of morbidity for many chronic conditions, it appears that the activity-limiting effects of these or other conditions have significantly lessened, supporting the hypothesis that management of chronic conditions has improved sufficiently to allow Canadians to continue to work and play for longer than they used to. The costs of this achievement are not revealed by the data. Indeed, what we cannot determine from these or any data is the extent to which these changes have affected the need for health expenditures or have come about as a result of health expenditures. More important, the data cannot tell us what effect trends in population health will have on expenditures, so it seems clear that Canadians cannot rely on these trends to generate significant savings.

The Cost-of-Dying Effect
Reductions in mortality may flatten the relationship between age and health expenditures. Specifically, health expenditures appear to increase with age not simply because of a direct age effect but because most such expenditures on an individual occur in the last year or two of life. If this is so, then future reductions in mortality rates will not cause an increase in the fraction of the population that is expensive, even though they will cause an increase in the fraction of the population that is elderly.

Hogan and Pollock (2001) estimate the extent of the cost-of-dying effect in the past. If their estimated ratios between the amount spent on those who are in their last year of life and those who are not were to continue into the future, then most of the impact on health expenditures of population ageing due to reductions in mortality would disappear. An optimistic conclusion is, however, unwise. First, Hogan and Pollock's estimates, inferred indirectly from aggregate data rather than being based on direct observation, are subject to wide confidence intervals and are almost certainly overestimates.[4] Second, in any event, as we saw above, the projected impact on health expenditures of population ageing from reduced mortality is fairly small relative to the baby-boom effect – a point often overlooked in discussions about the effect of so-called compression of morbidity on projections of expenditure pressures caused by ageing.

The cost-of-dying effect will tend to offset the effect on projections if mortality rates fall by more than expected. That is, the existence of a cost-of-dying effect will tend to reduce the sensitivity of the projection to unexpected falls in mortality.

Generation-Specific Capital Investments
Data on per-capita health expenditures for different age groups probably underestimate the future cost of providing health care to the baby-boom generation as it ages. This is because the temporarily increased absolute number of elderly people will necessitate investment in additional health-care infrastructure and human capital, the need for which will have diminished before that capital has fully depreciated. This is probably only a small issue, but it does raise a caution when one is considering the proposition that the overall effect of ageing on public expenditures will be small, as savings in education on the young will offset the increased costs of health-care for the elderly. Such claims, based on per-capita expenditure figures, probably understate the cost of servicing the baby-boom generation as it ages and overstate the savings available from post-baby-boom age groups, as they implicitly assume that schools can be costlessly converted into health-care facilities, teachers into physicians, and so on. One might be tempted to argue that there exists an unused stock of hospitals and other health-care facilities that were shut down during recent fiscal cutbacks and that it might be easy to simply recommission these facilities. But many of the shut-down facilities were closed because the population that they served was not sufficient to justify the operating costs or because the buildings were old and deemed substandard. Despite worthy indi-

vidual cases for reversing past decisions, it seems unlikely that this would be worthwhile on a large scale.

Technological Change

In what follows here, we refer to technological change in the economists' sense. That is, we mean any change in the way of producing a given output and does not necessarily involve a move to using more modern or sophisticated technologies, although such change is a major component of technological change in the health sector.

Technological change is often the wild card in any projection. It has obviously spurred both health expenditures and health outcomes, but there is currently no good or accepted measure of it, so quantifing its overall impact in the past is difficult. Furthermore, by its very nature of being the discovery of previously unknown ways of doing things, it is impossible to predict, so even if we did have backward-looking measures of it, they would be of little use for predicting the future. Another problem is that any future technological change that may affect healthcare in Canada could save money or cost money for the health sector. Savings could arise if technological progress generated cheaper ways of delivering particular health outcomes (for example, if the discovery of new techniques for preventing heart disease seriously reduced the need for treatment or if a new, less expensive treatment were developed). Similarly, expenditures could increase if an expensive new treatment became available and it proved irresistible to the health system – a new cure for cancer, for example – or if wages in the health sector increased as technological progress in other sectors pushed up wages in the economy in general.

One form of technological change that seems particularly relevant to discussions of ageing, because of its importance to elderly patients, and that illustrates the difficulty in quantifying and predicting effects is developments in pharmaceuticals. Expenditures on drugs (prescribed and over-the-counter) now exceed those on physicians and are second only to hospitals among health expenditures in Canada. There are different interpretations of this trend. Perhaps the increase in expenditures represents the development of newer and better drugs leading to increases in both total health expenditures and in health outcomes, but technological progress in pharmaceuticals may have lowered expenditure overall, by allowing reductions in hospitalization. In contrast, Evans et al. (2001a) contend that the trend in expenditures on drugs simply represents a tendency for physicians to prescribe newer and more expensive products that do not provide a significant therapeutic advantage over older and cheaper drugs.

Given these conflicting claims about the past, the difficulty of predicting future advances, and the uncertainty as to whether the prescribing effect described by Evans et al., if it is real, will be reversed in the future, it is impossible to predict whether further technological change in the pharmaceutical industry will strengthen or weaken the relationship between health expenditures and age.

Policy-Induced Changes
Obviously, population ageing does not have to affect public expenditures in the way suggested by the projection because governments can choose to respond by restricting expenditures, particularly on the elderly. If governments in fact restrict expenditures when faced with pressures, the conclusions from using a projection based on an assumption of no change in service levels would still be valid, but they would imply that the costs of ageing would be absorbed as a reduction in service rather than as an increase in expenditures, not that the costs were non-existent. In other words, if governments do not allow health expenditures to increase as much as ageing pressures would require, the difference between actual future expenditures and the projections in this paper would represent a monetary estimate of the reduction in per-capita service levels. This might be felt more tangibly as longer waiting lists or decreased quality of care.

However, the possibility of governments choosing to restrict expenditures despite significant pressures (or, similarly, to spend more in the absence of real pressure to do so) does affect the interpretation of data. There simply do not exist reliable expenditure data that separate out price from level of service, since both are measured in dollars and there is no general unit of measurement for health services. It is therefore not possible to distinguish between the cost of achieving a particular health outcome and the policy decisions that change the quantity of health services provided. For example, age-expenditure data from Health Canada show a striking fall in relative expenditures on the 85+ age group in the mid- to late 1990s. Did expenditures on this group drop because the cost of achieving a given health outcome fell or because the health status of this group was allowed to fall in order to reduce costs? It is tempting to attribute the reduction in expenditures to the former, but there is also some anecdotal evidence that hospitals responded to fiscal restraints by cutbacks in quantity and quality that hit elderly patients hardest. As unreliable as anecdotal evidence may be, the data do not refute the claim. The difficulty in improving the data is clear when one considers how one might calculate the cost of achieving a given health outcome when that cost may vary significantly from one person to the next.

Similarly, since governments in other countries may also make policy decisions that affect health expenditures and their data also do not allow for the isolation of price from level of service, little useful information can be gained by looking at international data to see how other governments have adjusted to the expenditure pressures of ageing. The ageing issue in Canada requires a policy response that cannot be drawn from the past or from elsewhere.

General Cost Increases Attributable to Ageing
The final source of deviation from the baseline projection is that ageing, by increasing the overall demand for health services, might raise the price of scarce health resources and thus cause an increase in the cost of providing health care to all age groups. The area where this is a particular concern is health workers. Data from McMaster University[5] reveal that the aged use physicians' services more intensively than do younger people, and an even stronger relationship between age and service levels of nursing seems likely.

Concern intensifies when one considers that demographics also affect labour supply. Research at Health Canada using data from the Southam Medical Database has estimated that, given the current rates at which physicians of different ages and sexes enter and leave the profession, we would expect to see a 30 per cent reduction in the number of physicians in Canada over the next 50 years. About half of that reduction should derive from baby-boom physicians reaching retirement age, and half from the smaller fraction of the population in the age groups that tend to enter the profession.[6]

The data also show that, although demographics will significantly affect the excess demand for physicians, a return to the rates at which physicians entered and exited the profession in Canada in the early 1980s would more than compensate for the demographic effect on both the demand for and supply of physicians. It is doubtful, however, that the required increase in health workers could be obtained without raises in their relative wages and salaries. Indeed, Chan (2002) decomposes the reduced entry rate of physicians into the profession in the early 1990s and finds that most of the decline resulted from physicians spending more time in postgraduate training and from a slower inflow of foreign doctors and that only a small fraction was due to cuts in medical-school enrolment. Increasing the supply of physicians therefore is not simply a matter of returning to former enrolment levels.

Recognition that wage and salary rates in the health sector are not fixed but respond to changes in this sector is relevant to one common suggestion for lowering the costs of treating elderly patients – a greater use of home care as an alternative to hospitalization or residential care facilities. A study by Hollander and Chappell (2001) suggests that home care is a cheaper way of caring for seniors with low or moderate levels of disability, even if one takes into account the burden imposed on family members. Based on this and other studies, and noting that home services account for only 2 to 6 per cent of provincial health budgets, Hébert (2002) concludes that a 'real shift in resources is needed to reverse the traditional hospital-centred approach.' It is not clear, however, that home care would continue to be cost effective under such a real shift in resources, because a substantial increase in the number of home-care workers might necessitate a real increase in wage rates in the sector.

Policy Implications

The baseline projection suggests that, based on the current relationship between age and health expenditures, ageing will probably lead to pressure for increased real per-capita expenditures on health, but that this pressure is also likely to be small relative to historical rates of growth of expenditures attributable to non-ageing factors. It is important to keep this perspective in mind when discussing the implications of ageing for the Canadian health system. However, the fact that population ageing is likely to be a secondary driver of health expenditures is not in itself a reason for dismissing it as a major public-policy issue in the health sector. We still have to ask whether the projected 0.9 per cent average annual growth in real per-capita expenditures due to ageing requires an immediate policy response.

Furthermore, the previous subsection suggests a very large band of uncertainty around any forecast of future health expenditures caused largely by inherent uncertainties, not just by lack of data or empirical analysis. The key conclusion from this situation is not that we need more research, but that we must accept the wide band of uncertainty and focus policy conclusions on risk management – that is, on taking uncertainty into account when planning. It is also a caution against accepting demagogic analysis that selectively considers only the best-case or the worst-case scenarios, and then derives policy conclusions from them.

The other main implication concerns the need for planning about health workers, since the biggest risk of a greater-than-projected ageing-derived pressure on expenditures arises from shortages there. We discuss these implications in more detail in the next section.

Policy Proposals

This section considers the appropriate approach to the issue of population ageing for governments in areas where they have direct jurisdiction – that is, principally provincial governments, except in some specific areas of federal jurisdiction such as First Nations and Inuit health. The next section considers some cross-jurisdiction implications for the federal government. There are four main policy directions in this section:

- *System reform?:* Population ageing does not represent a justification in and of itself for reforming the health system. The system can always benefit from improvements in efficiency, but population ageing should not be used to excuse advocates of reforms from justifying proposed changes on their own terms.
- *Pre-funding:* Expected health liabilities from population ageing should be pre-funded. Governments should be building up a dedicated fund to cover the impact of ageing on future expenditures. That is, the likely impact of ageing on fiscal balances is manageable, given the current fiscal outlook, but it would be serious if fiscal management turns to 'pay-as-you-go' thinking.
- *An ageing strategy:* Governments should deal with ageing as a public-finance problem and avoid the temptation to put in place 'an ageing strategy' of current health expenditures on programs and projects designed to reduce future demand.
- *Human-resources planning:* To retain the flexibility needed to deal with future problems, governments should direct current funding towards increasing labour supply in the health sector.

System Reform?

As we saw above, commentators who advocate reform of the health system in Canada in order to constrain expenditures – usually those who favour greater use of private funding or delivery – often invoke the spectre of ageing. The issue of ageing as a cost driver, however, is misplaced in discussions of general system reform.

First, even under the most pessimistic scenario imaginable from the considerations presented above, ageing represents mostly a one-time pressure on expenditures (admittedly over an extended period of about 30 years), not ongoing growth. If one were to make an argument that the system needs to be reformed to deal with that 30-year pressure, then the same argument would suggest a return to the old health system after 30 years. For a one-time increase in needs, it would be simpler and probably less costly to absorb the expenditure increase by diverting resources from other uses, in contrast to an ongoing pressure, where there might be a real imperative for system reform.

Second, and more important, ageing and the associated expenditure pressures will occur whatever the system – that is, the fiscal pressures associated with ageing are not *caused* by the system. The increased pressures on expenditures likely as the population ages are associated with real needs, caused by the inherent nature of ageing, that will increase regardless of the type of system, not with some distorted way in which the current system is unnecessarily generous with the aged. Unless one argues that the current system is providing too much health care to the aged, reforming the system cannot be the key to reducing expenditure pressures.

Of course, if there are reforms that can help reduce costs and hence offset the fiscal pressures of ageing without causing a serious reduction in service levels, they should be implemented, but such efficiency enhancers would be desirable even if there were no fiscal pressures from ageing. That is, reforms need to be justified on their own terms, not piggy-backed onto concerns over ageing. Such efficiency reforms would have been and will always be desirable and should have their own debate rather than being treated as a subsection of the ageing debate.

The conclusion that cost pressures associated with ageing cannot justify system reform does *not* derive from the result seen above – that ageing is likely to be only a secondary driver of health-expenditure growth; rather, the link between ageing pressures and system design is a non sequitur. Ultimately, population ageing is an issue of public finance rather than of the health system. Should we cover future costs by diverting resources from other uses or absorb the impact of population ageing by reducing service? This choice is the subject of the following subsection.

Pre-Funding

The analysis of the previous subsection is that governments should not look to system reform to avert the pressures created by ageing. Instead, they have three options to respond to the resulting increased demand for services: reducing the extent and generosity of publicly funded health care at the time of the increased demand; funding the increased demand when it occurs by raising taxes or cutting back on other public expenditures; or funding the increased demand over time by running larger budget surpluses in advance.

The system for financing public health in Canada, in which current tax revenues pay for current health expenditures, involves an implicit social contract between governments and citizens, whereby working-age Canadians pay taxes to fund health care that goes disproportionately to older people in the expectation that they will receive the same higher share of public-health expenditures when they reach their senior years. Cutting back on health services when the baby boom is in its years of high health expenditure would violate this implicit contract and hence not be good public policy.

How then should governments ensure that they can meet their implicit contractual obligations to fund a reasonable level of health care to an increasingly elderly population? The policy debate here hinges on whether future liabilities should be met partially from current taxes (i.e., by 'pre-funding' future health care) or by maintaining a pay-as-you-go health system. We argue for pre-funding. This could imply treating health in a way similar to the Canada Pension Plan, by setting up a fund into which government would initially pay while the population was still relatively young and on which it would then draw to help fund public health in later years.

Of course, pre-funding is possible simply by having governments run budget surpluses without bearing the administrative costs of a separate trust fund. The advantage of a formal trust fund is that it would create a mechanism whereby governments could credibly commit themselves to carrying over some tax revenues to pay for future expenditures. The main issue here is not the institutional form of government savings, but the idea that governments should seek to finance future health expenditures now. The remainder of this sub-section, addresses three common arguments against any form of pre-funding.

Argument no. 1 against pre-funding: *The increase in expenditures caused by ageing will be small relative to likely economic growth and will therefore not require a change in funding style.* This argument for continuing to pay as we go assumes that the increase in health-care costs attributable to ageing is small relative to other historical drivers of health expenditures, hence not important enough to justify moving away from 'paying as we go.' The statement about the relative role of ageing is true (as the simple projection above shows), but one can draw too optimistic a conclusion from this. For one thing, population ageing is an expenditure driver that does not fund itself. Consider two other expenditure drivers: increases in demand associated with higher gross domestic product (GDP) and increases in the cost of labour in the health sector. Much of the increase in real per-capita health expenditures over time is closely related to increases in real per-capita GDP. This occurs for two reasons. First, higher GDP leads to an 'income-effect' increase in the demand for health services; that is, as GDP growth leads to higher individual incomes and government tax revenues, demand for health services, along with other goods and services, rises. Second is the phenomenon known as Baumol's 'cost disease' (Baumol and Bowen 1966), whereby general economic growth tends to lift wages and salaries in the economy as a whole and hence pushes up costs in labour-intensive industries such as health and education, as workers will not continue to enter those sectors if their wage and salary levels fall behind those available elsewhere. As Baumol (1993) points out, increases in the demand for public-health expenditures that are caused by increases in GDP do not present a funding dilemma for governments, as they are essentially self-funding. On the other hand, the same analysis suggests that Canada cannot rely on future GDP growth to fund the costs of ageing, as increased demand for health services or increased wages and salaries from the 'cost disease,' have already spoken for that growth.

Baumol's cost disease relies on the assumption that productivity gains will be lower in the labour-intensive sector than in the rest of the economy, so that increases in wages and salaries there will not be offset by employing less labour to produce a given output. Evans et al. (2001b) criticize this line of analysis in the health sector because there is evidence of huge productivity changes in that sector. Productivity growth, however, negates Baumol's 'cost disease' only to the extent that it permits reduced employment in the sector, rather than simply allowing a greater range of health services with the same labour input. It would be a very high-risk strategy for governments to assume that they can contain expenditures by delivering the current range of services with fewer doctors and nurses in the future – the implied policy prescription of Evans et al.

In the 18 years to 1997, the average annual increase in real per-capita health expenditures caused by factors other than ageing, *in excess of GDP growth*, was only 0.7 per cent. The projected 0.9 per cent average annual growth caused by ageing is not small relative to this number.[7]

An alternative form of the argument about the minimal costs of ageing accepts some of the more optimistic scenarios for predicting lower increases in expenditures than in the baseline projection. As noted above, these scenarios cannot be dismissed, but cannot be relied on. The uncertainty involved is simply too great. It would therefore be more prudent to indulge in precautionary savings rather than relying too heavily on optimistic projections.

Argument no. 2 against pre-funding: Simultaneous downward pressures in other areas will offset increased pressures in the health sector. This argument suggests that when all age-related expenditures are looked at as a whole, there is no serious financing issue, since at the same time as ageing is putting upward pressure on health-care budgets and public pension plans, other demographic changes will create offsetting downward pressure on other areas of public expenditures, notably education. This point has been made by Denton and Spencer (1995), among others.

Again, the basic premise is correct: if, as we have argued, the pressures on health-care budgets from ageing should be viewed as a matter of public finance rather than of health, one needs to look at all aspects of ageing and public expenditures, not just at health, when discussing the implications for public finance. There are, however, three problems with using this line of argument. First, one cannot assume that resources can be transferred at no cost from one activity to another or even that they can be transferred at all. (Can teachers simply retrain as physicians? Blackboards and school gymnasiums transformed into hospital beds and palliative-care units? Decrepit, unused hospitals renovated and put back into use at a reasonable cost?) Second, one cannot assume that governments will be prepared to make the offsetting reductions in education or other expenditures; that is, even if it is economically feasible to substitute resources away from education towards health, it may not be politically feasible to do so, as these other sectors may well have good uses for the extra resources that become available. Finally, even if the savings from some areas were to offset most or all of the projected increases in health expenditures over time, they cannot be expected to do so each year, so that, if reduced expenditures on education are to pay for increased expenditures on health, the savings from the former would need to be hoarded until the need for the latter arises. Pre-funding into a dedicated public trust fund provides a mechanism for doing so. With such a fund, if the political will exists to make offsetting reductions in education, these can become a source of revenue for the fund at the time they arise.

Argument no. 3 against pre-funding: Canada's fiscal position is such that population ageing will not require pre-funding. This argument, like the previous one, considers other aspects of the overall fiscal position to address whether the impact of ageing on health expenditures will be a problem. Although ageing may, on balance, place expenditure pressures on governments, current debt and deficit levels in Canada imply that, given all future explicit and implicit liabilities (interests on government debt, expenditures on health and CPP for an ageing population, and so on), there would be no need to increase taxes or reduce other expenditures in the future to meet those obligations, given current trends. This argument is alluded to by Mérette (2002), who notes that future implicit liabilities of Canadian governments for age-related expenditures are offset to a large extent by the implicit asset of deferred taxes that will be paid as retirees cash in their RRSPs.

It is beyond the scope of this paper to assess the overall fiscal position of Canadian governments, but even if the country is in a position of fiscal balance (i.e., future liabilities can be met without increasing taxes or reducing services), ageing is still a fiscal concern. Specifically, if Canada is in fiscal balance, the concern is not that it will be difficult to meet obligations to future generations of elderly Canadians. Rather, there is a risk that, by not making the financial liability of those obligations explicit through pre-funding, governments will take Canada out of fiscal balance by devoting budget surpluses to current rather than to future priorities. Pre-funding of the health system would be not so much a way of starting now to bear the costs of ageing, but a mechanism for ensuring that the necessary resources are available for health care in the future and are not spent now or devoted to other uses.

Furthermore, although the country as a whole may be in fiscal balance, this is not necessarily true of every province, and it is at the provincial level that most public funding of health arises.

An Ageing Strategy

The key message of the sensitivity analysis is that, although ageing is predictable, the future relationship between age and health needs and the future of medical technology are not. In such an environment, the most important thing that governments can do is to make sure that the financial resources will be available as ageing puts pressure on the system and not invest in high-risk strategies such as programs to promote healthy ageing as a means to avert the pressure.

This is not to say that there are no programs or services involving the aged that would be worth funding, just as there will always be potential for improvements or innovations in the delivery of health services to any age group. Rather, governments should not look to current expenditures as an *investment* – that is, as an alternative to saving to meet the future needs of an ageing population – because the high level of uncertainty regarding the efficacy of such programs implies that this would be a very high-risk investment strategy.

There is an inevitable tendency for democratic governments to spend immediately on programs that are purported to generate great benefits in the future, rather than saving resources, because the latter means that a different government may benefit from a predecessor's saving efforts and may be seen as failing to spend on important programs. To reconcile the interests of government with those of the Canadian population, the former must find some way of making the public understand why resources must be put away for the future. Given the high level of public awareness of the ageing issue, this should not be difficult. In fact, awareness is so high that if governments *fail* to save for the future they may well be seen as irresponsible.

Human-Resources Planning

Although it would be unwise to assume that an ageing strategy can bring about the best-case scenario of ageing pressures on expenditures, governments should try to avert the worst-case scenario – costs and service levels generated by chronic shortages of health-care workers. Such shortages would affect the entire population, not just the aged. It would be felt as a significant deterioration in service and quite possibly in the health status of Canadians of all age groups, but particularly of the aged and of those whose need for health care is greatest. Furthermore, a shortage of personnel will affect workers already in the system, pressing them to extend their hours and subjecting them to additional stress. In turn, the health sector could lose even more human resources, and the performance of people who remain may suffer. It could well trigger a vicious downward spiral in the quality of care and level of service.

Of course, the picture painted here is grim, but there is a serious risk that it is not far from the truth. Quite apart from the issue of an ageing population, Canada has had difficulty retaining and recruiting workers in the health sector for at least a decade. The downward spiral could therefore be a challenge for Canada even without population ageing. Once ageing is added to the problem, increasing the demand for physicians and decreasing their supply through retirement, a grim scenario may be possible. Even if the probability is slim, if it does occur it could well be the biggest challenge that the Canadian health system has ever faced. And turning things around once they have begun to spiral downward will be much more difficult than avoiding the scenario in the first place.

But because labour supply reacts slowly to changes in working conditions, because of the time it takes to train more people or to attract them from other countries, conditions must begin to change *now* in order to ensure sufficient personnel in the future. It would probably be prudent therefore for governments to make one of the major uses of current funding an increase in the remuneration of health-care providers, rather than trying to provide more health services. Because of the time required to change the supply of labour, if governments wait until the situation is desperate, it will take years before Canadians feel a turnaround, and that wait would take place while unacceptable conditions in the health sector persist. Clearly, it would be better to start waiting now, before serious pressures are felt.

Of course, as we saw above, it is unclear how much wages and salaries would need to rise to generate sufficient change, but, given the consequences of underestimating the required increase, it would be prudent to err on the high side, leaving room for adjustment later.

Federal Implications

We have considered the policy implications for governments that are directly responsible for the provision of health services to Canadians. Given that health is mostly a provincial jurisdiction in Canada, these policy implications are most relevant to provincial governments, but they also relate to the federal government in areas coming under its jurisdiction, such as First Nations and Inuit health. In contrast, this subsection considers some cross-jurisdictional implications.

This subsection operates from the framework known as 'fiscal federalism'; that is, it asks what is the essential federal interest in ageing in areas of health that are under provincial jurisdiction. What are the criteria in this framework that can justify federal involvement in provincial areas?

As is so often the case in economics, there are twin, but sometimes opposing criteria of efficiency and equity. The equity justification for government involvement in areas of provincial jurisdiction is to seek an equitable distribution of publicly provided goods among Canadians of all provinces. This is the motivation behind equalization payments, which seek to compensate for interprovincial differences in the tax base and hence minimize the extent to which Canadians living in poorer provinces have less access to public services than those in richer provinces.

There are two aspects to the efficiency criteria. First, federal intervention should seek to minimize the extent to which a provincial government has an incentive to take action that would benefit its own province by imposing greater costs on others. Second, it should seek to promote efficient interprovincial migration, in which citizens choose the province where they will live based on their own preferences and on the underlying opportunities available in each province, rather than on distortions created by an unequal distribution of government 'goodies.'

Fiscal federalism often involves trade-offs between equity and efficiency. For instance, equalization payments to poorer provinces can promote interprovincial equity, but they reduce the incentives for those provinces to implement policies promoting economic growth (as higher provincial GDP will lead to an automatic reduction in federal transfers to the province), and they create a disincentive at the margin for residents to relocate where their productivity would be higher.

Now let's consider these criteria in the context of federal policy with respect to ageing and the public health system.

First, through equalization payments, the Canada Health and Social Transfer (CHST), and the Canada Health Act, the federal government is involved in the implicit contract that Canadian governments have made with the population to provide pay-as-you-go health care. That is, working-age Canadians have paid federal taxes to fund transfers to provinces that help finance health-care that goes disproportionately to older Canadians, so they can expect similarly to receive the benefit of such federal spending as they age. Second, age distribution varies across provinces, and the differences are expected to widen. For instance, Saskatchewan and Manitoba have a relatively old population, but one that is not ageing quickly. In contrast, Newfoundland has a relatively young but rapidly ageing population. Such geographical differences in demographics are discussed in more detail in Moore and Rosenberg (1995) and Robson (2001).

By the equity criterion for federal involvement, the first of these points suggests that Ottawa should be increasing the CHST to provinces as the country's population ages, over and above any other increases that would be justified by increasing costs, rising incomes, and so on, because to do otherwise would deny current taxpayers the health care that they have been led to expect for their senior years, thereby violating the implicit contract. The second point then suggests that, again by the equity criterion, these transfers should be tied in some way to the demographic situation of the province, with larger transfers being made to provinces with a relatively old population.

One can also justify a policy of demographically determined federal transfers by the efficiency criterion. A situation in which there was no federal involvement in financing provincial health expenditures would create incentives for individuals to locate in low-tax, low-health-expenditure provinces during their working years and live their retirement years in high-tax and high-health-expenditure provinces. This distortion would probably be small and not sufficient to justify demographically determined federal transfers, but, in this context, efficiency complements equity rather than implying a trade-off.

If we accept the argument in the sections above for some amount of pre-funding for the health system, then the federal government must pre-fund future increases in transfers to the provinces and relate these transfers to demographics in some way. This recommendation, which has also been made by Robson (2001), among others, implies a major overhaul of the CHST. Robson also observes that, in the absence of a pre-funded, demographically based form of federal transfer, federal transfers for health could become highly efficiency-reducing in the face of ageing. In Robson's words, 'One danger is that, as provinces get into trouble one by one (from the health expenditure pressures created by ageing), the federal government will make repeated *ad hoc* deals for enriched transfers, creating incentives that discourage longer-term reforms.'

A final point: the federal government is currently in a stronger fiscal position than many provinces and so is in a good position to lead by example in initiating some degree of pre-funding of the health system.

Concluding Remarks

The analysis presented in this paper has led to a fairly simple conclusion about how best to deal with population ageing and its impact on the health system – a conclusion that points to a course of action that is not as revolutionary as some who raise the spectre of ageing might recommend, but still implies taking the issue seriously and acting now to forestall future problems. Insofar as the required course of action is not revolutionary, accomplishing it should be possible with a minimum of disruption. What disruption there may be, however, will probably be more political than economic, because the problems that arise from population ageing are certainly manageable from the point of view of Canada's finances, but they require governments to behave in a way that is not usually expected of them.

Specifically, the governments of Canada – and the voting public – must be convinced of the need to put future needs ahead of short-term consumption by dedicating current savings to future health expenditures and by investing in health workers rather than increasing current service levels. If governments fail to do so, population ageing may have a severe impact on the health system. The resulting downward spiral in the health system that could occur if Canada fails to prepare for the years to come could take decades longer to reverse and be far more costly than prevention. If governments succeed in preparing for the future, the system should have enough flexibility to cope with the uncertainty that lies ahead, and thus they will have ensured that Canadians can count on their health system to see them through the next forty years and beyond.

Overall, the conclusion of this paper is that the pressures likely to be placed on the health system by population ageing are real, but small enough to be easily managed. The notion that ageing is likely to cause the system to collapse has been thoroughly rebutted many times. The biggest danger is that, in rejecting the apocalyptic scenarios of those who see ageing as a major problem requiring systemic reform, advocates of the ageing-is-not-a-problem view might encourage governments and the public to become too complacent and avoid taking action now at a time when it would be relatively easy to do so.

NOTES

1 Provincial and Territorial Ministers of Health 2000.
2 The data on health expenditures used in this paper come from the National Health Expenditures Database compiled by Health Canada.
3 The projection used here is one that we were involved in constructing at Health Canada. It is described in the briefing notes that constitute Health Canada 2002. We use this projection rather than a more widely cited one such as CIHI 2000 partly because the results presented here rest on a common set of demographic assumptions and are internally consistent and partly because the Health Canada projection includes a decomposition of the ageing effect into fertility and mortality components, which is important for the policy implications one draws from the results. However, all demographic projections of current expenditure patterns produce pretty much the same numbers: The debate about the significance of ageing involves how the expenditure patterns themselves are expected to evolve and the interpretation of the results of a simple projection, not the projections themselves.
4 Direct evidence from U.S. Medicare data suggests that expenditures on people in their last year of life are between 4 and 11 times that on non-decedents (Scitovsky 1994). This is about a quarter of the magnitude estimated by Hogan and Pollock.
5 The data come from the System for Health Area Resource Planning (SHARP) model.
6 These results are contained in Srivastava 2002 – a supply-side analysis. The demand-side analysis of Denton, Gafni, and Spencer 2002 looks at the effect of demographics on physician demand in Ontario. Their conclusion is that the increase in demand is likely to slow down in the coming decades as the effect of ageing is more than compensated for by a slowdown in the rate of population growth, which is unlikely to alleviate pressures on the labour market, as it is also a key determinant of labour supply.
7 For an analysis of the role of GDP growth in wage and salary increases in the health sector and its relative importance in total health-expenditure growth, see Ariste and Carr 2001.

REFERENCES

Ariste, Ruolz, and Jeff Carr. 2001. 'Health Human Resources: Cost Driver of the Canadian Health Care System.' Paper presented to the Canadian Economics Association Annual Meetings, June.

Baumol, William J. 1993. 'Health Care, Education and the Cost Disease: A Looming Crisis for Public Choice.' *Public Choice* 77: 17–28.

Baumol, William J., and William G. Bowen. 1966. *Performing Arts: The Economic Dilemma*. New York: Twentieth Century Fund.

Canadian Institute for Health Information (CIHI). 2000. *National Health Expenditure Trends, 1976–2000*. Ottawa: Canadian Institute for Health Information.

Chan, Ben. 2002. *From Perceived Surplus to Perceived Shortage: What Happened to Canada's Physician Workforce in the 1990s?* CIHI Report. Ottawa: Canadian Institute for Health Information.

Chen, J., and W.J. Millar. 2000. 'Are Recent Cohorts Healthier Than Their Predecessors?' *Health Reports* 11, no. 4: 9–24.

Denton, Frank T., Amiram Gafni, and Byron Spencer. 2001. 'Population Change and the Requirements for Physicians: The Case of Ontario.' *Canadian Public Policy / Analyse de politiques* 27, no. 4: 469–85.

Denton, Frank T., and Byron G. Spencer. 1995. 'Demographic Change and the Cost of Publicly Funded Health Care.' *Canadian Journal on Aging* 14, no. 2: 174–92.

Evans, Robert G., et al. 2001a. 'Apocalypse No: Population Aging and the Future of Health Care Systems.' *Canadian Journal on Aging* 20 Suppl 1: 160–91.

– 2001b. 'Apocalypse Regained – A Note to Accompany Apocalypse No: Population Aging and the Future of Health Care Systems.' www.chspr.ubc.ca/misc /Apocalypse-Regained.htm

Health Canada. 2002. *Briefing Notes on Aging*. www.hc-sc.gc.ca, forthcoming.

Hébert, Réjean. 2002. 'Research on Aging: Providing Evidence for Rescuing the Canadian Health Care System – Brief Submitted to the Commission on the Future of Health Care in Canada,' 28 May. Forthcoming in *Canadian Journal on Aging*, Sept. 2002.

Hogan, Sarah. 2002. 'Chronic Conditions in an Aging Society.' In Health Canada 2002.

Hogan, Seamus, and Allan Pollock. 2001. 'Why Does Health Care Utilization Increase with Age: The Cost of Living or the Cost of Dying?' Paper presented to the Canadian Economics Association Annual Meetings, June. Earlier version at www.chera.ca/program.html

Hollander, M.J., and N.L. Chappell. 2001. *Final Report of the Study on the Comparative Cost Analysis of Home Care and Residential Care Services*. Victoria: National Evaluation of the Cost Effectiveness of Home Care.

Martel, Laurent, and Alain Bélanger. 1999. 'An Analysis of the Change in Dependence-Free Life Expectancy in Canada between 1986 and 1996.' *Report on the Demographic Situation in Canada: Current Demographic Analysis*. Ottawa: Statistics Canada, 164–83.

Mérette, Marcel. 2002. 'The Bright Side: A Positive View on the Economics of Aging.' *Choices* (Institute for Research on Public Policy) 8(1):

Moore, E.G., and M.W. Rosenberg, with D. McGuinness. 1997. *Growing Old in Canada: Demographic and Geographic Perspectives*. Ottawa: Statistics Canada and ITP Nelson.

Provincial and Territorial Ministers of Health. 2000. *Understanding Canada's Health Care Costs: Final Report*. Aug. www.gov.on.ca/health/english/pub/ministry/ptcd/ptcd_doc_e.pdf

Robson, William. 2001. 'Will the Baby Boomers Bust the Health Budget? Demographic Change and Health Care Financing Reform.' *Commentary* (C.D. Howe Institute) 148:

Scitovsky, A. 1994. '"The High Cost of Dying" Revisited,' *Milbank Quarterly* 72: 561–91.

Srivastava, Divya. 2002. 'Aging and the Future Supply of Physicians in Canada.' In Health Canada 2002.

3 Medical Malpractice, the Common Law, and Health-Care Reform

TIMOTHY CAULFIELD

Health professionals face growing pressure to serve ends that fit awkwardly with the ideal of fidelity to patients.

— Bloche 1999, 268

This paper provides an overview of the possible application and ramifications of malpractice jurisprudence in the context of health-care reform in Canada.[1] The changing nature of Canadian health care has shaped, and will continue to influence, the practice environment for most professionals in the field. But, as we see throughout this paper, much of this change does not fit comfortably with existing principles of common law. This is largely because cost containment and reform of health care challenge well-established legal obligations. Because tort law and fiduciary law focus largely on the interests of the patient and on the maintenance of the legal standard of care, they usually ignore broader social concerns, such as social equity. This emphasis may create tension between the pressures associated with malpractice law, such as the incentive to provide more care and to focus strictly on the needs of the particular patient, and the broader goals of health-care reform.

This paper begins with an overview of the purpose of malpractice law and how it relates to health-care reform. There follows a discussion of several specific areas of the common law, including the establishment and application of the legal standard of care, informed consent obligations, and fiduciary law. We see that, in general, existing common law principles do little to facilitate reform of health care and may in some circumstances act as a significant barrier. The paper then looks at other malpractice issues and suggests policy options to address the issues raised here.

Context: Tort, Common, and Malpractice Law

Alhough other areas of the common law are obviously relevant to the practice of health care in Canada (such as contract, fiduciary, administrative, and even property law), tort law has dominated jurisprudence in health law. When one considers health law, one usually thinks of malpractice litigation – which is, to a large degree, simply the application of tort law in the context of health care. Indeed, many of the basic legal duties and responsibilities of health-care providers in Canada – be they in relation to informed consent, confidentiality, or the provision of an appropriate level of care – have emerged in the context of malpractice litigation. Much of this paper therefore deals with the relevance and impact of tort principles. In addition, it focuses on physicians, although much of the analysis applies to other health-care providers.

In general, tort law 'provides a legal means whereby compensation, usually in the form of damages, may be paid for injuries suffered by a party as a result of the wrongful conduct of others' (*Hall v. Hebert* 1993; Klar 1996, 1). Tort law addresses and defines responsibility for harm and when and why a specific harm is worthy of compensation (Mariner 2001, 258). Another goal of tort law, however, is to act as a deterrent and to help establish and maintain a given standard of conduct (Klar 1996). That is, the fear of liability will cause individuals, such as physicians, to practise a certain level of care – although the validity of this assumption continues to be debated (Prichard 1990; Jacobi and Huberfeld 2001). One well-known Canadian study, the Report on Liability and Compensation Issues in Health Care (Prichard 1990), concluded that 'on balance, the threat of tort litigation against health care providers for negligence contributes in a positive way to improving the quality of health care provided and reducing the frequency of avoidable health care injuries' (Prichard 1990, executive summary. See also Studdert and Brennan, 2001). However, there remains little actual evidence to support the use of tort law as a means of ensuring a high quality of health care (Bovbjerg, Miller, and Shapiro 2001, 369).

Because the common law helps define the rights and duties of health-care providers and patients and creates an incentive to perform in a certain manner, it is highly relevant to health-care reform. Malpractice lawsuits are determined case by case. They focus on the rights and legal duties of individual physicians and patients. While the principles of tort law obviously have social utility, the rights and duties of patients and doctors are rarely subordinated to the needs of the broader health-care system. For example, as we see more fully below, jurisprudence on informed consent flows directly from the application of the ethical principle of autonomy (*Ciarlarliello v. Schacter*, 1993), and the needs of third parties are rarely, if ever, considered.

But many reform initiatives will necessarily involve a weighing of the needs of the general population against those of individuals. And because physicians remain a central and controlling element in the use of health-care resources, reform will also inevitably implicate them (Perkel 1996, 266). But the more doctors are asked to play an active role in cost containment, the greater the potential to strain existing legal norms – particularly if reform alters the existing physician–patient dynamic. As Marc Rodwin notes, '[Health-reform] trends and views encourage the idea that rather than strive to promote only the welfare of individual patients, doctors and medical organizations must also act in the interest of the population they serve' (Rodwin 1995, 254). While there are undoubtedly strong policy justifications for such an approach, Canadian malpractice law is not, as least currently, equipped to handle this shift.

Although it remains unclear whether fear of malpractice liability is a constructive influence on physicians' behaviour and the quality of care (Prichard 1990), it affects the way they practise. Numerous studies have found that doctors are conscious of liability concerns. In general, they seem to believe that malpractice pressures encourage them to provide more care – a practice often known as 'defensive medicine.'

To cite but a few examples of survey data on this point, a 1994 survey of Canadian physicians found that 70 per cent thought the 'risk of malpractice suits forces physicians to order tests that may not be required' (*Medical Post* 1994). In another study, 91 per cent of the doctors surveyed 'believed their test-ordering behaviour was affected by [a] perceived risk of litigation' (Salloum and Franssen 1993). And in a study done for the Royal Commission on New Reproductive Technologies, 62 per cent of Alberta physicians said that they believed that fear of lawsuits leads to more PND than is medically required (Renaud et al. 1993).

Medical Malpractice and the Legal Standard of Care

In this section, I explain how the legal standard of care is established in Canada and explore the possible interactions between reform initiatives for health care and the legal standard (including the possibility of local exemptions).

Establishing the Standard

As in many common law jurisdictions, the legal standard of care is determined in Canada by examining what 'could reasonably be expected of a normal, prudent practitioner' (*Crits v. Sylvester* 1956, 508). The Supreme Court of Canada affirmed this rule in *ter Neuzen v. Korn* (1995) when it held that doctors 'have a duty to conduct their practice in accordance with the conduct of a prudent and diligent doctor in the same circumstances' (588). National and even international guidelines for clinical practice are becoming more common – particularly in this era of evidence-based medicine. However, regardless of how well formulated, practice guidelines remain only one piece of evidence in the formulation of the legal standard of care. Case-by-case analysis remains the norm. Thus the standard of care is re-examined in each lawsuit and is generally established by the profession itself via expert testimony.

Because of constant innovation and improvements in clinical practice, the standard of care has generally moved forward and become increasingly stringent (Mohr 2000). As Robertson observes: 'Medical knowledge and technology are constantly evolving, and what was reasonable medical practice a few years ago may not necessarily be so today' (Robertson 1999, 87). Only rarely has a Canadian court suggested easing of the existing legal standard of care. There have been situations where courts have had to consider whether the standard, as established by the profession, was inappropriately low (for example, *Anderson v. Chasney* 1950; *ter Neuzen v. Korn* 1995) or whether, in the circumstances, the standard was attainable (*Bateman v. Doiron* 1991, 291), but seldom has it been deemed too high (however, see *Elofson v. Davis* 1995, discussed below).

Given that quality control is, rightly or not, one of the understood goals of tort law, this adherence to established standards makes sense. To allow a slippage in the standard of care would be to deem a lower quality of care appropriate. Moreover, because the standard is established case by case, judges seem reluctant to have a specific injured plaintiff bear the burden of broader health-policy concerns.

Reform and Liability

Of course, the judicial trend of reinforcing an established standard of care could affect any reform initiative that places pressure on physicians to provide less (or even different) care. The potential effect of existing tort principles is well illustrated by the British Columbia decision of *Law Estate v. Simice* (1994; see also Irvine 1994), one of the few Canadian cases where a court has had to consider the impact of cost-containment pressure on a physician's clinical decision.

In this case, a patient arrived in the emergency room with a headache. The patient later died of an aneurism. One of the critical issues was why a CT scan was not provided in a timely fashion. In response, the defendant physician invoked constraints imposed by the provincial insurance scheme on the use of such diagnostic tools. In this regard, Justice Spencer stated as follows: 'If it comes to a choice between a physician's responsibility to his or her individual patient and his or her responsibility to the Medicare system overall, the former must take precedence in a case such as this. The severity of the harm that may occur to the patient who is permitted to go undiagnosed is far greater than the financial harm that will occur to the Medicare system if one more CT procedure only shows the patient is not suffering from a serious medical condition.'

More than in any other Canadian case, this judicial statement dramatically exemplifies the dilemma that physicians and health-policy decision makers face in this context. In the eyes of this judge, physicians should ignore calls for economic restraint and address the needs of the individual patient. Cost containment will not excuse substandard care.

We see a similar examination in the Newfoundland case of *McLean v. Carr* (1994), which also dealt with the withholding of a CT scan. Although the judge here comes to a conclusion similar to that in *Law Estate*, he implies that information concerning the costs of providing CT scans may have influenced his decision concerning the appropriate standard. 'The question is one of the cost effectiveness of precautions which could have been taken. It was allegedly too costly in 1987 to do a CT Scan on all head-injured patients. I was not, however, provided any evidence to establish that the cost would be prohibitive to scan, not all, but just patients whose skulls had considerable force applied and who had a resulting skull fracture' (*McLean v. Carr* 1994, 289).

An Economic 'Locality Rule'?

Though controversial vis-à-vis health-care reform, the conclusions in *Law Estate* and *McLean* are entirely consistent with existing tort theory and case law. The idea of using cost containment as an 'excuse' for substandard care is not unlike the legal issues associated with practising medicine in a rural setting. Physicians in rural settings have often had to contend with fewer resources. In such situations, the courts have always been sympathetic to the less-than-ideal circumstances. In general, they will not find a doctor negligent for substandard care if he or she did his or her best with the resources available.

Though not involving a rural setting, *Bateman v. Doiron* (1991) stands as a good example of how the courts handle situations of actual scarcity. In this case it was alleged that the hospital was negligent for staffing its emergency room with family physicians instead of specialists. The plaintiff was admitted to a Moncton hospital's emergency room with chest pains, and the plaintiff claimed that the defendant – a family physician – did not handle the situation properly. The court held that the hospital was not negligent for using family doctors if that was all that was available. In other words, because there was an actual scarcity of the needed resource – emergency specialists – the hospital could not be held liable for not meeting the legal standard of care. 'The non-availability of trained and experienced personnel, to say nothing of the problems of collateral resource allocation, simply makes this standard unrealistic, albeit desirable' (*Bateman v. Doiron* 1991, 291).[2]

However, Canadian courts have been very hesitant to allow external circumstances, such as lack of resources, to result in an actual decrease in the standard of care. For example, they have largely rejected the idea of a 'locality rule' – that is, varying the standard of care to accommodate those practising in rural settings. In the malpractice case of *Sunnucks v. Tobique Valley Hospital* (1999), for example, the court summarized current thinking on the matter: 'The experts called by the defendant doctors referred often to the problems facing doctors in rural areas such as a lack of specialists to refer to, lack of facilities, and the long periods of being on-call, and generally being overworked. This so-called "locality rule" has been roundly criticized by both the courts and in various legal texts. The rule simply establishes that the standard of the profession depended on the acceptable conduct of the community or similar communities. The danger is that the rural–urban distinction might create a double standard based on geography allowing inferior health care to be considered adequate in some areas. The standard of care Dr. Wecker owed to the plaintiff is exactly the same as that expected of an urban doctor' (280–1).[3]

This general reluctance to reduce the standard of care permeates much of tort law. For example, note the strict approach taken to setting the standard of care for novices practising in the health-care professions. Although it is important to encourage and promote new health-care professionals, common law courts will not reduce the standard of care in order to soften trainees' liability exposure. John Fleming nicely summarizes the rationale for this stance: 'While it is necessary to encourage [beginners], it is equally evident that they cause more than their proportionate share of accidents. The paramount social need for compensating accident victims, however, clearly outweighs all competing considerations, and the beginner is, therefore, held to the standard of those who are reasonably skilled and proficient in that particular calling or activity' (Fleming 1983, 105).

Implications

The existing malpractice regime will create challenges to the implementation of physician-focused reform. As we saw above, there seems little doubt that fear of liability affects how health-care providers practice. In general, tort law encourages the provision of more care, thus increasing the cost to the system. More important, however, if it remains the case that health-care providers will be held accountable for injuries associated with reform initiatives, physicians may understandably resist (consciously or unconsciously) cost containment that requires them to integrate economic factors into their clinical decisions.

Liability concerns may also have other, more subtle effects on cost-containing initiatives. For example, delisting currently covered services is one suggested mechanism (though highly criticized) to help control costs (for example, Alberta 2002). Because tort liability generally encourages the provision of care, it may also encourage physicians to diagnose patients in a manner that ensures continued public coverage – thus again frustrating cost-containment goals. This 'diagnostic drift' was noted as one of the problems with the well-known 'Oregon Plan' (McPherson 1991).

In addition, tort law leads perhaps to more aggressive practices in health care (for instance, more diagnostic tests and more medication). It may thus increase the number of iatrogenic injuries, which in turn costs money – although there are few data on this point (see Studdert and Brennan 2001).

In sum, the interaction between health-care reform and malpractice law may create unique legal and policy dilemmas. It seems unlikely, at least in the short term, that Canadian courts will allow reform to erode the existing legal standard of care. Although the judiciary will undoubtedly remain sympathetic to actual scarcities of resources, it will view conscious decisions to provide substandard care with suspicion. Physicians may feel legally compelled to ignore (consciously or unconsciously) requests to contain costs and may seek ways to provide care within the publicly funded system – thus frustrating efforts to save money through initiatives such as delisting of services.

There is an important caveat to this conclusion, however. As we saw above, there are only a few cases directly on this point, and so, we can only guess how the courts will respond to such cases in future.[4] Most relevant jurisprudence tells us that they will continue to emphasize maintenance of the standard of care and the physician's focus on the best interest of the patient. Eventually, however, tort law will need to respond to the changing environment. As one author recently suggested, 'courts may be reluctant at first to support such a decline in the medical standard, but ultimately, negligence law must adjust to the realities of health care economics' (Walker 2002).

Nevertheless, given the tone of the existing law, I suspect that any future change will continue to distinguish between actual scarcity and conscious decisions to contain costs. Such a distinction fits most comfortably with the existing negligence jurisprudence. Finally, speculation about how tort law may accommodate health-care reform is not terribly relevant to the immediate efforts to reform the system. Until there are more relevant cases to provide physicians with much-needed guidance (Walker 2002), providers of health care will need to work with the current legal uncertainty and liability concerns.

Informed Consent and Health-Care Reform

Law on consent and informed consent is a major part of Canadian health-law jurisprudence. It is a manifestation of society's deep reverence for the ethical principle of autonomy and helps define the physician–patient relationship. In this section, I review basic law on informed consent and explore its relevance to and effect on reform of health care.

Standard of Disclosure

Canada has a rich body of jurisprudence touching on all aspects of the consent process (Nelson 1999; Dickens 1999; and Picard and Robertson 1996). In some jurisdictions, the basic consent principles have been codified in legislation (see Health Care Consent Act, SO 1996 s. 11[1]). Except in a few circumstances, such as an emergency, health-care providers must get a patient's consent before providing any procedure. For the consent to be legally valid, providers must give patients all material information regarding the procedure. In other words, the consent must be informed. The seminal Supreme Court of Canada case of *Reibl v. Hughes* (1980) defined material information as anything that a reasonable person in the patient's position would want to know. Failure to provide this information constitutes negligence on the part of the physician.

Since *Reibl,* Canadian courts have had many opportunities to interpret the scope of the physician's duty. In general, this jurisprudence has consistently expanded the physician's duty of disclosure, partly because of the dominant role that the principle of autonomy has played in the evolution of consent jurisprudence. In *Ciarlarliello v. Schacter* (1993), for example, the Supreme Court of Canada declared that 'the concept of individual autonomy is fundamental to the common law and is the basis for the requirement that disclosure be made to a patient.' This emphasis on autonomy has destroyed the paternalistic approach to disclosure decisions and allowed courts to focus on what a reasonable patient would want to know (Dickens 1999, 131). External factors rarely, if ever, mediate the scope of the disclosure obligation. Even the withholding of information for the patient's welfare – a practice known as 'therapeutic privilege' – has been largely overwhelmed by the judicial respect for autonomy (*McInerney v. MacDonald* 1992).

Disclosure Obligations and Health-Care Reform

Reform initiatives in health care may have an unusual impact on the process of informed consent. First, it is arguable that physicians have a legal obligation to disclose information about any cost-containment initiatives that may press them to provide less, or different, procedures (Caulfield and Ginn 1994; Miller 1992; Picard and Robertson 1996, 131–2). For example, a doctor may have an obligation to tell patients of a regional health authority's policy of using fewer diagnostic procedures. Although such information does not involve the traditional 'medical risk' data often associated with the consent process, clearly a reasonable person in the patient's position would want to know about it. Wolf notes that 'it is hard to imagine information more material' than that relating to factors that may affect the clinical decision-making process (Wolf 1999, 1661). Likewise, physicians should report on any additional risks that may be associated with health-care reform or cost containment (for example, the risks, if any, associated with being on a waiting list).

Second, physicians may also be required to tell patients about services that are a reasonable alternative but not available within the public system. For example, the recent Report of the Premier's Advisory Council on Health (Alberta 2002) recommended delisting of a number of procedures. If the government delists services that a health-care provider would have normally considered a treatment option, this option should still be disclosed (see Seney v. Crooks 1998). This may also mean that physicians have a duty to disclose information to patients about the existence of private options that may be available both within and outside a given jurisdiction if it can be conceived as something that a reasonable person in the patient's position would want to know. Private options that are not substantially different, faster, or more convenient may not have to be disclosed. However, if a private option is available that would allow access to a procedure that would provide treatment in a manner that would lower the risks to the patient or speed access to a medically necessary service, that private option should probably be disclosed. Again, this is something that a reasonable person in the patient's position would want to know. As Dickens suggests, 'If patients have the means to obtain indicated care in another hospital, town, province or country, physicians may be obliged to inform them, because the option may be material to patients' choice between accepting the lesser care or seeking superior care elsewhere. Physicians who do not know whether patients have such means should ask them' (1999, 133).

At least one group of doctors has decided to address this consent issue formally. Recently, the Calgary Regional Medical Staff Association circulated to all its members a form letter (Lightstone 1999) in the form of an information sheet (on file with author) that they could give to patients who have been placed on a waiting list for a variety of medical services (such as MRIs and consultations with specialists). The letter warned patients that 'the waiting time for [the particular] procedure involves some risk' and states, 'You may also wish to contact other centres in Alberta or the rest of Canada to determine whether the necessary services is available there sooner. You have the option of leaving the country and possibly getting the service immediately.' Likewise, in January 2000 the Canadian Press (2000, A9) reported that a number of hospitals in Toronto asked patients to sign waivers 'spelling out the dangers of long waiting lists for care' and that the 'waiver would establish, in writing, that the patient was fully aware of the health risk of joining a lengthy queue.'

Although the provision of information on the existence and impact of health-care reform initiatives may seem like an extreme application of informed consent, it is clearly within the tenor of existing jurisprudence. This is information that a reasonable person in the patients' position may want to know. Moreover, there are a number of legal policy justifications for such disclosure. First, this information 'can empower consumers' and 'encourage dialogue among consumers, physicians [and] local regulators' (Khanna, Silverman, and Schwartz, 1999, 292). Second, in some circumstances, such information may help patients choose between different providers. A patient may wish to find a doctor who is not under the same constraints or who does not, for example, have a long waiting list. As Lewis et al. note, 'A patient may languish on a particular physician's waiting list for a long time without ever knowing that another physician could provide the needed service much sooner' (2000, 1299). Having to disclose resource information may in turn encourage physicians to be more efficient in their management of resources (for example, the management of waiting lists). Third, and most important, to withhold information that is potentially relevant to the provision of a health-care service is to adopt a paternalistic approach that would contrast starkly with the current philosophical and legal trend.

Implications

The application of informed-consent law in this context has the potential to create a number of policy dilemmas. For example, requiring physicians to provide information about private options may facilitate the development of a 'second tier.' This may be particularly offensive to health-care providers who are strong supporters of the public system. For patients, hearing about private facilities from their doctor could certainly be viewed as an 'advertisement' for a treatment option that they may not have been considering. In addition, some patients may not have the financial resources to pay for private options. For this sector of society, being told about unattainable private options might seem cruel and ethically inappropriate.

These are all valid concerns. However, they do not alter the physician's legal-disclosure obligations. As we saw above, doctors can only rarely withhold information for the good of the patient – 'therapeutic privilege.' In the case of *Meyer Estate v. Rogers* (1991), for instance, a physician intentionally withheld information about the risks associated with contrast media. The court stated that the 'therapeutic privilege' should not be part of Canadian law because it may erode the requirement of informed consent (see also *McInerney v. MacDonald* 1992; Picard and Robertson 1996, 147–9). It is unlikely that a Canadian court would characterize the fear that a low-income patient may become upset about his or her inability to purchase private options as a justification for the exercise of therapeutic privilege. On the contrary, the physician should not presume to know how the patient would react or use such information. Likewise, personal concern about the social consequences of providing information will probably do little to limit disclosure duties. As with other value-laden issues, such as abortion, physicians must be careful not to allow personal views to interfere with their legal and ethical obligations.

Another interesting policy issue relates to what is known as 'the causation hurdle.' Although Canadian consent law has placed increasingly onerous disclosure obligations on health-care providers, it is still difficult for plaintiff/patients to win lawsuits on informed consent. This is because plaintiffs must satisfy the court that 'but for' the nondisclosure they would not have had the treatment (or would have had a different treatment) and therefore would not be injured. It has been very difficult for patients to satisfy this test (Robertson 1991; *Arndt v. Smith* 1997; Nelson and Caulfield 1998).

This causation dilemma may have a particularly odd effect on cases relating to 'health-care reform.' Let us consider how one of these cases may actually play out. If, for instance, a person is injured while on a waiting list, he or she may argue that had the physician explained the risks associated with being on a waiting list and the existence of private options, the injury would not have occurred. In this context, the court must be satisfied that 'a reasonable person in the patient's position' would have chosen the private option. Applying the controversial 'modified objective' test, the court would need to investigate whether the patient had the financial resources to cover the private option. Given the causation hurdle, Canadian courts could reasonably conclude that only plaintiffs who can afford private services can succeed in such cases.

Although this conclusion may seem perversely unjust (indeed, it compounds the inequities already present in a two-tiered system), it is entirely consistent with existing case law. For example, in cases such as *Mickle v. Salvation Army Grace Hospital Windsor Ontario* (1998) and *Arndt v. Smith* (1997) the courts have used very personal characteristics, such as the religious beliefs of the plaintiff, to determine this causation issue. In *Mickle*, for example, the court held that, because the child's disabilities were not severe, a reasonable woman in Mickle's position would not select abortion (1998). Given this case law, it seems entirely possible that a Canadian court could use the fact that a patient/plaintiff had a low income to conclude that the plaintiff could not satisfy the causation test – that is, that a reasonable person in the patient's position would not have taken the private alternative.

To date, there is no Canadian informed-consent case directly on this point. However, in other jurisdictions, particularly the United States, this controversy has already led to a great deal of academic debate, case law, and even legislation compelling disclosure of cost-containment mechanisms and incentives to provide less care (Khanna, Silverman, and Schwartz 1999; Miller and Sage 1999). In addition, it seems that Canadian policy makers are already beginning to take formal action to comply with their perceived consent obligations, as evidenced by the approach mentioned above taken by the Calgary Regional Medical Staff Association.

As with tort law generally, principles of informed consent will do little to facilitate the implementation of health-care reform based on broader notions of social equity. More than any area of health law, informed consent is a manifestation of a society's deep reverence for personal autonomy. As such, it is concerned with providing patients with relevant information in order to permit autonomous decisions. Withholding or tailoring the provision of information in order to meet a broader social agenda conflicts directly with the ethical principles that underlie Canadian consent jurisprudence.

Fiduciary Obligations

Fiduciary law is another area that has tremendous significance in the context of health-care reform. Fiduciary obligations flow from the relationship of trust between physician and patient. Indeed, fiduciary law compels providers of health care to concentrate almost exclusively on the best interests of the patient. 'Loyalty is the core value of fiduciary relationships and hence the focus of fiduciary law' (Litman 2002, 91). As such, fiduciary law is clearly relevant to any scheme of health-care reform that explicitly or implicitly challenges the nature of this loyalty.

Fiduciary Obligations in Canada

Canada places particularly onerous fiduciary obligations on health professionals. Unlike in some jurisdictions, such as Australia, in Canada physicians are clearly in a fiduciary relationship with their patients – at least in most situations. In *McInerney v. MacDonald* (1992), a case dealing with a patient's right of access to her health care record, the court held that the physician–patient relationship is fiduciary in nature and that 'certain duties do arise from the special relationship of trust and confidence between doctor and patient' (423). In *Norberg v. Wynrib* (1992), Justice McLachlin stated that 'the most fundamental characteristic of the doctor–patient relationship is its fiduciary nature' (see also *Henderson v. Johnston* 1956).

Fiduciary principles also dictate that health-care providers 'must avoid an appearance of conflict of interest, even when there is neither actual nor potential conflict in the classic sense' (Litman 2002, 95). For example, in *Cox v. College of Optometrists of Ontario* (1988) the court held that even though there were no actual conflicting financial pressures, merely having an office in an optical company's retail space was enough to lead the court to conclude that there was an inappropriate conflict of interest. Litman believes that extending the application of fiduciary principles to situations where there is a mere appearance of conflict can be justified. He argues that 'it has the effect of maintaining and perhaps even enhancing public confidence in the integrity of an important health-service institution where both loyalty and a perception of loyalty are essential to the efficacy of the institution' (Litman 2002, 96).

Focus on the Patient's Best Interests

Fiduciary principles create clear barriers for health-care reform that seeks to integrate broader social concerns into the physician's decision-making process. This is particularly so if there are economic incentives in place that encourage a specific pattern of use. Numerous authors have noted this dilemma. For example, in the United States, Perry noted: 'The economic benefits and hazard of today's practice of medicine provide sundry and frequently subtle opportunities for fiduciary conflicts of interest' (1994). Recently, my colleague Litman observed: 'From the perspective of an individual patient, treatment decisions driven or influenced by cost-containment considerations are highly improper because they violate the basic fiduciary tenet that fiduciaries may consider only the interests of their beneficiaries in the discharge of their fiduciary responsibilities' (2002, 110).

The clear conflict created by many models of health care-reform has not dissuaded legal commentators from calling for an even more vigorous application of fiduciary principles in this context. Indeed, many legal scholars view fiduciary law as a needed protection against the inappropriate influences of financial incentives. 'It is part of a court's traditional function to correct for market imperfections by defining fiduciary duties to curb betrayals of trust. Despite physicians' own best efforts, pressure to curb cost may lead to erosion of their professional norm of loyalty to individual patients' (Cahill and Jacobson 2001, 431).

Disclosure of Conflicts of Interest

Fiduciary law also heightens the disclosure obligations of health-care providers, particularly vis-à-vis any possible or apparent conflict of interest. For example, in the well-known U.S. case of *Moore v. Regents of the University of California* (1990) it was noted that, because doctors are fiduciaries, they are legally required to inform their patients of any conflicts of interest in their treating of the patient, including disclosure of 'personal interests unrelated to the patient's health, whether research or economic, that may affect [the doctor's] medical judgment' (1990, 485).

Although there are no Canadian fiduciary-law cases dealing with health-care reform, disclosure of conflicts is a well-understood and classic component of fiduciary law. It is certainly possible that an application of fiduciary principles in this context would compel providers of health care to disclose information about incentive schemes, such as capitation programs, that create conflicting pressures affecting treatment decisions. As Martin and Bjerknes note: 'Pursuing a claim for breach of fiduciary duty, particularly in conjunction with a claim for violation of informed consent, is likely to succeed based on the long history of judicial regulation of economic conflicts of interest in fiduciary relationships' (1996, 457).

Implications

The impact of fiduciary law in this context is obvious. At a minimum, it compels the disclosure of all relevant conflicts. And, if strictly applied, it may also prohibit physicians from providing care in situations where they are in a clear conflict of interest – such as when they may financially benefit from the provision of a privately funded 'enhanced service' (Caulfield, Flood, and von Tigerstrom 2000). However, it may also make it difficult to implement a wide variety of cost-containment schemes. Although, again, it is difficult to predict how a Canadian court may interpret fiduciary principles in the context of formal health-care reform, I believe that, as with the tort principles outlined above, physician-initiated 'bedside rationing' – an inevitable component of many cost-containment schemes – will be viewed with a degree of suspicion by Canadian courts. Indeed, some commentators, particularly in the United States, have suggested that all incentive mechanisms aimed at physician's utilization behaviour be banned. 'Patent financial incentives that reward overcare or undercare weaken patient–physician and patient–nurse bonds and should be prohibited' (Policy Perspective 1997, 1733). But, given the key role of health-care providers, especially physicians, in the control of health-care budgets, how can costs be contained without such incentive schemes?

Other Malpractice Issues

Because of the limited space available, this paper has dealt mainly with the effect of malpractice law on physicians' behaviour in relation to health-care reform in Canada. However, common-law malpractice principles will also affect a number of other relevant areas. Below is a brief sampling of five other malpractice issues that should be considered in this context.

Group Practice, Shared Responsibilities?

Historically, the 'buck stops' with the physician. That is, the majority of legal responsibilities in the delivery of health-care services have generally fallen on the physician. For example, although physicians can delegate aspects of the informed-consent process to a variety of other health-care professionals, they remain responsible for ensuring that the patient was properly informed and actually understood the information provided. In *Ciarlarliello v. Schacter* (1993) the Supreme Court of Canada noted that 'it is appropriate that the burden should be placed on the doctor to show that the patient comprehended the explanation and instructions given' (140). Will the fact that doctors remain the focal point of legal responsibility impede attempts to create interdisciplinary health-care teams?

Confidentiality Issues

Although a number of Canadian jurisdictions are introducing specific legislation to protect the confidentiality and privacy of patient health information (for instance, Alberta's Health Information Act), in many provinces the common law remains a dominant aspect of the law in relation to the handling of health-care information (see *Canadian AIDS Society v. Ontario* 1995; *R. v. Osolin* 1993; *R v. O'Connor* 1995; and *McInerney v. MacDonald* 1992). In general, this jurisprudence places a strong and clear obligation on providers of health care to maintain the confidentiality of health-care information (for example, *Peters-Brown v. Regina District Health Board* 1995). Will this law, and the emerging legislation on health information, make it more difficult to implement population health initiatives? For example, such projects often require access to a large amount of identifiable health-care information. If consent is needed for access to all such data, as mandated by the common law, this work will be feasible?

Medical Error

The past few years has seen rising interest in the health and cost implications of 'medical error.' A 1999 report by the U.S. Institute of Medicine suggested that as many as 44,000–98,000 U.S. deaths per year resulted from medical error (Leape 2001, 146; Bovbjerg, Miller, and Shapiro 2001). Comprehensive health-care reform will need to address this critical issue. Many commentators have argued that malpractice law may both contribute to the incidence of medical error and make it more difficult to address. For example, a number have suggested that fear of litigation may cause physicians to be less forthcoming regarding their involvement in a possible medical error, thus hurting efforts to gather detailed information about the incidence and nature of errors. 'Data on the incidence of harmful mistakes suggests that the supposed deterrent effect of medical suits alone has not been sufficient to address the problem. On the contrary, litigation may well stifle efforts to reduce error' (Studdert and Brennan 2001, 227).

Contributory Negligence of Patients for 'Unhealthy' Behaviour

There have been a number of Canadian decisions where patients have been found contributory negligent as a result of their unhealthy behaviour. For example, in *Dumais v. Hamilton* (1998), a physician was found liable for not appropriately disclosing the risks associated with a 'tummy tuck' operation. However, because the patient continued to smoke, the court found that she had failed to mitigate her damages and as such was 50 per cent liable for her injuries. Given the increasing emphasis (as a way of reducing health-care costs) on encouraging Canadians to lead healthy lives (Alberta 2002), will the courts place more and more weight on patients' behaviour in their assessment of malpractice claims?

Liability of Hospitals, Regional Health Authorities, and Government

While I believe that Canadian physicians will probably bear much of the liability exposure in relation to health-care reform, many other entities, such as hospitals, regional health authorities (RHAs), and provincial governments will obviously be involved. Although 'bedside rationing' will remain an inevitable component of almost any health-care reform (Ubel 2002), it can be argued that these middle- and upper-level decision makers most profoundly affect what is available to patients and therefore should be held liable for any decisions that result in substandard care.

Again, Canada has very few cases directly on this point. Hospitals and PHAs can be found directly negligent if they breach a well-established duty (for example, selecting competent staff) and vicariously liable for the negligence of their personnel acting within their scope of employment (Picard and Robertson 1996). And, as they do vis-à-vis doctors, the courts will probably remain sympathetic to RHAs and hospitals that have an actual scarcity of resources (for instance, *Bateman v. Doirin* 1991). However, the extent to which they will hold middle- and upper-level decision makers liable for decisions on allocation remains unclear.[5] Likely factors to be considered in this context include the degree to which the decision truly involved 'policy,' thereby rendering a public authority immune from liability, and the extent to which the harm was 'forseeable' (see, for example, *Brown v. British Columbia* 1994). In general, I believe that Canadian courts will probably display some deference to public entities making broad decisions on allocation, as have both British and U.S. courts (Caulfield 1994; Jacobson 1999; Cahill and Jacobson 2001).

This issue is beyond the scope of this paper (see Mariner 2001), but the policy implications of extending liability to middle- and upper-level decision makers should inform any initiative on tort reform. For example, as with physicians' liability, imposing liability on these authorities could inhibit implementation of effective programs of cost containment. As Jacobson observes: 'The success of managed care cost containment innovations depends on many factors, including how courts decide litigation challenging various cost containment initiatives' (Jacobson 1999, abstract). Moreover, 'such claims may deter vigorous decision making' by public officials (*Decock v. Alberta* 2000, para. 37).

A Uniquely Canadian Dilemma?

As I have touched on throughout this paper, a number of countries have already struggled with many of these issues. And while this malpractice dilemma has led to controversy, it has not had the dramatic impact that it may in Canada. This is because these legal dilemmas may be particularly problematic in Canada.

First, as compared to many other common-law jurisdictions, Canadian health law is especially 'patient focused.' For example, in Britain and in many U.S. states the standard of disclosure for informed consent remains that of a 'reasonable professional' (the Canadian standard is that of a 'reasonable patient'). In addition, Canada's strong emphasis on fiduciary principles, perhaps the strongest in the common-law world, also heightens this patient-centred ethos. As we saw above, it is this stress on the patient that, rightly or not, may cause many of the legal challenges associated with health-care reform.

Second, in the United States, much of the relevant common law is clouded by the complex organizational nature of HMOs/MCOs and the application of the federal Employee Retirement Income Security Act (ERISA) (Mariner 2001; Anderlik 1998). ERISA limits the type of action that beneficiaries may bring against many MCOs. Its application was a key issue in many of the most relevant U.S. decisions (*Wickline* 1986; *Pegram* 2000).

Finally, unlike in the Britain, in Canada many of our current legal standards emerged decades ago in an era of fee-for-service remuneration and minimal administrative interference with professional decision making. The adoption of new forms of remuneration, new incentive schemes, or new organizational frameworks will represent a significant shift for Canadian physicians. As I have noted throughout this paper, there is currently little Canadian jurisprudence that is capable of easily accommodating a radical shift in this area.

Possible Reform Options

The common law, specifically malpractice law, is not the best tool for changing health care. The goals of malpractice law – compensating injured patients and maintaining a high standard of care – are not necessarily congruent with, for example, containing costs. For instance, because malpractice law continues to reinforce the paramountcy of a physician's duty to his or her patients, it does little to facilitate the introduction of broader health-care reform initiatives. To put the matter simply, tort law is not designed as a tool for effectuating broadly based social reform.

However, malpractice law is a powerful social force. Given its impact on health-care providers and their behaviour, policy makers must consider whether some degree of tort reform is necessary and/or desirable. For example, reform that reduced physicians' liability exposure would make cost-containment initiatives easier to implement. However, what other social goals would such a reform scheme compromise? This section outlines three reform options and suggests the need for more research.

Court-Initiated Reform

One option is to leave the policy concerns outlined in this paper to the Canadian courts. Case-by-case evolution of malpractice principles might permit the judiciary to develop new methods of resolving the policy concerns linked to health-care reform. As Walker (2002) noted above, some type of judicial accommodation is inevitable, as Canadian courts must, at some level, respond to changes in health care.

Although a case-by-case approach may lead to a radical change in the law, it seems highly unlikely. Malpractice principles – and tort law in general – have, over the years, remained tremendously consistent (Mariner 2001, 258). Incremental change, not radical revisions or paradigm shifts, is the norm. As Mariner suggests in relation to U.S. health-care reform, we are 'not likely to find salvation in new theory' (270). This is not to say that the courts are unaware of the relevant policy issues. In one U.S. study of over 480 cases involving managed care, the authors found that in 56 per cent of the cases the courts raised at least one policy issue: 'Judges are actively considering the policy implications of their decisions. This does not mean that the courts are actually formulating health care policy. But it does suggest that the judiciary is well aware of the policy conflicts at stake and is willing to consider them in the decision-making process' (Jacobson, Selvin and Pomfret 2001, 286).

However, even in the United States, which has seen many health-care reform cases, no radical shift in tort law has emerged. It is true that courts throughout the world have shown substantial degree of deference to those entities making broader allocation decisions, including U.S. MCOs, but there has been little or no change in the basic malpractice principles as they apply to individual health-care providers. Moreover, as we saw above, there are to date few Canadian cases on this issue. Despite numerous headline-grabbing stories about possible liability concerns (Priest 2000) and oft-cited cases, such as *Law Estate v. Simice* (1994), Canadian courts have yet to grapple with many of the issues raised in this paper. Thus the evolution of Canadian tort law in response to health-care reform, if it is going to happen at all, has not even begun.

Finally, the common law will inevitably lag behind broader social change. It is largely a reactive mechanism. Before a specific issue can be addressed it must be brought before the courts by an individual seeking compensation. Case-by-case evolution of malpractice law will not generate broad-based, comprehensive reform. Though a rich and complex source of legal principles, malpractice jurisprudence develops in a largely ad hoc manner. There is no nationally co-ordinated approach.

Specific Legislated Responses

Of course, legislation can alter the common law. Policy makers concerned about the impact of the common law on health-care reform could thereby minimize or alter malpractice liability. For example, though not intended to facilitate reform of health care, ERISA has greatly limited the liability exposure of U.S. MCOs. Similarly, a number of U.S. jurisdictions have also passed laws to protect patients from the effects of aggressive cost containment. For instance, 'requirements to disclose financial incentives have been enacted in many states and are included in recent reforms to Medicare and Medicaid' (Miller and Sage 1999, 1424).

Such an approach faces a number of challenges in Canada. First, because this type of legislation would probably be considered a provincial matter, each province would need to craft and enact its own legislation. There are ways to co-ordinate such efforts, but variation in political philosophy and in methods of health-care reform would probably result in a patchwork of regulatory responses (as in emerging provincial legislation on health information).

Second, limiting liability exposure through legislation has serious policy implications. As we saw above, a number of scholars have suggested that the accountability associated with malpractice law helps to maintain a high standard of care and encourages all health-care decision makers – from physicians to RHAs – to consider the needs of individual patients (Litman 2002; Cahill and Jacobson 2001; Prichard 1990). In addition, legislation to limit liability exposure would make it even more difficult for patients to receive compensation. The Prichard Report concluded that 'only about 250 injured patients annually receive any compensation from the liability and compensation system and that this represents only a modest percentage (less than 10 percent) of those suffering negligent injury' (Prichard 1990, principle finding 5). Legislation that further inhibited patients' ability to obtain compensation would only make this situation worse.

Comprehensive Tort Reform

The most dramatic option would be to address health-care reform as part of a broader overhaul of tort law. Over the past few decades, many authors have noted the general failings and inefficiencies of existing medical malpractice (for example, Jacobi and Huberfeld 2001; Report of the Harvard Medical Practice Study 1990). A number of countries, such as New Zealand and Sweden, already have medical no-fault systems (Elgie, Caulfield, and Christie 1993). And, as a result, the adoption of a no-fault system continues to be considered by a variety of international commentators. 'The central premise of this model is that patients need not prove negligence to access compensation. They must prove only that they have suffered an injury, that it was caused by medical care, and that it meets whatever severity or other threshold criteria apply' (Studdert and Brennan 2001).

The cost of medical malpractice insurance, though still not as high in Canada as in the United States, is also relevant to this discussion. For some medical disciplines, such as obstetrics, its cost can be extremely high, and some jurisdictions pay for it, at least partly, through public dollars, thus adding to the overall cost of health care.

By dealing with the malpractice issues associated with health-care reform within a broader tort-reform initiative, policy makers could facilitate health-care reform, public-health work, and a reduction of medical error while increasing the opportunity for patient compensation. Given the concerns outlined in this paper, emerging worries about medical error, the rising cost of malpractice insurance, and the ambivalent evidence about tort law as a mechanism of quality control, some form of no-fault scheme may well be timely.

There are, of course, numerous challenges to implementing such a plan. For example, as with almost any legislative initiative affecting private law, it would have to be done province by province, reducing prospects for national consistency. In addition, issues surround the economic and administrative efficiencies of a no-fault system (which could be at least as efficient as the existing, fault-based approach) (Bovbjerg and Sloan 1998; Elgie, Caulfield, and Christie 1993). Finally, despite a lack of strong data supporting the deterrent effect of tort law, there is concern that we would lose the quality-control benefits currently associated with the malpractice system. Indeed, this seems to be the primary reason why Prichard recommended that we maintain tort actions against health-care providers (Prichard 1990).

The Need for More Research

While tort law may not be an effective tool for health-care reform, existing common-law principles should not be viewed simply as a barrier to constructive social change. There are good reasons why tort law and fiduciary law have placed such a strong emphasis on the health-care provider's obligation to the patient. And the judiciary's continued deference to the ethical principle of autonomy, which lies at the heart of much of this common law, is the result of centuries of socio-political development. Before steps are taken to erode or alter these well-established social norms – for example, through a no-fault scheme – Canadian society needs carefully to consider the long-term trade-offs. Do we really want to reduce the impact of autonomy in health-care decision making? Would a lessening of the physician's fiduciary obligations harm the relationship of trust so essential to health care? Of course, there is already a large body of literature considering medical ethics in this context (Caulfield and von Tigerstrom, 2002, 272), but I believe that more Canadian work is essential, particularly in relation to tort reform.

We also need more research on the actual social benefits and harms of malpractice jurisprudence. Since the Prichard Report of 1990, very little empirical work has been done on this tremendously expensive system. 'Given how much reliance society places on legal mechanisms to promote safety and the very large expense of liability systems, it is rather stunning that there is so little scientific evidence on how effectively liability and discipline perform' (Bovbjerg, Miller, and Shapiro 2001, 369).

NOTES

1 I have considered many of the issues discussed in this paper in a variety of articles and book chapters, including T. Caulfield, 'Malpractice in the Age of Health Care Reform,' in Barbara von Tigerstrom and Timothy Caulfield, eds., *Meeting the Challenge: Health Care Reform and the Law* (Edmonton: University of Alberta Press, 2002); T. Caulfield and K. Siminoski, 'Physician Liability and Drug Formulary Restrictions,' *CMAJ* 166 (2002), 458; T. Caulfield and G. Robertson, 'Cost Containment Mechanisms in Health Care: A Review of Private Law Issues,' *Manitoba Law Journal* 27 (1999), 1; and T. Caulfield and D. Ginn, 'The High Price of Full Disclosure: Informed Consent and Cost Containment in Health Care' *Manitoba Law Journal* 22 (1994), 328. This paper has been informed by and builds on these previous publications. I do not reference them again in this paper.

2 However, even if physicians are not liable for cost containment that causes an actual scarcity of resources, such situations may create other legal challenges. For instance, doctors may need to become increasingly sensitive to

the lack of resources available within a given jurisdiction. As Robertson comments: 'Lack of resources or equipment is also relevant in the context of the doctor's duty to refer. A doctor who does not have access to particular equipment or testing may be negligent in failing to refer the patient to another facility which does, or possibly in failing to inform the patient that it is available in another facility' (Robertson 1999, 89).

3 However, see *Elofson v. Davis* (1997). To my knowledge, this is the only recent case where the locality rule has been explicitly accepted – largely in the hope that a reduced standard of care will encourage more physicians to practice in rural communities. 'The law recognizes and reflects public policy that a less stringent standard applies to a rural medical general practitioner ... The rural general practioner is badly needed in the rural areas of Canada, and in this case rural Alberta; and it is likely that if the rural practitioner was held to a higher standard, it would seriously increase the existing deterrent to rural practice' (para 56 [QL]). The case represents one of the rare examples of a Canadian court, at least in a malpractice setting, lowering the standard of care in order to address a specific population health concern. Given the tone of recent jurisprudence relevant to the locality rule, this case seems an exception to the general rule reflected in *Sunnucks* (1991). Nevertheless, the case illustrates how external policy concerns may persuade a court to alter the legal standard.

4 The lack of relevant jurisprudence is quite surprising. *Law Estate* (1994) and *McLean* (1994) are the only cost-containment decisions. Given the huge cuts to the health-care system in the mid-1990s, I expected many similar decisions. It is possible that the relevant cases have been litigated but settled prior to trial.

5 It is certainly possible to sue government officials in relation to allocation decisions. In the well-publicized case of *Decock v. Alberta* (2000), the Alberta Court of Appeal held that Premier Ralph Klein and Minister of Health Shirley McClellan could be named in a malpractice lawsuit. In the case, the plaintiffs allege that 'Klein and McClellan had a duty to ensure that they [the plaintiffs] were provided with reasonable and proper medical care, attention and treatment, which duty was breached' (*Decock* 2000, para. 6). Of course, it is far from clear whether the plaintiffs will succeed.

REFERENCES

Alberta. 2002. *Report of the Premier's Advisory Council on Health*. Edmonton: Government of Alberta, 8 Jan. 2002.

Anderlik. 1998. *A New Weapon against Managed Care Organizations: ERISA Perspective in Health Law, Health Law and Policy Institute, University of Houston.* www.law.uh.edu/LawCenter, 29 July 2002.

Bloche, M.G. 1999. Clinical Loyalties and the Social Purposes of Medicine. *JAMA* 281: 268–74.

Bovbjerg, Randall, R. Miller, and D. Shapiro. 2001. Paths to Reducing Medical Injury: Professional Liability and Discipline vs. Patient Safety – and the Need for a Third Way. *Journal of Law, Medicine and Ethics* 29: 369–80.

Bovbjerg, Randall, and Frank Sloan. 1998. No-Fault for Medical Injury: Theory and Evidence. *University of Cincinnati Law Review* 67: 53–123.

Cahill, M., and P. Jacobson. 2001. Pegram's Regress: A Missed Chance for Sensible Judicial Review of Managed Care Decisions. *American Journal of Law and Medicine* 27: 421–38.

Canadian Press. 9 Jan. 2000. 'Treatment Wait May Harm Health, Cancer Centre Warns.' *Edmonton Journal,* p. A9.

Caulfield, Timothy. 1994. Suing Hospitals, Health Authorities and the Government for Health Care Allocation Decisions. *Health Law Review* 3: 7–11.

Caulfield, Timothy, Colleen Flood, and Barbara von Tigerstrom. 2000. 'Comment: Bill 11, Health Care Protection Act.' *Health Law Review* 9: 22–5.

Caulfield T., and D. Ginn. 1994. The High Price of Full Disclosure: Informed Consent and Cost Containment in Health Care. *Manitoba Law Journal* 22: 328–44.

Caulfield, T., and B. von Tigerstrom, eds. 2002. *Health Care Reform and the Law in Canada: Meeting the Challenge.* Edmonton: University of Alberta Press.

Dickens, Bernard. 1999. 'Informed Consent.' In Jocelyn Downie and Timothy Caulfield, eds., *Canadian Health Law and Policy.* Toronto: Butterworths, 117–41.

Elgie, Robert, T. Caulfield, and M. Christie. 1993. Medical Injuries and Malpractice: Is It Time for 'No-Fault'?' *Health Law Journal* 1: 97–117.

Epstein, R. 1994. 'The Social Consequences of Common-Law Rules.' In S. Levmore, ed., *Foundations of Tort Law.* Oxford: Oxford University Press.

Fleming, John. 1983. *The Law of Torts.* 6th ed. Toronto: Carswell.

Health Care Consent Act, 1996, SO, 1996, c. 2.

Irvine, John. 1994. 'Case Comment: *Law Estate v. Simice.*' CCLT 21: 259.

Jacobi, John, and Nicole Huberfeld. 2001. 'Quality Control, Enterprise, Liability, and Disintermediation in Managed Care.' *Journal of Law, Medicine and Ethics* 29: 305–22.

Jacobson, Peter. 1999. Legal Challenges to Managed Care Cost Containment Programs: An Initial Assessment: Are the Courts Willing to Hold Health Plans Accountable for the Delay or Denial of Care? *Health Affairs* 18, no. 4: 69–85.

Jacobson, P., E. Selvin, and S. Pomfret. 2001. 'The Role of the Courts in Shaping

Health Policy: An Empirical Analysis.' *Journal of Law, Medicine and Ethics* 29: 278–89.

Khanna, V., H. Silverman, and J. Schwartz. 1999. 'Disclosure of Operating Practices by Managed Care Organizations to Consumers of Health Care: Obligations of Informed Consent.' *Journal of Clinical Ethics* 9: 291.

Klar, L.N. 1996. *Tort Law.* Toronto: Carswell.

Leape, L. 2001. 'Preventing Medical Accidents: Is "System Analysis" the Answer? *American Journal of Law and Medicine* 27: 145–8.

Lewis, S., et al. 2000. 'Ending Waiting-List Mismanagement: Principles and Practice.' *CMAJ* 162: 1297–1300.

Lightstone, S. 1999. 'Waiting-List Worries Cause Calgary MDs to Prepare Letter for Patients.' *CMAJ* 161: 183–4.

Litman, Moe. 2002. 'Fiduciary Law and For-Profit and Not-for-Profit Health Care.' In Timothy Caulfield and Barb von Tigerstrom, eds, *Health Care Reform and the Law in Canada.* Edmonton: University of Alberta Press, 85–130.

Mariner, Wendy. 2001. 'Slouching toward Managed Care Liability: Reflections on Doctrinal Boundries, Paradigm Shifts and Incremental Reform.' *Journal of Law Medicine and Ethics* 29: 253–77.

Martin, J., and L. Bjerknes. 1996. 'The Legal and Ethical Implications of Gag Clauses in Physician Contracts.' *American Journal of Law and Medicine* 22: 433–76.

McPherson, A. 1991. The Oregon Plan: Rationing in a Rational Society. *CMAJ* 145, no. 11: 1444–5.

Medical Post. 1994. 'Physician Survey.'

Miller, F. 1992. 'Denial of Health Care and Informed Consent in English and American Law.' *American Journal of Law and Medicine* 18: 37–71.

Miller, T., and W. Sage. 1999. 'Disclosing Physician Financial Incentives.' *JAMA* 281: 1424–30.

Mohr, J. 2000. American Medical Malpractice Litigation in Historical Perspective. *JAMA* 283: 1731–7.

Nelson, Erin. 1999. The Fundamentals of Consent. In Jocelyn Downie and Timothy Caulfield, eds., *Canadian Health Law and Policy.* Toronto: Butterworths, 101–16.

Nelson, Erin, and T. Caulfield. 1998. 'You Can't Get There from Here: A Case Comment on *Arndt v. Smith.*' *University of British Columbia Law Review* 32: 353–64.

Perkel, R. 1996. 'Ethics and Managed Care.' *Medical Clinics of North America* 80: 263–78.

Perry, C. 1994. 'Conflicts of Interest and the Physician's Duty to Inform.' *American Journal for Medicine* 96: 375–80.

Picard, E., and G. Robertson. 1996. *Legal Liability of Doctors and Hospitals in Canada*. Toronto: Carswell.

Policy Perspective. 1997. 'For Our Patients, Not for Profit.' *JAMA* 278: 1733.

Prichard, R. 1990. 'A Report of the Conference of Deputy Ministers of Health of the Federal/Provincial/Territorial Review on Liability and Compensation Issues in Health Care.' In *Liability and Compensation in Health Care*. Toronto: University of Toronto Press.

Priest, L. 2000. 'ER Crisis May Bring Rash of Suits.' *Globe and Mail*, 17 Jan. A1.

Renaud, M., et al. 1993. 'Canadian Physicians and Prenatal Diagnosis: Prudence and Ambivalence.' In *Royal Commission on New Reproductive Technologies* 13: 235–507.

Report of the Harvard Medical Practice Study to the State of New York. 1990. *Patients, Doctors, and Lawyers: Medical Injury, Malpractice Litigation and Patient Compensation in New York*. Cambridge, Mass.: President and Fellows of Harvard College.

Robertson, Gerald. 1991. 'Informed Consent Ten Years Later: The Impact of *Reibl v. Hughes*.' *Canadian Bar Review* 70: 423–47.

– 1999. 'Negligence and Malpractice.' In Jocelyn Downie and Timothy Caulfield, eds., *Canadian Health Law and Policy.* Toronto: Butterworths, 91–109.

Rodwin, Marc. 1995. 'Strain in the Fiduciary Metaphors: Divided Physician Loyalties and Obligations in a Changing Health Care System.' *American Journal of Law and Medicine* 11: 241–57.

Salloum, S., and E. Franssen. 1993. 'Laboratory Investigation in General Practice.' *Canadian Family Physician* 93: 1055.

Studdert, David, and Troyen Brennan. 2001. 'Toward a Workable Model of "No-Fault" Compensation for Medical Injury in the United States. *American Journal of Law and Medicine* 27: 225–52.

Ubel, P. 2002. 'Physicians, Thou Shalt Ration: The Necessary Role of Bedside Rationing in Controlling Healthcare Costs.' *Healthcare Papers* 2: 10–21.

Walker, A. 2002. 'The Legal Duty of Physicians and Hospitals to Provide Emergency Care.' *CMAJ* 166: 465–9.

Wolf, S. 1991. Toward a Systematic Theory of Informed Consent in Managed Care. *Houston Law Review* 35: 1631.

Case Law

Anderson v. Chasney, [1950] 4 DLR 223 (SCC).

Arndt v. Smith (1997), 148 DLR (4th) 48 (SCC).

Bateman v. Doiron (1991), 8 CCLT 284 (NBQB); aff'd (1993), 18 CCLT 1 (NB CA).

Brown v. British Columbia, [1994] 1 SCR 420.

Canadian AIDS Society v. Ontario (1995), 25 OR (3d) 388 (Ont. Gen. Div.).

Ciarlarliello v. Schacter, [1993] 2 SCR 119.

Cox v. College of Optometrists of Ontario (1988), 65 OR 461 (Ont. High Ct).

Crits v. Sylvester (1956), 1 DLR 502 (Ont. CA); affd [1956] SCR 991.

Decock v. Alberta, [2000] AJ No. 419 (Alta CA).

Dumais v. Hamilton, [1998] AJ No. 761 (Alta CA).

Elofson v. Davis (1997), 49 Alta. LR (3a) 327 (Alta QB).

Hall v. Hebert (1993), 15 CCLT (2d) 93 at 118 (SCC), cited in L. Klar, *Tort Law* (Toronto: Carswell, 1996), 1.

Henderson v. Johnston (1956), 5 DLR (2d) 524 (Ont. High Ct).

Law Estate v. Simice (1994), 21 CCLT (2d) 228 (BCSC) at 240, aff'd [1996] 4 WWR 672 (BC CA).

McInerney v. MacDonald (1992), 93 DLR (4th) 415 (SCC).

McLean v. Car (1994), 363 APR 271 (Nfld. TD).

Meyer Estate v. Rogers (1991), 78 DLR (4th) 307 (Ont. Gen. Div.).

Mickle v. Salvation Army Grace Hospital Windsor Ontario, [1998] OJ No. 4683 (Ont. Crt Justice).

Moore v. Regents of the University of California 793 P. 2d 479 (Cal. 1990).

Norberg v. Wynrib (1992), 92 DLR (4th) 449 (SCC).

Pegram v. Herdrich (2000), 120 S. Ct 2143 (2000).

Peters-Brown v. Regina District Health Board, [1995] SJ No. 60 (Sask. QB).

R. v. O'Connor (1995), 130 DLR (4th) 235 (SCC).

R. v. Osolin (1993), 109 DLR (4th) 478 (SCC).

Reibl v. Hughes (1980), 114 DLR (3rd) 1 (SCC).

Seney v. Crooks, [1998] AJ No. 1060 (QL) (Alta CA).

Sunnucks v. Tobique Valley Hospital (1999), 216 NBR (2d) 201 (NB QB).

ter Neuzen v. Korn (1995), 127 DLR (4th) 577 (SCC).

Wickline v. State of California, 228 Cal. Rptr 661 (Cal. App. 2 Dist. 1986).

4 Section 7 of the Charter and Health-Care Spending

MARTHA JACKMAN

Section 7 of the Canadian Charter of Rights and Freedoms states: 'Everyone has the right to life, liberty and security of the person and the right not to be deprived thereof except in accordance with the principles of fundamental justice.' With the Supreme Court of Canada's decision in *Eldridge v. British Columbia* (1997), the applicability of section 7, and of the Charter generally, in the health-care context has expanded significantly (Jackman 2000). In the *Eldridge* case, the court held that the actions not only of governments, but of hospitals and other non-governmental health-care providers planning and delivering publicly funded health-care services, are subject to Charter scrutiny. The *Eldridge* decision has generated renewed interest from commentators on legal and health-care policy in the possible impact of the Charter on the future direction of Canadian health care (Laverdière 1998–9; Karr 2000; von Tigerstrom 2002; Hartt and Monahan 2002; Manfredi and Maioni 2002). While the full parameters of section 7 have yet to be established, three principal questions emerge from the case law to date. These are, first, whether section 7 guarantees a right to refuse unwanted health care; second, whether it establishes a right to receive care; and third, whether it guarantees the right to provide health-care services free of governmental restrictions. The answers have potential significance for health-care spending.

This paper examines the relevant case law in each of these areas in order to consider what this impact might be. The first section reviews the claim that section 7 guarantees the right to refuse unwanted health care. The second considers the argument that it guarantees the right to receive health care. The third section examines the claim that it guarantees the right to provide health-care services. The fourth section considers the potential impact of section 7 on health-care spending in the light of the requirement that decision making respect the 'principles of fundamental justice.' The fifth section considers the cost implications of section 7 in view of the recognition, under sections 7 and 1 of the Charter, that interference with individual rights must be balanced against the interests of Canadian society generally.

The Right to Refuse Health Care

Although the Supreme Court of Canada has only begun to address the issue of whether the Charter protects health or other welfare-related interests, it has recognized the profound impact of health-care decisions on an individual's right to 'life, liberty, and security of the person' in a number of cases. In *R. v. Morgentaler* (1988) the court was called on to assess the constitutionality of the provisions on therapeutic abortion in section 251 of the Criminal Code. In his majority judgment, Chief Justice Dickson held that 'forcing a woman, by threat of criminal sanction, to carry a foetus to term unless she meets certain criteria unrelated to her own priorities and aspirations, is a profound interference with a woman's body and thus a violation of security of the person' (*R. v. Morgentaler* 1988, 56–7). He also concluded that delays faced by women seeking abortions, which increased the level of complication and risk in the procedure, amounted to an infringement of both the physical and the psychological aspects of the right to security of the person (60).

In her concurring judgment, Justice Wilson agreed that the right to security of the person under section 7 protects an individual's physical and psychological security, and she noted: 'State enforced medical or surgical treatment comes readily to mind as an obvious invasion of physical integrity' (173). Justice Wilson held that a pregnant woman's section 7 rights were violated by the therapeutic abortion provisions because the control exercised by the state over her reproductive capacity and choices 'is not ... just a matter of interfering with her right to liberty in the sense ... of her right to personal autonomy in decision-making, it is a direct interference with her physical "person" as well' (173).

The Supreme Court's decision in *Rodriguez v. British Columbia* (1993) also has particular relevance to health care. At issue was the constitutionality of the prohibition against assisted suicide under section 241 of the Criminal Code. In her dissenting opinion, Justice McLachlin argued that the right to security of the person under section 7 of the Charter protects 'the dignity and privacy of individuals with respect to decisions concerning their own body' and that 'it is part of the persona and dignity of the human being that he or she have the autonomy to decide what is best for his or her body' (*Rodriguez* 1993, 618). In his majority decision, Justice Sopinka noted that 'a right to choose how one's body will be dealt with, even in the context of beneficial medical treatment, has long been recognized by the common law' (588). Justice Sopinka agreed with Justice McLachlin's conclusion that, by interfering with an individual's ability to make autonomous choices about his or her own bodily treatment, the prohibition against assisted suicide violated the right to security of the person under section 7 (588–9).

In *B. (R.) v. Children's Aid Society of Metropolitan Toronto* (1995) the issue of whether section 7 guarantees the right to refuse unwanted medical treatment was raised indirectly. The appellants challenged a wardship order under which the Children's Aid Society authorized blood transfusions for their infant daughter, against their religious beliefs as Jehovah's Witnesses. The appellants claimed that the wardship order and the child-welfare legislation on which it was based violated their right to parental liberty under section 7 of the Charter. In his judgment for a plurality of the Supreme Court, Justice La Forest found that section 7 included the right to make fundamental personal decisions without interference from the state and, in particular, that 'the right to nurture a child, to care for its development, and to make decisions for it in fundamental matters such as medical care, are part of the liberty interest of a parent' (*B. [R.]* 1995, 370). In their dissenting judgment, Justices Cory, Iacobucci, and Major held that 'although an individual may refuse any medical procedures upon her own person,' section 7 of the Charter does not give a parent the right to deny a medical treatment which is necessary to preserve the child's life or health (432).

The question of whether section 7 provides a barrier against unwanted medical care was squarely addressed by the Ontario Court of Appeal in *Fleming v. Reid* (1991), a case dealing with the rights of involuntary psychiatric patients to refuse treatment. In reviewing the provisions of the Ontario Mental Health Act, which allowed the prior wishes of a mentally competent patient to be overridden by a government appointed review board, the court argued: 'The common law right to bodily integrity and personal autonomy is so entrenched in the traditions of our law as to be ranked as fundamental and deserving of the highest order of protection. This right forms an essential part of an individual's security of the person and must be included in the liberty interests protected by s. 7. Indeed, in my view, the common law right to determine what shall be done with one's own body and the constitutional right to security of the person, both of which are founded on the belief in the dignity and autonomy of each individual, can be treated as co-extensive' (*Fleming v. Reid* 1991, 88).

The Court of Appeal went on to find that psychiatric patients do not, by reason of their mental illness, lose their section 7 right to be free from non-consensual invasions of their person, including the administration of unwanted drugs.

If the right to refuse health care is recognized as an aspect of the right to life, liberty, and security of the person under section 7, it follows that decisions that impinge on that right must respect the 'principles of fundamental justice.' An infringement of a section 7 right will offend the principles of fundamental justice if it violates 'basic tenets of our legal system' (*Re B.C. Motor Vehicle Act* 1985, 503). These tenets 'may be reflected in the common-law and statutory environment which exists outside of the *Charter*, they may be reflected in the specific and enumerated provisions of the *Charter*, or they may be more expansive than either of these' (*R. v. S. (R.J.)* 1995, para. 49). Principles of fundamental justice include those recognized both in domestic law and under international human-rights conventions (*Re B.C. Motor Vehicle Act* 1985, 512; *United States v. Burns* 2001, paras. 79–81). As Justice Sopinka explained in *Rodriguez* (1993, 594), the principles of fundamental justice also require a balancing of the interest of the individual and of the state: 'Where the deprivation of the right in question does little or nothing to enhance the state's interest ... a breach of fundamental justice will be made out. '

Thus, in Justice Dickson's view in *R. v. Morgentaler* (1988, 70), the arbitrariness, vagueness, and unfairness of the decision-making and administrative procedures put in place by section 251 of the Criminal Code, including the failure to define the concept of 'health,' violated section 7 principles of fundamental justice. Justice Wilson found that section 251 violated the principles of fundamental justice because it interfered with other Charter guarantees, particularly with the right to freedom of conscience under section 2 (*Morgentaler* 1988, 180). While, in *Rodriguez* (1993, 624), Justice McLachlin found that the prohibition on assisted suicide was arbitrary and therefore fundamentally unjust, Justice Sopinka held that the prohibition reflected the fundamental value of respect for the sanctity of life and thus accorded with the principles of fundamental justice (608).

In *B.(R.)* (1995, 377), Justice La Forest found that, because the appellants were able to participate in the judicial proceedings in which the wardship determination in relation to their child was made, the principles of fundamental justice had been met. In *Fleming v. Reid* (1991), however, the inadequacies of the hearing process provided for under Ontario's Mental Health Act led the Court of Appeal to conclude that the principles of fundamental justice had been violated. In particular, the court found: 'A legislative scheme that permits the competent wishes of a psychiatric patient to be overridden, and which allows a patient's right to personal autonomy and self-determination to be defeated, without affording a hearing as to why the substitute consent-giver's decision to refuse consent based on the patient's wishes should not be honoured, in my opinion, violates "the basic tenets of our legal system" and cannot be in accordance with the principles of fundamental justice' (93).

In summary, the decision – that involuntary medical treatment infringes the right to liberty and security of the person – is consistent with the Supreme Court's interpretation of section 7 as a general guarantee against threats to, or interferences with, individual bodily integrity.

In the light of the reasoning in *Morgentaler* (1988), *Rodriguez* (1993), and *B. (R.)* (1995), it is probable that when this issue does come directly before it, the Supreme Court will confirm that section 7 guarantees the right to refuse unwanted medical treatment and that any interference with this right must respect the principles of fundamental justice.

The Right to Receive Health Care

While it seems clear that the right to refuse medical treatment is protected under the Charter, the issue of whether section 7 also guarantees a right to receive health care, and what the scope of such a right might be, remains to be resolved. In *Irwin Toy Ltd. v. Québec* (1989, 1003–4), the Supreme Court of Canada expressly left open the possibility that 'economic rights fundamental to human life or survival,' such as the social and economic rights included under international human-rights treaties ratified by Canada, might be protected under section 7. In his decision in *Rodriguez* (1993, 585), Justice Sopinka held that 'security of the person is intrinsically concerned with the well-being of the living person.' In discussing the scope of the right to security of the person in *Singh v. Canada* (1985), Justice Wilson cited the Law Reform Commission of Canada's assertion, in its working paper on *Medical Treatment and the Criminal Law* (1980, 6), that 'the right to security of the person means not only protection of one's physical integrity, but the provision of necessaries for its support.' Justice Wilson also referred to the Federal Court's decision in *Collin v. Lussier* (1983), in which the transfer of a federal inmate suffering from heart disease from a medium- to a maximum-security penitentiary, where emergency medical services were limited, was found to infringe the section 7 right to security of the person. In his judgment, Justice Decary held that 'increasing the applicant's anxiety as to his state of health, is likely to make his illness worse and, by depriving him of access to adequate medical care, is in fact an impairment of the security of his person' (239). Justice Wilson's subsequent judgment in *Stoffman v. Vancouver General Hospital* (1990, 544) underscored the fact that 'government has recognized for some time that access to basic health care is something no sophisticated society can legitimately deny to any of its members.'

In many cases, however, lower courts have been unsympathetic to health-related challenges brought forward under section 7. Such claims have been rejected on the grounds that the legislative history of the Charter precludes recognition of 'economic' rights of this kind and that a reading of section 7 that recognizes individual rights to health would lead to unwarranted judicial interference in the health-care system. For example, in *Ontario Nursing Home Association v. Ontario* (1990, 177), the Ontario High Court rejected the plaintiffs' argument that the level of provincial funding to nursing homes was inadequate and that this under-funding violated the residents' rights to security of the person, on the basis that section 7 does not deal with property rights or guarantee 'additional benefits which might enhance life, liberty or security of the person.' Similarly, in *Brown v. British Columbia (Minister of Health)* (1990, 467–9), the British Columbia Supreme Court rejected the plaintiffs' challenge of the province's decision not to subsidize the costs of the AIDS drug AZT, on the grounds that section 7 did not protect against economic deprivations or guarantee benefits that might enhance life, liberty, or security of the person. And, in *Cameron v. Nova Scotia* (1999a), which involved a challenge to Nova Scotia's failure to fund in vitro fertilization under the provincial health-insurance plan, the province's Supreme Court concluded that 'finding the public fund-ing of particular medical services to be considered an element of the right to life, liberty or security of the person would expand the param-eters of judicial review, well beyond its present scope' (para. 160).

In three recent cases, however, the courts have shown greater recep-tivity to the claim that section 7 guarantees access to health-care ser-vices. In *Sawatzky v. Riverview Health Centre Inc.* (1998), the Manitoba Court of Queen's Bench granted an interlocutory injunction preventing the Riverview Health Centre from imposing, against his spouse's wishes, a 'do not resuscitate' order on an elderly patient suffering from advanced Parkinson's disease and pneumonia, based in part on the argument that such an order might violate section 7 rights to life, lib-erty, and security of the person. In *R. v. Parker* (2000), the Ontario Court of Appeal found that the Criminal Code prohibition on the possession and cultivation of marijuana violated the accused's section 7 right to liberty and security of the person because it prevented him from obtaining marijuana as a medical treatment for his epilepsy. Justice Rosenberg found that, akin to the situation in *Fleming v. Reid* (1991), 'the choice of medication to alleviate the effects of an illness with life-threatening consequences is a decision of fundamental personal importance,' falling within the liberty interest protected under section 7 (*Parker* 2000, para. 102). In terms of the accused's right to security of the person, relying on the Supreme Court's reasoning in *Morgentaler* (1988) and *Rodriguez* (1993), Justice Rosenberg held that preventing the accused from using marijuana to treat his medical condition by threat of criminal prosecution constituted an unconstitutional interference with his physical and psychological integrity (*Parker* 2000, para. 110).

In the Quebec Superior Court case of *Chaoulli v. Québec* (2000), the issue of whether section 7 of the Charter creates an affirmative right to receive health care was raised directly. The plaintiffs alleged that lack of timely access to provincially insured health-care services, because of constraints on financial and human resources within the public sys-tem, coupled with legislative restrictions on access to private care, amounted to a violation of the section 7 right to life, liberty, and secu-rity of the person. In addressing the plaintiffs' claim, Justice Piché reviewed the evidence brought forward by the parties on the issue of the accessibility and efficiency of private *versus* public systems of health-care delivery. After examining the evidence at length, she con-cluded that the development of a parallel private health-care system would have deleterious effects on the existing public one. In this regard, she cited U.S. health economist Ted Marmor's testimony that: 'allowing private insurance to be available as an alternative to Medicare would have profound negative impacts on the public system rather than none as is assumed. It would not increase availability of services in the public sector or reduce waiting lists. Instead, it would divert resources from the publicly financed program to be available to private activities and it would increase total Canadian expenditures on health. It would also give those able to secure private coverage an advantage over others' (*Chaoulli* 2000, para. 107).

After reviewing Supreme Court case law on the scope of section 7, Justice Piché concluded that the court had left the door open to recognizing economic rights intimately connected to life, liberty, or personal security. In answer to the question whether access to health-care services was such a right, she concluded in the affirmative. In her view: 'S'il n'y a pas d'accès possible au système de santé, c'est illusoire de croire que les droits à la vie et à la sécurité sont respectés' (If there is no access to the health-care system, it is illusory to think that the rights to life and security are respected) (para. 223). On the further matter of whether the right to purchase full-coverage private health insurance or to contract privately for hospital services, currently restricted under provincial health insurance legislation, was also protected under section 7, she also found the answer was 'Yes.' To the extent that legislative restrictions on private insurance rendered private health care uneconomical, and access to private health care illusory, she held that section 7 rights were affected. In her view, however, limits on access to private services would violate section 7 only where the public system was unable effectively to guarantee access to similar care: 'Le Tribunal ne croit pas par contre qu'il puisse exister un droit constitutionnel de choisir la provenance de soins médicalement requis' (The Court does not think, however, that there is a constitutional right to choose the source of medically required health care) (para. 227).

On appeal, Justice Piché's decision was upheld by the Quebec Court of Appeal in three concurring judgments (*Chaoulli* 2002). Justice Delisle found that access to publicly funded health care was a fundamental right under section 7. However, he held that the right to purchase private health insurance was an economic claim, which was not fundamental to human life, and was not therefore protected under section 7 (*Chaoulli* 2002, para. 25). Justice Forget agreed with Justice Piché that, while the plaintiffs' health rights were threatened by the limits placed on private health services, the province's decision to favour the collective interest in the public health-care system was in accordance with the principles of fundamental justice (*Chaoulli* 2002, para. 63). Justice Brossard found that the evidence failed to show that the statutory restrictions on private health care had in fact imperilled the plaintiffs' rights to life or health (para. 66).

As discussed above in the context of unwanted medical treatment, once the right to receive health care is recognized as an aspect of the right to life, liberty, and security of the person, measures limiting access to such care must respect the principles of fundamental justice. In *Collin v. Lussier* (1983), the Federal Court found that, by failing to provide the plaintiff with notice of the decision that would adversely affect his ability to receive medical treatment, by failing to provide him with an opportunity to make representations about his particular circumstances, and by failing to ensure that the relevant decision-making authority would render an impartial decision on the basis of all the evidence presented to it, the decision-making process at issue did not conform with the principles of fundamental justice (240). In *Parker* (2000), Justice Rosenberg found that the blanket prohibition on possession and cultivation of marijuana was contrary to the principles of fundamental justice for a number of reasons, including because it did little or nothing to promote state interests (para. 144), was irrational in its adverse impact on the health of those affected, and was inconsistent with the principle of the sanctity of life (para. 137), and because 'the right to make decisions that are of fundamental importance includes the choice of medication to alleviate the effects of an illness with life threatening consequences. It does not comport with principles of fundamental justice to subject that decision to unfettered ministerial discretion' (para. 188).

In summary, while a number of lower courts have rejected the claim that section 7 guarantees the right to health services, others have seen access to health care as a necessary component of the right to life, liberty, and security of the person. Where health care has been recognized as a section 7 right, decisions affecting access have been subject to scrutiny for conformity with the principles of fundamental justice. As in other section 7 contexts, the principles of fundamental justice applicable in the health-care setting include guarantees of due process of such as the requirement to provide the person whose health is at issue with an opportunity to be fully and fairly heard by an impartial decision-maker (*Collin v. Lussier* 1983). Fundamental justice has also been held to impose substantive requirements, such as respect for the principle of the sanctity of life (*Parker* 2000) and for domestic and international human rights guarantees (*Morgentaler* 1988). Finally, courts have balanced the interests of the individual claiming a right to receive health care against the state interests involved in limiting access to such care (*Parker* 2000; *Chaoulli* 2002).

The Right to Provide Health Care

A third issue raised by section 7 of the Charter is whether the right to life, liberty, and security of the person guarantees the right to provide health-care services. In its decision in *Irwin Toy* (1989, 1004), the Supreme Court held that section 7 protects the life, liberty, and personal security of human beings, and not of corporate or other non-human entities. Based on a reading of the legislative history, the court also rejected the argument that economic rights of a corporate or commercial nature are entitled to protection under section 7. Government control over the activities of institutional health-care providers will be subject to constitutional scrutiny where it interferes with other Charter rights that corporations do enjoy, such as the right to freedom of commercial expression under section 2(b) (*Rocket v. Royal College of Dental Surgeons* 1990; Shirreff 2000). As we saw above, such limits may also be subject to Charter review where the section 7 rights of individual patients are directly affected. However, the court's reasoning in *Irwin Toy* makes it clear that institutional or corporate providers of health care will not be able to invoke section 7 to challenge governmental limits on their own ability to provide health care (Jackman 1995).

In the case of individual health-care providers, the Charter's potential as a basis for challenging government regulation and control also appears to be limited. In *Wilson v. British Columbia (Medical Services Commission)* (1988), the appellant physicians challenged the validity of the British Columbia Medical Services Act Regulations, which enabled the province to restrict the types and geographical locations of doctors' practices covered by the provincial health insurance plan, through the allocation of billing numbers to practitioners. In its decision, the British Columbia Court of Appeal invalidated the regulations on the grounds that 'denying doctors the opportunity to pursue their profession falls within the rubric of 'liberty' as that word is used in section 7' (*Wilson* 1988, 189). In response to the suggestion that the appellants' claim involved a purely economic interest, the court maintained that 'denial of the right to participate under the plan is not the denial of a purely economic right, but in reality is a denial of the right of the appellants to practise their chosen profession within British Columbia' (187).

The soundness of the court's conclusion was put into serious doubt by Justice Lamer's concurring judgment in *Reference Re the Criminal Code* (1990). Justice Lamer held that while the non-economic or non-pecuniary aspects of work are important to the individual, the rights under section 7 do not include the right to exercise one's chosen profession (1179). By his reasoning, government restrictions on the activities of individual health-care providers, including on the ability of physicians or other health-care professionals to provide health-care services, would not be subject to section 7 review.

In several recent decisions, lower courts have taken the view that the *Wilson* (1988) decision has been overturned by the Supreme Court. In *Waldman v. British Columbia* (1999), the appellant physicians challenged a series of post-*Wilson* billing restrictions imposed by the British Columbia Medical Services Commission to control the number and distribution of physicians within the province. The British Columbia Court of Appeal upheld the trial court's conclusion that *Wilson* (1988) had been overruled and that, while physicians' interprovincial mobility rights under section 6 of the Charter were affected, section 7 had no application in the case (*Waldman* 1997, para. 293; *Waldman* 1999, para. 52). In *Rombaut v. New Brunswick* (2001), the New Brunswick Court of Appeal rejected the plaintiff's attempts to distinguish the *Wilson* (1988) case and concluded that a provincial plan designed to regulate the number and distribution of physicians in the province by controlling billing numbers did not engage physicians' liberty or other section 7 rights (*Rombaut* 2001, para. 104). Justice Piché came to a similar decision in *Chaoulli* (2000) – that section 7 did not guarantee physicians' rights to provide health-care services. In this regard, she asserted: 'l'article 7 de la *Charte* ne protège pas le droit d'un médecin d'exercer sa profession sans contrainte dans le domaine privé. Ceci est un droit purement économique' (section 7 of the Charter does not protect physicians' right to practise their profession without constraint in the private domain. This is a purely economic right) (para. 226).

This case law suggests that the likelihood of individual health-care providers being able to claim successfully a section 7 right to provide services, within or outside the publicly funded system, is doubtful, inasmuch as the courts have characterized government control over the supply of health care as affecting economic interests that fall outside the scope of section 7.

Potential Implications of Fundamental Justice as a Standard for Decision Making in Health Care

If section 7 guaranteed an unqualified right to refuse, to receive, or to provide health-care services, the implications for health-care spending would be enormous. However, as discussed above, the rights under section 7 are not absolute. It is not every interference with the right to life, liberty, or security of the person that is objectionable, but rather those violations that do not conform with the principles of fundamental justice. As outlined in the preceding section of the paper, the principles of fundamental justice identified by the courts are both procedural and substantive in nature. At the level of due process, the case law (*Collin v. Lussier* 1983; *Singh* 1985; *Morgentaler* 1988) suggests that decisions that are likely to have a significant impact on an individual's health will fail section 7 scrutiny unless certain procedural safeguards are provided. These safeguards include the right to adequate notice of a decision, the right to respond, and the right to be heard by a fair and impartial decision-maker. Such due-process guarantees are designed to ensure not only that the decision-maker has all the information needed to make an accurate and appropriate decision, but also that the decision-making process itself respects the dignity and autonomy of the person whose life, liberty, or security is at stake.

An individual whose health rights are threatened, either by non-consensual treatment or because he or she is being denied care, would therefore have the right to know that a treatment decision was being made, and on what basis. He or she would have the right to discuss the treatment decision with the person responsible for making it, to understand and assess all the available treatment options, and to convey his or her particular priorities and concerns. A person whose health was at risk would have the right to fairness and open-mindedness on the part of the ultimate decision maker. It would have to be shown that any decision made was not the result of inadequate or arbitrary standards and that the standards that did exist were not applied in an irrational or unfair way. In short, the principles of fundamental justice would require physicians and other health-care providers not only to state what treatments were being offered and their attendant risks, but to treat patients as active participants in their own care.

In order effectively to protect the life, liberty, and security interests at issue in health-care decision making, however, respect for the principles of fundamental justice would have to extend beyond the individual treatment setting. Otherwise, the entire burden of ensuring Charter compliance would rest on those most immediately and directly dependent on the health-care system and on the decision makers operating within it. Limiting the requirements of fundamental justice to individualized decision-making would also fail to address the fact that primary care decisions are frequently the product of resource allocation and other considerations beyond health-care providers' immediate control (Caulfield 1994). A person whose health is threatened by an individualized treatment decision has the right to participate in the decision-making process. As the reasoning in *Singh* (1985) and *Morgentaler* (1988) suggests, where a more general health-care policy or regulatory decision threatens to have a similar impact on life, liberty, and personal security, but on a larger scale, the same requirements of due process should apply (Canadian Bar Association 1994; Jackman 1995–6).

Thus, when governments or other publicly funded health-care providers make policy or regulatory decisions affecting the allocation of health-care resources and services, they should ensure that those whose fundamental interests are at risk are adequately involved. As in the individualized treatment setting, in order for regulatory decisions that adversely affect health-related interests to be characterized as fundamentally just within the meaning of section 7, decision making must become more inclusive and accountable. The individualized service-delivery setting can meet requirements of due process relatively easily by providing an opportunity for individual patients to participate in decisions about their care on a case-by-case basis. In the policy and regulatory setting, due process can be met by ensuring that decisions relating to the allocation of health-care resources and services are publicly debated before they are put in place.

Possible mechanisms for securing collective input into making of health policy include public hearings and other forms of public consultation. Public consultation should extend to such matters as the restructuring of delivery models, the development of treatment criteria, the design of cost-containment and rationing mechanisms, the elaboration of practice guidelines, the design and implementation of consent-to-treatment standards, and the listing and delisting of services under public health-insurance plans. Alternative mechanisms for broadening participation in decision making might include better dissemination of information; effective representation for the public, patient, and advocacy groups on decision-making bodies about health policy, whether at the governmental or service-delivery levels; and greater decentralization of decision making (Abelson et al. 2002).

Aside from responding to concerns at a procedural level, increased individual and collective participation in health-care decision making is also consistent with the more substantive dimensions of fundamental justice identified by the Supreme Court. The court has referred in particular to international human-rights treaties ratified by Canada as a source of section 7 principles of fundamental justice (*Re B.C. Motor Vehicle Act* 1985; *United States v. Burns* 2001). Over the past 50 years, Canada has assumed extensive international obligations to protect and promote individual health and welfare and to ensure universal access to health-care services in the event of illness (von Tigerstrom 2002). These international health-related rights have not been directly incorporated into Canadian law and so cannot be claimed at the domestic level. However, the Supreme Court has held that Canada's international human-rights obligations are a clear source of guidance in interpreting not only the Charter, but federal and provincial laws and policies (*Baker* 1999).

Of particular force, article 25(1) of the Universal Declaration of Human Rights (1948), adopted by Canada along with other members of the United Nations General Assembly, provides that 'everyone has the right to a standard of living adequate for the health and well-being of himself and his family, including ... medical care.' Article 12(1) of the International Covenant on Economic, Social and Cultural Rights (1966) (ICESCR), ratified by Canada in 1976 after lengthy discussions with the provinces, recognizes 'the right of everyone to the enjoyment of the highest attainable standard of physical and mental health.' And article 12(2)(d) of the ICESCR sets out the obligations of Canada and other parties that have ratified the treaty to take all steps necessary for 'the creation of conditions which would assure to all medical service and medical attention in the event of sickness.'

The International Convention on the Elimination of all Forms of Racial Discrimination (1969), the International Convention on the Elimination of All Forms of Discrimination against Women (1979), the International Convention on the Rights of the Child (1989), and more recent international agreements such as the Vienna Declaration and Programme of Action (1993) all contain anti-discrimination and other substantive provisions designed to ensure that the health rights recognized under the Universal Declaration and the ICESCR are enjoyed equally by all members of society, including the most vulnerable

(Sholzberg-Gray 1999; von Tigerstrom 2002). Given the status and scope of the right to health at the international level (Toebes 1999), and Canada's clear international treaty obligations in this area, failure to recognize and protect individual and collective rights to participate in health-care decision making at the domestic level would not conform with section 7 principles of fundamental justice.

Respect for other Canadian Charter and domestic human-rights norms has also been identified by the Supreme Court as a requirement of fundamental justice (*Morgentaler* 1988). Of special significance in health law are the substantive equality principles set out under section 15 of the Charter, and under federal and provincial human-rights laws. As discussed below in relation to *Eldridge v. British Columbia* (1997), health-care decision making that has a disparate impact on the basis of gender, race, disability, or other prohibited grounds of discrimination will violate principles of fundamental justice, whether or not the discriminatory effects were intentional. In individual treatment, for example, compelled medical treatment of a pregnant woman in the interests of her foetus would clearly offend the principles of fundamental justice on grounds of sex equality (Jackman 1993; Rogers 2002). Similarly, limiting eligibility for treatment on the basis of gender (*J.C. v. Forensic Psychiatric Service Commissioner* 1992), disability (*Cameron* 1999b), or age (Canadian Bar Association 1994, 59; Gilmore 2002) would constitute a fundamentally unjust deprivation of section 7 rights.

At the broader policy or regulatory level, whatever the mechanisms adopted to increase public participation in health-related decision making, the principles of fundamental justice would require affirmative steps to guarantee the representation of historically disadvantaged groups, such as aboriginal peoples (Royal Commission on Aboriginal Peoples 1995, 247–60) and people living in poverty (Swanson 2001; Raphael 2001), who are lacking in resources and influence and do not have a history of inclusion in health-care decision making. Such additional measures are necessary to ensure that increasing collective participation in decision making actually results in a more equitable distribution of decision-making authority and health-care resources and doesn't simply reinforce existing decision-making patterns and structures that are inconsistent with principles of equality rights (Abelson et al. 2002, 72).

Assessed in the light of these broader procedural and substantive concerns, the cost implications of section 7 principles of fundamental justice are mixed. On the cost side, a significant consequence of increasing due process in health-care decision making relates to the additional time that is required to make decisions. At the individual level, most decisions about health-care treatment are made by physicians whose time is expensive, in both opportunity and dollar terms. While doctors must currently meet private-law standards of informed consent (Caulfield 2002), requiring them to spend more time ensuring patients' meaningful participation in health-care decision making will probably result in higher short-term costs. To fully inform and involve patients in decision making about their own care may also require other types of health-care expertise – for example, counselling or education about non-medical or non-traditional treatment options about which physicians have limited knowledge or interest (Haigh 1999). Expanding patients' interaction with a wider range of health-care providers may also result in additional costs.

The requirements of fundamental justice may also mean that decision-making at the broader policy or regulatory level becomes more time-consuming, and therefore more costly. An example of this is provided in the facts of the *Eldridge* case (1997). The appellants were deaf residents of British Columbia who had all experienced problems within the provincial health-care system because of their inability to communicate with health-care providers in the absence of sign-language interpretation services. For example, one of the appellants underwent an emergency Caesarean delivery without the attending medical and nursing staff being able to communicate with her because interpretation services were not available in the hospital. In 1990, a non-profit agency that had been providing free medical interpretation in the lower mainland applied to the British Columbia Ministry of Health for funding to continue the service. Following a brief discussion, the ministry's executive committee turned down the funding request on the summary explanation, set out in an internal ministry memorandum, that 'it was felt [that] to fund this particular request would set a precedent that might be followed up by further requests from the ethnic communities where the language barrier might also be a factor' (*Eldridge* 1992, para. 75). Given the centrality of effective communication to the delivery of health-care services, the Supreme Court concluded that the province's failure to provide interpretation services denied the deaf equal benefit of the law relative to the hearing, in violation of section 15 of the Charter (*Eldridge* 1997, para. 80).

Apart from its discriminatory character, the Ministry of Health's refusal to fund interpretation services in the *Eldridge* case was also deficient in terms of section 7 principles of fundamental justice. It made the decision without receiving any meaningful input from those whose life, liberty, and security were directly affected – deaf residents of the province who were unable to communicate with health-care providers in the absence of interpretation services. The refusal to fund medical interpretation services was based not on any evidence presented to the executive committee, but rather on factors totally unrelated to the health-care needs of the deaf. Finally, there was no opportunity for those affected to address the committee's concerns either before or after the decision was made. In each of these regards, the decision-making structure in *Eldridge* violated the due-process requirements of section 7. To remedy these deficiencies, a more inclusive and account-able process would have been required. By increasing the time needed for each funding decision, reforming the decision-making process in *Eldridge*, like the procedure for insuring and de-insuring health-care services in other provinces, would probably have meant increased expenditures.

As for the financial implications of fundamental justice as a standard for decision making in health care, while respecting due process may increase process-related costs at both the individual and the broader regulatory levels, savings achieved through more effective health-care decisions may outweigh such expenditures. At the collective level, a lack of inclusiveness and accountability in decision-making may lead to irrational and ineffective spending. For example, in *Eldridge* the Ministry of Health was unable to provide any evidence that its refusal to fund interpretation services, at a projected cost of $150,000 a year, or 0.0025 per cent of the provincial health-care budget (*Eldridge* 1997, para. 87), was economically rational. The appellants raised the question whether, by forcing deaf patients to make longer and more frequent visits to doctors and hospitals in the absence of interpretation services, and in view of the mis- or delayed diagnoses of health conditions likely to result from their inability to communicate effectively with health-care providers, the actual costs to the public health-care system of the refusal to fund interpretation services may have been much greater than any purported savings.

In *Auton v. British Columbia* (2000), the British Columbia Supreme Court came to the same conclusion with respect to the provincial Ministry of Health's refusal to fund autism treatment for children as a medically insured service. Having concluded that that failure was discriminatory on the basis of mental disability, Justice Allan considered the province's section 1 argument that health-care funds were limited and that providing treatment for autistic children would divert resources away from other health-care priorities. In the light of the evidence presented, Justice Allan concluded: 'It is apparent that the costs incurred in paying for effective treatment of autism may well be more than offset by the savings achieved by assisting autistic children to develop their educational and societal potential rather than dooming them to a life of isolation and institutionalization' (*Auton* 2000, para. 147). On that basis, Justice Allan found that the violation of the rights of children deprived of autism treatment could not be justified under section 1.

Similarly, at an individual level, where patients are more fully informed and involved in health-care decisions, they and the providers advising them may make better and more effective long-term treatment choices. In some cases, this may result in additional treatment being requested, with the associated increase in health-care expenditures. However, in other cases, greater information and patient involvement may result in the choice of less costly alternative treatments or in the choice not to be treated at all (Haigh 1999; Royal Commission on New Reproductive Technologies 1993, 94–5).

Providing patients with a meaningful opportunity not only to decide what treatments they want, but to decide against receiving any treatment at all, is particularly important at the end of life (Canada, Senate, 2002). A decision to terminate treatment against a patient's wishes, such as was at issue in the *Sawatzky* (1998) case, must clearly respect all procedural and substantive requirements of fundamental justice. However, as the facts of the *Rodriguez* (1993) and *Nancy B.* (1992) cases illustrate, life-prolonging treatment may not always be consistent with the patient's own interests and wishes. While health-care providers may feel an imperative to treat in order to prolong life, patients who are fully informed of their health status and prognosis and who are given a meaningful opportunity to direct their own care may make different choices. Irrespective of any financial considerations, as the Supreme Court underscored in *Rodriguez* (1993), ensuring an individual's full and informed involvement is equally, if not more, important to human dignity and autonomy in end-of-life decision-making as it is in other health-care contexts (Sneiderman 2002; Manitoba Law Reform Commission 2002).

In summary, decisions within the health-care system that impinge on individual life, liberty, and security, including the threat of non-consensual treatment or the denial of care, must respect the principles of fundamental justice. Decisions that are procedurally defective, or that offend the substantive principles of fundamental justice reflected in domestic and international equality and other basic legal norms, will fail a section 7 review. As outlined above, respecting the procedural and substantive requirements of fundamental justice may result in higher immediate costs to the health-care system, because of the increased time required for decision making and because additional treatments may be made available. However, to the extent that more rational and effective decisions are made, increased participation and accountability may also lead to reductions in spending, both within and beyond the health-care system.

Balancing Individual and Collective Interests under Section 7 and Section 1

In *Rodriguez* (1993, 594–5), Justice Sopinka held that, in order to determine whether a violation of the right to life, liberty, and security of the person conformed with the principles of fundamental justice under section 7, the interests of the individual had to be balanced against those of the state. As Justice La Forest expressed it in *Godbout v. Longueuil* (1997, 900), the idea that 'individual rights may, in some circumstances, be subordinated to substantial and compelling collective interests' is a basic tenet of Canada's legal system. In *Chaoulli* (2000), having found that section 7 guarantees a right to health-care services and that the right to life, liberty, and security of the person was affected by provincial statutory restrictions on access to private care, Justice Piché went on to consider whether such measures were in conformity with the principles of fundamental justice. Applying the balancing-of-interests test articulated by Justice Sopinka (*Rodriguez* 1993), Justice Piché pointed out that the province designed its health-insurance legislation to create and maintain a public health-care system, universally accessible to all residents of the province without barriers related to individual economic circumstances, and that it placed restrictions on private care to prevent a transfer of resources out of the public system (*Chaoulli* 2000, para. 259). As she explained: 'La preuve a montré que le droit d'avoir recours à un système parallèle privé de soins, invoqué par les requérants, aurait des répercussions sur les droits de l'ensemble de la population ... L'établissement d'un système de santé parallèle privé aurait pour effet de menacer l'intégrité, le bon fonctionnement ainsi que la viabilité du système

public. Les articles [contestés] empêchent cette éventualité et garantis-
sent l'existence d'un système de santé public de qualité au Québec'
(para. 263). (The evidence has shown that the right, claimed by the
plaintiffs, to use a parallel, private health-care system would have
repercussions on the rights of the general population ... The creation of
a parallel, private health-care system would threaten the integrity,
proper operation and viability of the public system. The [challenged]
sections prevent such an occurrence and guarantee the existence of a
quality, public health-care system in Quebec).

   This balancing of interests in favour of the collective benefit of preserving a viable and effective public health-care system, Justice Piché
found, was in conformity with the principles of fundamental justice: 'le
gouvernement limite les droits de quelques-uns pour assurer que les
droits de l'ensemble des citoyens de la société ne soient pas brimés'
('government restricts the rights of a few to ensure that there is no
interference with the rights of all citizens) (*Chaoulli* 2002, para. 262).
Thus restrictions on access to private health care under provincial
health-insurance legislation did not, Justice Piché concluded, violate
section 7.

   The balancing exercise that the courts have engaged in at the funda-
mental-justice stage of section 7 analysis is similar to what is required
under section 1 of the Charter. Section 1 provides that the Charter
'guarantees the rights and freedoms set out in it subject only to such
reasonable limits prescribed by law as can be demonstrably justified in
a free and democratic society.' In *R. v. Oakes* (1986), the Supreme Court
proposed a framework for deciding whether an infringement of an
individual right can be justified under section 1. First, the government
must show that the objective in violating the individual rights is 'pressing and substantial.' Second, it must prove that the means adopted to
achieve this objective are 'proportionate' in the sense of being rationally connected to their objective, of impairing the individual right as
little as possible, and of producing benefits to society that outweigh the
harm to the rights of the individual.

   Section 1 provides an additional opportunity for governments and
other health-care providers to introduce considerations relating to the
cost of health-care services, and the fiscal sustainability of the health-
care system, into the analysis of whether the violation of individual
rights is constitutionally permissible. In *Cameron* (1999b), for example,
the Nova Scotia Court of Appeal accepted the province's argument
that its failure to fund in vitro fertilization (IVF) and intra-cytoplasmic

sperm injection (ICSI) as a treatment for infertility was justified in view of the severe financial constraints facing the provincial health-care system. Justice Chipman accepted the government's evidence that, given the costs, the limited success rate, and the risks of IVF and ICSI, it was not yet ready to accept them as insured services. Justice Chipman concluded: 'The evidence makes clear the complexity of the health-care system and the extremely difficult task confronting those who must allocate the resources among a vast array of competing claims ... The policy makers require latitude in balancing competing interests in the constrained financial environment ... We should not second guess them, except in clear cases of failure on their part to properly balance the Charter rights of individuals against the overall pressing objective of the scheme under the Act' (paras. 234, 236).

In *Eldridge* (1997), however, the province (British Columbia) was unsuccessful in arguing that its actions were justified in view of the multiple competing demands that it faced for scarce health-care resources. Assuming, without deciding, that the province had shown that its refusal to fund medical interpretation services for the deaf was rationally connected to an important objective of controlling health-care expenditures, Justice La Forest found that the denial of interpretation services was more than a minimal impairment of the equality rights of the deaf. In coming to this decision, Justice La Forest pointed to the modest sum required to provide such services as a proportion of the total provincial budget for health care, and the fact that the ministry had failed to consider any other alternative that would have constituted a lesser limitation on deaf persons' rights. He also rejected the province's argument that, if compelled to fund interpretation services for the deaf, it would have to provide interpreters for non-English speakers, thereby severely straining the fiscal sustainability of its health-care system. Justice La Forest characterized this claim as speculative, given the province's failure to provide any evidence of the potential cost and scope of providing oral language interpretation services, in the event that they were found to be constitutionally mandated (*Eldridge* 1997, paras. 87–93). In concluding that the province's refusal to fund interpretation services could not be justified under section 1, Justice La Forest asserted: 'The evidence clearly demonstrates that, as a class, deaf persons receive medical services that are inferior to those received by the hearing population. Given the central place of good health in the quality of life of all persons in our society, the provision of substandard medical services to the deaf necessarily diminishes the overall quality of their lives. The government has simply not demonstrated that this unpropitious state of affairs must be tolerated in order to achieve the objective of limiting health-care expenditures' (para. 94).

The Supreme Court has underlined the fact that administrative convenience (*Singh* 1985) and the government's desire to save money (*Schachter v. Canada* 1992, 709) are not sufficient grounds for justifying a violation of rights under section 1. Rather, it has held that the cost of respecting a Charter right is relevant at the remedial stage. As Chief Justice Lamer expressed it in *Schachter* (1992, 709): 'Any remedy granted by a court will have some budgetary repercussions ... The question is not whether courts can make decisions that impact on budgetary policy; it is to what degree they can appropriately do so.' Where cost is a significant consideration, the court has shown considerable deference to the legislature in its choice of how to remedy the rights violation at issue. Even in *Eldridge* (1997), where the financial implications of its decision were held to be relatively modest, the Supreme Court did not order specific remedial measures, but instead issued a declaration that the province's failure to provide sign-language interpretation for the deaf was unconstitutional. As Justice La Forest explained: 'A declaration, as opposed to some kind of injunctive relief, is the appropriate remedy in this case because there are myriad options available to the government that may rectify the unconstitutionality of the current system. It is not this Court's role to dictate how this is to be accomplished' (*Eldridge* 1997, para. 96). The court also suspended its declaratory order for six months, with a further extension of twelve months, to allow the province time to formulate an appropriate response.

In principle, section 1 provides an opportunity for governments and other publicly funded health-care providers to defend decisions on health care that interfere with section 7 rights. However, because the section 7 principles of fundamental justice identified by the courts and the *Oakes* standard of section 1 review consider many of the same factors, such as the importance of the objective being pursued and the rationality of measures that interfere with a Charter right, it is difficult to conceive of a situation in which a decision found to violate the principles of fundamental justice would nevertheless be upheld under section 1 (Hartt and Monahan 2002, 24–5). Both section 1 and the procedural and substantive requirements of fundamental justice obligate decision makers to explain and justify their objectives and the means chosen to achieve them, in a principled way, supported by evidence. In the absence of any evidentiary basis, an allegation that a decision that violates individual rights is justified, because it furthers pressing public interests in the containment of health-care costs, is unlikely to succeed (*Eldridge* 1997; *Auton* 2000). Conversely, where it can be shown that a refusal to provide a particular health-care treatment or service was made carefully and fairly, in the light of all available evidence about its benefits, effectiveness, and cost, and in the light of competing health-care priorities and objectives, the decision is likely to be upheld (*Cameron* 1999a; *Chaoulli* 2000).

Conclusion

Equitable access to public health care is a pre-eminent value in Canadian society. It therefore stands to reason that fundamental health-related interests should be constitutionally recognized and that health-care decisions that are likely to have a significant adverse effect on human dignity, autonomy, and physical and psychological integrity should respect basic constitutional norms. Canadian courts have begun to recognize the right to refuse non-consensual treatment and the right to receive health care as aspects of the right to life, liberty, and security of the person under section 7 of the Charter and to hold that decisions impinging on these rights must conform with the principles of fundamental justice. In determining whether these principles have been met, the courts have considered both procedural and substantive concerns, including respect for fairness and due process and compliance with Canada's equality rights and other domestic and international human-rights obligations in relation to health. The courts have also found that the decision whether the right to life, liberty, and security has been violated requires a balancing of individual and societal interests, in accordance with section 7 principles of fundamental justice and under section 1.

As I suggested in the preceding section of the paper, the cost implications of recognizing and protecting health-related rights under section 7 of the Charter are mixed. One the one hand, the obligation to respect principles of fundamental justice will probably increase process-related costs of health-care decision making. To the extent that the refusal to provide health care cannot be shown to be fundamentally just, increased spending may also be needed. However, requiring health-care decision making to become more inclusive and accountable may generate better decisions at both the individual treatment and broader regulatory levels. As the facts of the *Eldridge* (1997) case illustrate, decision making that is more equitable and rational may also be more cost-effective in the immediate and longer terms. Seen from this perspective, rather than as a source of concern, the introduction of Charter values and principles into the Canadian health-care system is a positive development. Given the fundamental importance of health care to individual well-being and to the welfare of society as a whole, Canadians should be confident that health-care decision making respects basic constitutional values and, in particular, the values of security, dignity, and equality that are at the heart of the Canadian health-care system.

REFERENCES

Abelson, Julia, et al. 2002. 'Obtaining Public Input for Health-Systems Decision-Making: Past Experiences and Future Prospects.' *Canadian Public Administration* 45, no. 1: 70–97.
Auton (Guardian ad Litem of) v. British Columbia (Minister of Health) 2000. [2000] BCJ No. 1547 (BC SC).
B. (R.) v. Children's Aid Society of Metropolitan Toronto. 1995. [1995] 1 SCR 315.
Baker v. Canada (Minister of Citizenship and Immigration). 1999. [1999] 2 SCR 817.
Brown v. British Columbia (Minister of Health). 1990. (1990), 66 DLR (4th) 444 (BC SC).
Cameron v. Nova Scotia (Attorney General). 1999a. [1999] NSJ No. 33 (NS SC).
– 1999b. [1999] NSJ No. 297 (NS CA); leave to appeal to the Supreme Court of Canada denied, 29 June 2000.
Canada, Senate Standing Senate Committee on Social Affairs, Science and Technology. 2002. *Quality End-of-Life Care: The Right of Every Canadian.* www.parl.gc.ca/36/2/parlbus/commbus/senate/com-e/upda-e/rep-e/ repfinjun00-e.htm, 11 Sept. 2002.
Canadian Bar Association. 1994. *What's Law Got to Do with It? Health Care Reform in Canada.* Ottawa: Canadian Bar Association.
Caulfield, Timothy. 1995. Suing Hospitals, Health Authorities and the Government for Health-care Allocation Decisions. *Health Law Review* 3, no. 1: 7–11.
– 2001. 'Malpractice in the Age of Health Care Reform.' In Time Caulfield and Barbara von Tigerstrom, eds., *Health Care Reform and Law in Canada: Meeting the Challenge.* Edmonton: University of Alberta Press, 11–36.

Chaoulli v. Québec (Procureure générale). 2000. [2000] JQ no 479 (Cour supérieure du Québec – Chambre civile).
– 2002. [2002] JQ no 759 (Cour d'appel du Québec).
Collin v. Lussier. 1983. [1983] 1 FC 218 (Fed. C. Canada).
Eldridge v. British Columbia (Attorney General). 1992. (1992), 75 BCLR 68 (BC SC).
– 1997. [1997] 3 SCR 624.
Fleming v. Reid. 1991. (1991), 4 OR (3d) 74 (Ont. CA).
Gilmore, Joan. 2002. 'Children, Adolescents and Health Care.' In Jocelyn Downie, Timothy Caulfield, and Colleen Flood, eds., *Canadian Health Law and Policy*. Toronto: Butterworths, 205–49.
Godbout v. Longueuil (City). 1997. [1997] 3 SCR 844.
Haigh, Richard. 1999. 'Reconstructing Paradise: Canada's Health Care System, Alternative Medicine and the Charter of Rights.' *Health Law Journal* 7: 141–91.
Hartt, Stanley, and Patrick Monahan. 2002. 'The Charter and Health Care: Guaranteeing Timely Access to Health Care for Canadians.' *C.D. Howe Institute Commentary* 164: 1–29.
International Convention on the Elimination of All Forms of Discrimination against Women. 1979. 1249 UNTS 13; Can. TS 1982 No. 31.
International Convention on the Elimination of All Forms of Racial Discrimination. 1969. 660 UNTS 195; Can. TS 1970 No. 28.
International Convention on the Rights of the Child. 1989. 1577 UNTS, 3; Can. TS 1992 No. 3.
International Covenant on Economic, Social, and Cultural Rights. 1966. 993 UNTS 3; Can. TS 1976 No. 47.
Irwin Toy v. Quebec (Attorney General). 1989. [1989] 1 SCR 927.
Jackman, Martha. 1993. 'The Canadian Charter as a Barrier to Unwanted Medical Treatment of Pregnant Women in the Interests of the Foetus.' *Health Law in Canada* 14, no. 2: 49–58.
– 1995. 'The Regulation of Private Health Care under the *Canada Health Act* and Canadian Charter.' *Constitutional Forum* 6, no. 2: 54–60.
– 1995–6. 'The Right to Participate in Health Care and Health Resource Allocation Decisions under Section 7 of the Canadian Charter.' *Health Law Review* 4, no. 2: 3–11.
– 2000. 'The Application of the Canadian Charter in the Health Care Context.' *Health Law Review* 9, no. 2: 22–6.
J.C. v. Forensic Psychiatric Service Commissioner. 1992. (1992), 65 BCLR (2d) 386 (BC SC).
Karr, Andrea. 2000. 'Section 7 of the Charter: Remedy for Canada's Health-Care Crisis?' *Advocate* 48, nos. 3 and 4: 363–74 and 531–41.
Laverdière, Marco. 1998–9. 'Le cadre juridique canadien et québécois relatif au

développement parallèle de services privés de santé et l'article 7 de la Charte canadienne des droits et libertés.' *Revue de droit de l'Université Sherbrooke* 29: 117–221.

Law Reform Commission of Canada. 1980. *Medical Treatment and the Criminal Law*. Ottawa: Supply and Services Canada.

Manfredi, Christopher, and Antonia Maioni. 2002. 'Courts and Health Policy: Judicial Policy Making and Publicly Funded Health Care in Canada.' *Journal of Health Politics, Policy and Law* 27, no. 2: 213–40.

Manitoba Law Reform Commission. 2002. *Withholding or Withdrawing Life Sustaining Treatment: Discussion Paper*. Winnipeg: Manitoba Law Reform Commission.

Nancy B. v. l'Hôtel-Dieu de Québec. 1992. [1992] RJQ 361 (Cour supérieure du Québec).

Ontario Nursing Home Association v. Ontario. 1990. (1990), 72 DLR (4th) 166 (Ont. High Court of Justice).

Raphael, Dennis. 2001. 'From Increasing Poverty to Societal Disintegration: The Effects of Economic Inequality on the Health of Individuals and Communities.' In Hugh Armstrong, Patricia Armstrong, and David Coburn, eds., *Unhealthy Times: The Political Economy of Health and Health Care in Canada*. Toronto: Oxford University Press, 223–46.

Re B.C. Motor Vehicle Act. 1985. [1985] 2 SCR 486.

Reference Re ss. 193 and 195.1(1)(c) of the Criminal Code (Man.). 1990. [1990] 1 SCR 1123.

Rocket v. Royal College of Dental Surgeons. 1990. [1990] 2 SCR 232.

Rodriguez v. British Columbia (Attorney General). 1993. [1993] 3 SCR 519.

Rogers, Sanda. 2002. 'The Legal Regulation of Women's Reproductive Capacity in Canada.' In Jocelyn Downie, Timothy Caulfield and Colleen Flood, eds., *Canadian Health Law and Policy*, 2nd ed. Toronto: Butterworths, 330–65.

Rombaut v. New Brunswick (Minister of Health and Community Services) 2001. [2001] NBJ No. 243. (NB CA).

Royal Commission on Aboriginal Peoples. 1995. *Gathering Strength: Report of the Royal Commission on Aboriginal Peoples*. Volume 3. Ottawa: Supply and Services Canada.

Royal Commission on New Reproductive Technologies. 1993. *Proceed with Care: Final Report of the Royal Commission on New Reproductive Technologies*. Ottawa: Government Services Canada.

R. v. Morgentaler. 1988. [1988] 1 SCR 30.

R. v. Oakes. 1986. [1986] 1 SCR 103.

R. v. Parker. 2000. [2000] OJ No. 2787 (Ont. CA).

R. v. S.(R.J.). 1995. [1995] 1 SCR 451.

Sawatzky v. Riverview Health Centre Inc. 1998. [1998] MJ No. 506 (Man. QB).

Schachter v. Canada. 1992. [1992] 2 SCR 679.

Shirreff, Rhonda. 2000. 'Challenging Restrictions on Direct-to-Consumer Advertising of Contraceptive Drugs and Devices.' *University of Toronto Faculty of Law Review* 58, no. 2: 121–55.

Sholzberg-Gray, Sharon. 1999. 'Accessible Health Care as a Human Right.' *National Journal of Constitutional Law* 11, no. 2: 273–91.

Singh v. Canada. 1985. [1985] 1 SCR 177.

Sneiderman, Barry. 2002. 'Decision-Making at the End of Life.' In Jocelyn Downie, Timothy Caulfield, and Colleen Flood, eds., *Canadian Health Law and Policy*, 2nd ed. Toronto: Butterworths, 501–31.

Stoffman v. Vancouver General Hospital. 1990. [1990] 3 SCR 483.

Swanson, Jean. 2001. *Poorbashing: The Politics of Exclusion.* Toronto: Between the Lines.

Toebes, Brigit. 1999. *The Right to Health As a Human Right in International Law.* Antwerp: Intersentia.

United States v. Burns. 2001. [2001] 1 SCR 283.

Universal Declaration of Human Rights. 1948. GA Res. 217A (III), UN Doc. A/810 (1948).

Vienna Declaration and Programme of Action. 1993. UN Doc. A/CONF.157/24 (1993).

von Tigerstrom, Barbara. 2002. 'Human Rights and Health Care Reform: A Canadian Perspective.' In Timothy Caulfield and Barbara von Tigerstrom, eds., *Health Care Reform and Law in Canada: Meeting the Challenge.* Edmonton: University of Alberta Press, 157–85.

Waldman v. British Columbia (Medical Services Commission). 1997. (1997), 150 DLR (4th) 405 (BC SC).

– 1999. [1999] BCJ No. 2014 (BC CA).

Wilson v. British Columbia (Medical Services Commission). 1988. (1988), 53 DLR (4th) 171 (BC CA).

PART TWO

THE FINANCING AND DELIVERY OF HEALTH CARE

5 Financing Health Care: Options, Consequences, and Objectives

ROBERT G. EVANS

The Basic Options and the Predominance of Public Financing

In modern health-care systems people pay for the care of other people, not for their own. A relatively small proportion of total expenditures on health care is financed through payments by the users of care, consequent on their own use. People make contributions, in varying amounts and on varying terms, to 'third parties' – public agencies (through general taxation or social insurance) or private insurance companies that pool these contributions and disburse funds to the providers of care.

In Canada, for example, out-of-pocket payments by users accounted for $14.2 billion, or only 15.9 per cent, of the total of $89.5 billion spent on health care in 1999 (CIHI 2001, 18, 77). (This figure includes both purely 'out-of-pocket' transactions such as the purchase of non-prescription drugs ('over-the-counter,' or OTC) and various forms of user fees imposed by public or private third parties such as deductibles and coinsurance.) The corresponding percentage for the United States, generally regarded as the leading example of 'private' medical care, was actually slightly lower, at 15.0 per cent, in 2000 (Levit et al. 2002) – to all intents and purposes identical to 'socialized' Canada. (The U.S. share is of course much larger in dollar terms, because its health-care system is so much more expensive.) The point is general; Figure 5.1 shows the ratio of out-of-pocket to total health-care spending for a number of OECD countries.[1] In all, collective financing mechanisms raise the lion's share of the revenue used to fund the provision of health care.

Figure 5.1
Share of total health expenditures paid out of pocket, selected OECD countries, 1998

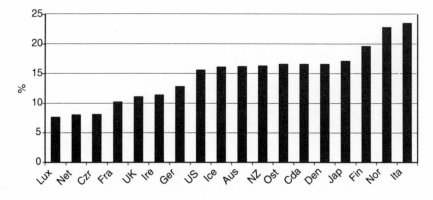

Moreover, as Figure 5.2 shows, in developed market economies these collective financing mechanisms are predominantly public, either governments or semi-independent 'social insurance' agencies. (Canada is actually towards the lower end of this range, contrary to public rhetoric alleging greater use of private finance in the European systems.) The latter are special-purpose quasi-state institutions for funding health care and sometimes other social benefits as well; the former simply reimburse health-care providers out of general tax revenue, typically through a government ministry.

Private insurance plays a minor role in financing health care outside the United States, with only a handful of OECD countries reporting more than 10 per cent of health expenditure from this source. Canada, at 11 per cent in 1999 (CIHI 2001), is among that handful.

Public Predominance, But Continuing Tension over the Mix

These four channels – general taxation, social insurance, out-of-pocket payments, and private insurance – effectively span the options for financing modern health-care systems. (In principle, the last are voluntary, 'private-market' transactions, although in practice this is not generally so – see below.) And while the predominance of public finance (either general taxation or, in a minority of cases, social insurance) is

Figure 5.2
Share of total health expenditures paid by public sector, selected OECD
countries, 1998

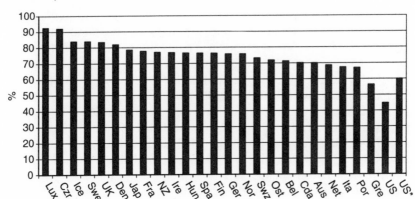

universal in the high-income, industrialized world,[2] the proportions of
these sources do vary from country to country (OECD 2001; see also
Wagstaff et al., 1999).

Moreover, in most countries, and certainly in Canada, the appropriate mix of these sources seems to be in more or less permanent contention. The debate over user charges, in various proposed forms, within
the publicly financed payment system for physicians and hospitals is
older than medicare itself, waxing and waning with fiscal cycles. Yet
prescription drugs, a rapidly increasing share of total health care
expenditures – 12 per cent in 2001, up from 8.2 per cent in 1991 and 6.4
per cent in 1981 (CIHI 2001) – are financed primarily from private
sources (at least ostensibly, but see below). Why are these essential
components of modern medical practice left out of the universal public
system?

Public debates over the mix of financing mechanisms typically take
place through competing claims about the general benefits from adopting one or other approach, or rather from shifting the mix in one direction or another. But any claim of universal benefit is necessarily false.
Any shift in the financing mix, in any system, will be beneficial to some
and will hurt others.[3] The choice of mix must involve a balance of benefits and harms, in which different people's interests are weighed differently. The very permanence of the controversy should tell us that it

arises from a permanent conflict of embedded interests, not from a simple inability to find the 'right' mix for everyone. In that sense, the choice of financing mechanisms is a matter of values, not a technical question.

But the technical questions matter a great deal, because participants in the debate over financing routinely make claims about the consequences of alternative mechanisms. The validity of these claims *is* a technical matter; are they supported by or inconsistent with known facts, with research findings and analysis, or even with simple logic? Such claims of consequence typically involve aspects of the health-care system that go well beyond the financing structure itself, concerning putative effects on the volume, mix, and distribution of services, their appropriateness, or the efficiency of their production. If we are to assess such claims, and thus to evaluate the probable effects of alternative financing mechanisms, it will be helpful not merely to describe alternative mechanisms but embed them in a logically consistent accounting structure tracing out the financial flows within any health-care system.

Financing Choices

Figure 5.3 inserts the four channels through which finances can be assembled into a framework adapted from the identity relationship underlying national income accounting.[4] There is a fundamental accounting identity based on the fact that, for the economy as a whole, the total of all incomes earned must be exactly equal to the total of all expenditures (on final demand) – every dollar of expenditure is simultaneously and always a dollar of someone's income. In the health-care sector, this identity expands to include a third term – total revenue. The revenues assembled, from whatever source, to finance health care must exactly equal the expenditures to fund providers of care, and these in turn must equal the total incomes earned by individuals from the provision of care:

total revenue ≡ total expenditure ≡ total income

This is an 'Iron Law,' a logical necessity, violated only by errors of arithmetic. Any change in one term must be matched by corresponding changes in the other two. In accounting, as in ecology, 'it is impossible to do only one thing.'

Figure 5.3
Alternative ways of paying for health care

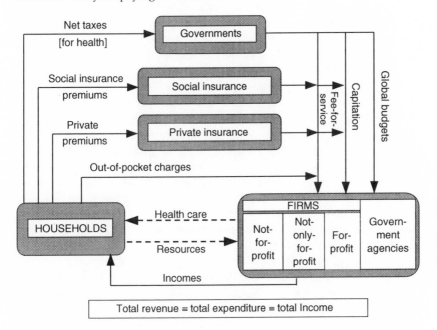

The box on the lower left of Figure 5.3 represents all the individual people in the system. They provide productive resources – labour and skills, raw materials, various forms of capital services, management and 'entrepreneurship' – to the institutions – hospitals, medical clinics, drug companies, and so on ('firms') – that produce health-care goods and services. As patients, they then 'consume' that care. They are also paid for the resources that they supply, in the form of wages, salaries, net income from professional practice, rent, interest, and dividends – all the ways in which people derive income from economic activity.

Figure 5.3 also makes clear the distinction between two issues often confused in the 'public–private' debates – private financing and private provision. The former refers to the way in which the revenues are raised; the latter, to the ownership and motivation of the organizations funded from these revenues. Logically, these questions are quite separate; a publicly owned and operated provider could raise part of its revenues through user fees – and does in Sweden, for example – and a public payment agency could provide full reimbursement for the services of private, for-profit providers, as the government of Alberta seems to propose in Bill 11, tabled in 2000.

In practice, however, the two questions are not so neatly separable. As Figure 5.3 indicates, the choice of financing mechanism may constrain the range of funding options. 'Single-payer' governments may choose (subject to public acceptance) to reimburse providers on a global budget basis (as hospitals are funded in Canada), or capitation (so much per period for each patient under care, as general practitioners are [mostly] funded in Britain), or per treated case (as are hospitals in the United States under the Medicare program for the elderly), or per item of service (as are physicians in Canada). Individual payments, by contrast, can be only by item of service. Private insurers have historically paid by item of service; in the United States, many have now transformed themselves into 'managed care' organizations (MCOs) paying by treated case or capitation. It is still unclear, however, whether these funding options are sustainable (and at what cost) in a multi-payer environment.

The mode of provider organization also tends to influence the mix of financing sources. 'Private' and 'public' are often treated rhetorically as if they were uniform categories, but this introduces a serious and potentially dangerous confusion.[5] There is a world of difference between a private medical practice and the Hospital Corporation of America. While both have a strong interest in the net revenues generated through their activities, only the latter is responsible to anonymous shareholders for whom share value is directly linked to the rate of growth of earnings. A self-employed practitioner can decide that he or she is earning an adequate income and focus solely on professional objectives. Capital markets do not permit this luxury for publicly traded corporations. If the rate of growth of earnings slows, share prices fall, and management typically falls with them.

The realities of capital markets thus set up a fundamental conflict between public objectives and private necessities. 'Cost containment,' which is essential to maintaining an efficient and effective system of public health care, cannot be reconciled with the growth requirements imposed by capital markets. Those pressures lie behind for-profit firms' continuing efforts to influence medical decision making in the direction of ever-increasing expenditure.[6] But they also lead to efforts to open up additional revenue sources by tapping private funds through 'added value' services over and above those reimbursed by public agencies – behaviour that might less politely be described as 'bait and switch.' The behaviour of eye clinics in Calgary, selling 'enhanced service packages' including foldable lens implants to cataract patients for extraordinary mark-ups over cost, fits into this category (Armstrong 2000).[7]

Pure Forms and Hybrid Financing Mechanisms

Figure 5.3 displays the four basic options – general taxation, social insurance, private insurance, user fees – as pure types, sharply distinct from each other, and in fact most revenue in most systems is raised in one or other of these ways. But there are also revenue-raising mechanisms – some merely proposed, others actually in use in some systems – that are hybrids of two or more of these pure types (Evans, 2000; 2002a). These are typically advocated as ways of mitigating the most obvious disadvantages of private financing mechanisms and thus of reducing political opposition to an expansion of their scope.

Public Health Insurance Premiums
The net effects of such hybrid mechanisms are usually not immediately transparent, at least to the general public, although they can be traced out with a bit of analysis. An even simpler source of confusion, however, is the mere mislabelling of a revenue source. The 'health care premiums' that the Alberta and British Columbia governments levy for physicians' services and (Alberta only) hospital care provide a leading example. The name suggests some form of 'insurance,' social if not private. But this impression is false. First, these premiums are compulsory and are paid directly into the provincial treasuries. Second, the premiums levied on an individual or household bear no relation to the payer's risk status, and the total collected has no necessary relation to program outlays. Third, perhaps most important (and largely unknown to the public), coverage does not depend on having paid one's premiums. To qualify for federal transfer payments, provinces must cover 100 per cent of their populations (net of special categories).

Accordingly, all students of health-care systems follow the practice of the national income accountants and treat these 'premiums' as a form of tax – in fact a poll tax. The level and even the existence of such a levy are a matter of general fiscal policy and tax incidence – they do not at this time exist in the other eight provinces of Canada – and have no relationship to the health-care system per se.

Subsidies for Private Insurance

Hybridized revenue sources, however, are both more interesting and a good deal less transparent. The form in most common use is the tax-expenditure subsidy, hybridizing taxation with private insurance through favourable tax treatment of private insurance premiums. In Canada, for example, an employer that pays the premiums of a private health-insurance plan covering employees can deduct the cost from taxable income as a business expense. But these premiums are not then taxed in the hands of the employees. An equivalent amount paid to employees as salary would of course be taxable income.[8] (Employer-paid 'premiums' for medicare are by contrast fully taxable in the hands of the employee.)

The fiscal effect is the same as if people with private insurance paid for it from after-tax income, as they would for any other commodity sold on the private market, and then received a rebate of part of the purchase price from the federal and provincial governments. Such a rebate would of course have to be financed from other tax sources, but the rebate amounts would show up in the public accounts and the identities of recipients would be matters of public record. Tax expenditure subsidies, by relieving some persons of taxation, require other tax sources to offset this revenue loss. But the process is not transparent, the amounts involved do not show up in the public accounts, and the beneficiaries are never identified.

Smythe (2001) estimates the cost of this subsidy to the Canadian federal and provincial governments in 1994 at $2.28 billion.[9] This subsidy amounted in that year to 3.1 per cent of total health-care expenditure of $73.1 billion (CIHI 2001, 77), or roughly 30 per cent of total health-care expenditures by private insurers.[10] Sheils and Hogan (1999) find a roughly similar proportion for the United States; just over one-third of private insurance payments are in fact 'rebated' through the government subsidy. Their estimate of the total cost of this subsidy to U.S. governments – $124.8 billion in 1998 – amounts to about 10.9 per cent of total health spending of $1,149.8 billion in that year.

Where private insurance enjoys this subsidy, the proportion of health care reportedly financed through that channel is in reality partly financed by governments. Private insurance plays a much larger role in financing health care in the United States than in Canada; official data report 34.2 per cent of the U.S. total flowing through this channel (in 2000). But accounting for the public subsidy would bring this share down to less than 25 per cent. This, plus adjusting for certain other accounting peculiarities, reduces the private share of U.S. health spending to about 40 per cent of the total (Fox and Fronstin 2000; Woolhandler and Himmelstein 2002). Hence the adjustment to the U.S. column in Figure 5.2; U.S.* is more accurate.

Tax-expenditure subsidies are as old as private insurance in North America and seem deeply rooted in financing structures. In 1981, Canada's federal minister of finance, Allan MacEachen, attempted to withdraw the subsidy and tax this particular employee benefit like any other. But he ran into heavy political opposition and withdrew the proposal. The pattern in other countries is more mixed; some provide such subsidies, others do not, and there are examples of subsidies being offered and later withdrawn – as in Quebec in 1993. But the constituency for such subsidies is smaller in most other countries, because private insurance is much less widespread.

The public subsidy to private insurance has three major effects. First, it expands the market for and the coverage of private insurance. Medical expenses paid out of pocket are paid with after-tax dollars; those covered by private insurance are paid for with before-tax dollars. Apart from the benefits of spreading risk, reimbursement through insurance is actually more expensive than out-of-pocket payment ('self-insurance') because of administrative overhead costs. The public subsidy reverses this disadvantage.[11] In its absence, the level of private coverage and the proportion of health-care costs paid through this route would surely decline (although it is hard to say by how much).[12]

Second, because the subsidy is available only for employer-paid premiums, it has contributed to the almost-complete dominance of the private insurance market by employee group contracts. It thus reinforces the natural dynamics of private health-insurance markets, in which asymmetric information and adverse selection severely limit the scope of individual contracting.[13] Private insurers discovered very early – at least fifty years ago – that individuals seeking to purchase coverage on a voluntary basis tended to be of higher than average risk status ('adverse selection') and that it was difficult or impossible for insurers to be as well informed about that risk status – current and expected future health – as individuals themselves (asymmetric information). By contracting with employee groups, in which individual participation was not optional but required, insurers could select a relatively low-risk population to cover. Thus, where private insurance exists, it covers a significantly lower proportion of health expenditures than of the population.

The fact that most private insurance in North America is purchased by employers and provided to workers as an employment benefit has led to the widespread belief that employers actually pay for the coverage of their workers. Most economists, however, argue that workers actually pay collectively for their coverage in the form of forgone wages. Thus the assembly of funds through the private insurance channel, net of the tax-expenditure subsidy, draws on wage incomes. The amount paid by the members of a particular employee group depends on the risk status of that group, but within the group the distribution of burden depends on the outcome of the wage-bargaining process.

Third, very significant but little-noticed, the tax-expenditure subsidy has a steeply regressive effect. The value to an individual of any tax exemption depends on his or her marginal tax bracket. The exemption of an employer-paid benefit costing $1,000 is worth $500 to someone in the 50 per cent marginal tax bracket, $250 to someone in the 25 per cent bracket, and nothing at all to someone whose income is too low to attract income tax. Accentuating this regressive effect, the extent of private coverage rises with income level.

A form of tax-expenditure subsidy is, of course, also provided for out-of-pocket medical expenses insofar as citizens can apply them to reduce liability for income tax. But the benefit, at least in Canada, is much less. Only expenses above 3 per cent of taxable income yield a federal tax credit – not an exemption – and this credit is based on the lowest tax bracket rate (in 2001, 16 per cent). Depending on the province of residence, this would gross up to about 25 per cent. Employer-paid premiums, by contrast, are fully exempt from taxation, and the value of the exemption rises with the taxpayer's marginal tax rate. For top-bracket earners in 2001, the value of the subsidy from the federal government would be 29 per cent of total premiums, with the provincial contribution (outside Quebec) bringing this up to about 45 per cent.[14]

Mandation
The tax-expenditure subsidy uses financial incentives to encourage the purchase of private insurance; mandation uses public authority to require it. Mandation has at various times been recommended in the United States in order to achieve universal coverage outside a public program (Pauly et al. 1991); Quebec has more recently adopted it to expand private drug coverage (Morgan 1998). In essence, mandation is

a form of taxation (legally required payments) in which the revenues are channelled directly to private insurers and so remain 'off-budget' for governments.

The coverage and pricing of mandated insurance nonetheless require close public regulation of the content of these 'private' contracts in order to suppress the natural forces of private insurance markets. Private, for-profit insurers, if they are to survive in competitive markets, must and do price coverage according to the risk status of the insured. The unhealthy pay more, the healthy pay less, whatever their income levels. Comprehensive private coverage is thus a much heavier financial burden for the unhealthy and unwealthy or is simply priced entirely out of their reach.

Governments must then restrict competition so as to permit or require private insurers to accept all comers at similar rates and cross-subsidize the unhealthy at the expense of the healthy. Alternatively, they can subsidize the coverage of the former from public funds or simply provide public coverage for the higher-risk segments of the population, the elderly, and the poor – as Quebec has done with its 'universal' program of drug insurance. This is also the pattern of health insurance in the United States, except that private coverage is not mandated among the general population, only heavily subsidized.[15]

Integrating User Charges with Income Tax
Other forms of hybridized revenue have received considerable attention recently but do not appear to have been put into practice on any significant scale, if at all. A proposal with a very long history – at least thirty years – is the combination of tax finance and user payments by linking an individual's income-tax liability to the public outlays for that individual's health care (Feldstein 1971; OEC, 1976; Gordon, Mintz, and Chen, 1998). Some portion of the costs associated with a person's care might be added directly to his or her tax bill; alternatively, some proportion of these costs might be treated as a 'taxable benefit' and added to taxable income before computation of tax liability.

The net effect, for any given level of total revenue raised, would be to lower the rate of taxation of income as normally defined and to associate a financial cost with the individual use of care – a user fee. But the user fee would look like a form of taxation and would vary according to the user's tax bracket. Those with higher taxable incomes ('those who can afford it') would pay a higher user fee for any given level of expenditure on their behalf. 'Those who can afford it' but generate no expenses would of course pay nothing extra and would in fact enjoy a lower rate of taxation on their net income. Such proposals attenuate somewhat the regressive nature of user fees unlinked to income, but only somewhat. They also make very explicit the central feature of all user fees – that they are inevitably 'taxes on the sick' (Lewis 1998).

Medical Savings Accounts

A much more recent proposal (at least in Canada) – so-called medical savings accounts – would be a hybrid of three different financing sources – the government, private insurance, and user-pay. Details vary, but in general individuals or households would be allocated a certain sum of money per period, either as a direct grant by government or through some form of favourable tax treatment such as tax exemption of individual contributions. From this account they would be required to pay for their own health care. People with surpluses in their accounts at period's end might be able to withdraw all or some part of the surplus for personal use or perhaps carry forward surpluses to apply against health expenditures later.

Those who overrun their accounts would be personally liable for all or some part of additional costs, up to some 'catastrophic' limit beyond which government would cover all costs; alternatively, individuals might wish or be required to purchase private insurance for these 'catastrophic' expenses. (Both the basic allowance and the catastrophic threshold could be adjusted to individual incomes.) Since severe illnesses are now primarily chronic, however, and high expenses in any one period are closely correlated with high expenses in the next, it is hard to see any significant role for voluntary private insurance. Coverage might be readily available to the healthy and low-risk population, but that is not the group using most of the health care and generating most of the costs.

There is ample room for adjusting the details, but the essence of such proposals is first, to increase the overall level of user charges and, second, to open up private market opportunities in health care by shifting the payment role from governments to individual 'consumers.' Tax exemptions for individual contributions to such 'savings' accounts would also shift the public contribution from direct, observable payments to indirect, tax-expenditure subsidies.

The user-fee aspect arises because individuals are liable for expenses beyond the amount in their account and is significantly extended if some part of account surpluses flows back to them as income. Credit for amounts not used is just as much a user fee as is liability for amounts used, even if the bookkeeping looks different. Either way, an individual's net economic position is affected by the use of care.

Consequences

Axes of Conflict in Financing Choices

The choice among, or the mix of, financing sources for health care will have three types of consequences affecting:

- Who pays?
- Who gets? and
- Who gets paid?

Who pays? reflects the fact that while collectively the residents of a country must pay the full costs of the care that they use, the distribution of the total bill will depend on the mix of financing sources used. Any changes in that mix will inevitably redistribute the burden, making some better off in straight financial terms, and others worse off. These redistributive patterns are in principle relatively transparent, though fairly little studied until the last decade.

Who gets? addresses the pattern of benefits, or at least the use of health-care services, that emerges from a particular health-care system. How the system is financed and how the revenues are raised may affect the pattern of access to services, where access includes not only what is provided to whom, but under what circumstances – quality, timeliness, convenience. To what extent is access responsive to 'need,' as viewed by either clinicians or patients, and how much is it conditioned by willingness/ability to pay for services? Can people with more money buy more or 'better' services and buy their way to the front of any queues?

Finally, *who gets paid?* refers to the levels and patterns of incomes associated with alternative financing arrangements. This includes the overall expenditures on health care for a given population, which are necessarily equal to the total incomes earned by those who provide resources for the production of health care. Some modes of financing are better adapted to achieving global cost control, if that is an objective. But total expenditures are the product of quantities of output multiplied by their relative prices. Cost control – or cost explosion –

may come about through constraining (or expanding) the quantity and range of services provided or through limiting (or enhancing) the relative incomes of those who supply resources to the sector – the wages of hospital workers, for example, or the fees of physicians, or the profits of drug-company shareholders.

To make these relationships more precise (if not necessarily more transparent), consider the revenue-expenditure-income identity diagrammed in Figure 5.3. We can write it as:

$$T+SI+PI+C \equiv P \times Q = W \times Z,$$

where T, SI, PI, and C represent the total amounts of money contributed for the reimbursement of health-care providers by all persons in the society (including those who work for or otherwise participate in health-care 'firms') through taxes (T), social insurance (SI), private insurance (PI), and out-of-pocket payments and user charges (C), respectively. $P \times Q$ represents the total expenditure on those services, where Q is a vector or string of amounts of different types of goods or services, and P is a corresponding string of their respective prices.

A provincial fee schedule for physicians, for example, identifies all the different medical acts for which physicians will be reimbursed and the corresponding string of fees, or prices, at which each is reimbursed. The components of Q are the numbers of each type of service that were actually provided in a particular jurisdiction and time period. Multiplying the number of each type of service or procedure actually performed by the corresponding price, and summing over all items, yields the 'vector product' $P \times Q$, or the total expenditure on (fee-practice) physicians' services. For services reimbursed other than by fee per item of service – global hospital budgets, for example, or capitated group practices – the breakdown of total expenditures into price and quantity components may be neither as simple nor as precise. But there will always be some implicit price associated with each product or service provided.

The total incomes earned can correspondingly be factored into $W \times Z$, where the elements of the string W represent the rates of reimbursement for particular resource inputs, and Z represents their amounts. An element of W might be the wage rate per hour of nursing services of a particular type, for example, or the net income per hour of a particular type of physician. The number of hours of skilled labour supplied by each would be the corresponding elements of the vector Z. But other inputs might be square feet of building space or amounts of capital invested. Levels of building rental and rates of return on invested capital, and shareholder profits, are also elements of W.

Thus, a negotiated increase in nurses' wages would be represented by a rise in the corresponding elements of W. If nursing employment (Z) remains constant, and there is no change in level of hospital activity (Q), then the effective price (P) of hospital care has risen, and in a publicly funded system T – the amount of tax revenues going to hospital budgets – must rise. If, however, hospital budgets are frozen, then Z must fall as W rises – fewer but more highly paid nurses or cuts in other parts of the hospital budget. This change could be reflected in a fall in hospital output Q and a corresponding rise in effective price, or it could result in greater 'efficiency,' with outputs staying the same as resource inputs decline – increased output per hour – so that increased wages are not passed on in higher prices. However, jobs will be lost if total budgets do not rise.

What has actually occurred will always be controversial, because hospital output is only partly linked to measurable quantities such as procedures performed, cases treated, and in-patient days. The quality of care and resulting patient outcomes are the real objectives, and there is always room for disagreement over whether or not 'quality' has changed. The identity does not say what will be the consequences of a change to any one of its component variables; what it does is to constrain the possible scenarios – the range of things that *can* happen – and ensure consistent stories. Whatever the consequences, they must add up correctly.

But the identity holds only at the aggregate level, for the whole society. For any one individual, revenues contributed may greatly exceed, or fall far short of, the total health-care expenditures on his or her behalf, and each of these may exceed or not reach the income received from the health-care system. The healthy surgeon will receive more in income than he or she contributes in public or private payments, and much more than the expenditures on his or her behalf. The wealthy and healthy businessperson will likewise contribute far more in revenue than he or she accounts for in expenditure but will (unless the business produces some form of health product or service) earn little in income from health care. (He or she might, however, own shares in a drug or medical-equipment company.) The elderly and chronically ill pensioner, however, may receive quite a large volume of services, costing far more than he or she puts in through any channel, while receiving little or nothing in the way of income from the health care sector.

These differently situated individuals represent, to a first approximation, the patterns of economic interests that are differentially affected by changes in the mix of financing mechanisms. Is one primarily a contributor to or a recipient from the financing of health care, and, among contributors, does one contribute more, or less, than the expenses generated on one's behalf? A priori, then, it seems plausible that the pattern of support for or of opposition to particular financing mechanisms will be influenced by the pattern of anticipated financial gains or losses. Not exclusively, of course, as we are all more than simply economic animals. But where one stands does tend to correlate, in part, with where one sits. Disagreements over health-care financing have roots in real, and permanent, conflicts of economic interests.

Who Pays (What Share of the Total Costs of Health Care)?

Everybody pays, of course. Except for the totally destitute and dependent, everyone in the lower-left-hand box of Figure 5.3 contributes some amount of money that will work its way into health-care expenditures and health-sector incomes. But how much, or what proportion of the total, will be paid by different individuals, or by individuals in different circumstances?

If health care is financed wholly from public general revenue, people contribute in proportion to their tax liabilities. Subject to some considerable complexity of detail, these contributions tend to be roughly proportionate to income. Conversely, in a system financed entirely from user charges, individuals' contributions would be proportionate to their use of care, which is more or less proportionate (again subject to qualifications in detail) to their need for care, or health status. Accordingly, any shift in the mix of financing sources towards (or away from) user-pay and away from (or towards) tax finance will lower (or raise) the share of burden borne by the wealthy and healthy and raise (or lower) that borne by the unhealthy and unwealthy. Equal and off-setting changes in T and C balance at the aggregate level, but not (except by accident) at the individual level.

Conceivably, if illness were highly (positively) correlated with income and if tax liabilities were not, a shift from tax finance to user-pay could raise the share of the burden borne by some higher-income people – the wealthy and unhealthy – while benefiting the healthy and unwealthy. But in all developed societies, the correlations go the other way; both health and tax liability are correlated with income.

Figure 5.4 illustrates the relationship between income level and contribution. This is derived from a Manitoba study (Mustard et al., 1998a, b) linking individual-level administrative records from the universal public programs covering hospital and physicians' services with census long-form records of family incomes and estimated tax liability for a large sample of the provincial population. The figure displays the distribution of public expenditures and of corresponding tax liability by income decile (scaled up to the whole provincial population of about a million), with the small but expensive institutionalized population as a separate category.

Panel 4a shows the dollar amounts spent by the public plans on the care of people in each income decile in 1994; panel 4b, the estimated amount of tax contributions. Panel 4c shows the difference, by income decile, between the total cost of care used and total taxes paid; panel 4d, this gain or loss as a share of total family consumable income. (The permanently institutionalized have no significant income.)

The scale of the transfers is quite striking, particularly from the top income bracket, making very clear the potential economic advantage to people in that group from shifting the financing mix away from (almost) complete tax finance to some form of private payment. Any such shift would shrink all the bars in panel 4d towards the X-axis, reducing the transfer of purchasing power from the more to the less wealthy that is embodied in the present (1994) financing system. But since those with very low incomes and large needs are unlikely to be able to bear a substantial portion of the costs of their own care, any shift in financing from taxation to private payment would presumably involve a transfer of funds primarily from the middle to the upper deciles of the income distribution.

This pattern of distributional effects is not at all mysterious; indeed, it should be intuitively obvious and beyond dispute. Whether one or other pattern of burden distribution is more or less 'fair' is of course a matter of personal values, about which rational people may legitimately disagree. But there seems to be no legitimate basis for disagreeing with van Doorslaer Wagstaff and Rutten (1993) on the basis of their detailed analysis of countries in the European Community: 'Out-of-pocket payments tend to be a highly regressive means of financing

Figure 5.4a

Expenditures on publicly financed health care, by income decile, Manitoba, 1994

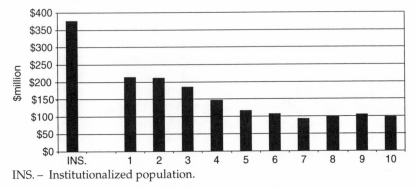

INS. – Institutionalized population.

Figure 5.4b

Tax contribution to health care, by income decile, Manitoba, 1994

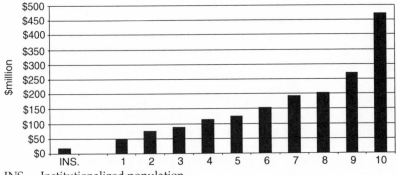

INS. – Institutionalized population.

health care' (42).[16] Subsequent analyses have confirmed this conclusion (van Doorslaer et al., 1999; Wagstaff et al., 1999).

Recognition of this regressivity, and of its inconsistency with prevailing notions of fairness, has motivated proposals mentioned above to integrate user payments with the income tax. If tax financed health-care costs became a taxable benefit, for example, in effect the proportion of medical bills paid out of pocket would vary by income class, and this would mitigate their regressivity. But the degree of mitigation depends on the number of income-tax brackets and the degree of difference between the bracket rates.

The federal income tax does have some progressivity built into it,

Figure 5.4c
Net transfer to/from income decile, public financing of health care,
Manitoba, 1994

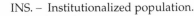

INS. – Institutionalized population.

Figure 5.4d
Net transfer by income decile, as share of consumable income, Manitoba, 1994

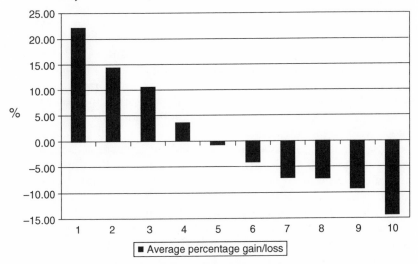

but not much. Consider, for example, a person whose use of health
care generated $1,500 in medicare outlays in 2001 (roughly the national
average), and suppose that these were added to his or her federal tax-

able income. With earnings of $25,000, he or she would have to pay $240 extra (16 per cent of $1500) or 0.96 per cent of before-tax income. At $50,000 the extra liability would be greater – 22 per cent of $1,500, or $330 – but only 0.66 per cent of income. At $75,000 the liability would rise to $390, or 0.52 per cent of income, and, entering the top bracket at $100,000, to $435, or 0.44 per cent. From then on, of course, the liability for extra contributions remains constant, dropping steadily as a share of income as income rises. At $250,000 one would pay only 0.17 per cent of income. Allowing for provincial taxation would raise all liabilities and percentages by roughly 50 per cent.

A so-called flat tax with a constant marginal tax rate regardless of income level would eliminate any mitigation of the regressivity of user fees. If everyone is required to pay the same proportion of income in taxes (after some basic exemption), then adding medical payments to the tax base would increase everyone's tax liability by the same proportion of their medical expenses, regardless of income. These liabilities would then be precisely as regressive as any other proportional user fee.

But the extra tax liability is only half the story. Amounts collected through this mechanism would permit lowering of other taxes or substitution for other increases. If we assume a tax system that is roughly proportionate overall, these alternatives would take (or return) four times as much from (to) the person at $100,000 as to the person at $25,000, compared to the 81.3 per cent difference in liability from taxing medicare expenditures. Above $100,000, the difference builds up rapidly; at $250,000, the difference in liability under a proportionate tax system is ten times. Comparing this mechanism for raising revenue with the alternative of general taxation demonstrates the point made graphically in Figure 5.4 – it is significantly more advantageous for people with higher incomes.

These calculations, however, pertain only to someone accounting for the *average* level of medicare outlays in any one year. But it is a universally observed pattern that care use is heavily concentrated among a relatively small proportion of the population. Reid et al. (2003) provide a comprehensive survey of studies showing this concentration for different countries, time periods, and types of care, while Forget, Deber, and Roos (2002) reveal the extraordinary concentration of physician and hospital expenditures in the Manitoba population over the period 1997–9. They found that the top 1 per cent of the population accounted for 26 per cent of expenditures, and the bottom 50 per cent, only 4 per cent. Since the average annual rate of expenditure was $730 per capita,[17] this implies an average expenditure of $18,980 among the top 1 per cent, and $58 among the lowest 50 per cent. Among the top decile of users, the average cost was about $5,000, and among the next decile, $1000. The addition of these sums to taxable income would have increased very substantially the liabilities of a small proportion of the population, while having little or no impact on the majority.

Most of the people who generated very high costs for health care were hospitalized one or more times during the period studied; hospital costs are particularly highly concentrated on a small (and presumably quite sick) proportion of the population. But Forget, Deber, and Roos (2002) also find that a large proportion of physicians' services is used by a relatively small proportion of the population, as do Reid et al. (2003) in British Columbia. In 1996–7, for example, 5.3 per cent of the adult population of British Columbia accounted for 33.7 per cent of total (non-obstetric) fee payments to physicians for adult care, or $2,640 each on average. Another 78.7 per cent accounted for the other 66.3 per cent, or an average of $350 each, while 15.9 per cent generated no medical billings. About half of the high users were over 60, compared with less than one-quarter of the low users and 10 per cent of non-users. Analysis of the diagnostic and procedural patterns shows that these high users are significantly sicker than the rest of the population – a conclusion that also emerges clearly from an analysis of Ontario data relating individual self-reports of health status to public expenditures for physicians' services (Finkelstein 2001). People who use a lot of health care are sick.

Thus the 'hybridized' tax and user-fee proposal is not only regressive, taking proportionately more from those with lower incomes and benefiting principally those with higher incomes, but it also imposes very substantial financial burdens on a relatively few, mostly very sick people. The relatively trivial-appearing numbers above – less than one percent of income paid in extra federal tax by the 'average' user earning $25,000 per year – look very different if we apply the ratios found by Forget, Deber, and Roos (2002).[18] Half the population in the $25,000 bracket will incur, on average, an increased federal tax liability of about $20, or 0.12 per cent of income, grossing up to about $30 or 0.18 per cent to allow for the provincial component of income tax. The top 10 per cent of users will see their federal liability increase by nearly $1,500, or 6 per cent of income, grossing up to about 9 per cent.

These 'back-of-the-envelope' calculations are illustrative only; a more precise analysis would require knowledge of the multi-year joint distribution of both hospital and physicians' services by income class and preferably by tax bracket, which would be a major research exercise. But no such data-intensive exercise is needed to support the general observation. Relative to financing from general taxation, the hybridized tax and user-fee approach is very little different in its distributional effects from the coinsurance form of user fee in which users pay some percentage of the costs incurred on their behalf. There is no getting away from the fact that user fees, whatever form they take, tax the sick. And relative to general taxation, they relieve the wealthy.

Private insurance adds some additional considerations to the question of 'who pays?' Universal private coverage, if it could be achieved, would be similar to tax finance in that contributions would not depend on the experience of illness and the use of care. Insofar as private insurers often require some degree of financial contribution by the user of care, a shift from public to private coverage might still involve some transfer of funds from the unhealthy to the healthy, but of course public programs may also impose such user payments, with the same distributional effects.

The major difference, however, is that private insurance, if sold by private, for-profit firms in a competitive market, carries premiums that are related to the expectation of illness, not to income level. (Higher-income people may pay greater premiums if they purchase more comprehensive coverage, but for the same package the price does not vary with income.) Accordingly, if the insurance market is functioning efficiently, the distribution of burden across the income spectrum should look very similar to that of average expenditures for care.

And indeed it does. Figure 5.5 is drawn from the work of Rasell, Bernstein, and Tang (1993; 1994), who analysed survey data for the non-institutionalized U.S. population. It reveals the distribution by income decile of total payments for health care (using a more comprehensive definition than in Figure 5.4) through each of taxes, private insurance, and out-of-pocket payments. Their results are shown for households with heads over and under age 65, because the former are covered, for hospital and physicians services, by the national Medicare program – national, universal, and tax financed.

Figure 5.5 portrays the contrast between the progressivity of U.S. tax finance and the regressivity of both out-of-pocket payment and private insurance. The similar pattern for both modes of private finance suggests that the U.S. private-insurance market does, in aggregate, link

Figure 5.5
Share of income spent on health care, United States (1987), by family-income decile and payment form

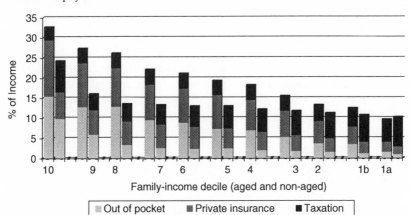

contributions quite closely to expected use. These highly regressive components of the financing mix overwhelm the progressivity of the tax-financed component and make the whole distribution highly regressive.

Perhaps surprisingly, however, this pattern occurs even among the elderly, covered by U.S. Medicare. The very substantial deductibles and co-payments built into the public program, ostensibly to control costs, help make the overall mix markedly regressive. Individuals can and do buy private Medigap coverage for these charges – as they do in France to cover the *ticket modérateur* in the statutory health-insurance scheme. But Medigap coverage, being private, is also regressive in its distribution of financing burden (premiums are based on risk status, not on income).

The U.S. Medigap industry also illustrates the link between user fees and private insurance in a system that is financed predominantly from public sources – as all systems in developed countries are. If private insurers are to have any market at all, the public system must embody substantial user fees and/or service exclusions – preferably both. Private insurers are therefore consistent advocates for such charges. Their arguments may be many and various, but the underlying objective is to open a market for their product.

There is, however, a second distributional aspect to the choice of private or public insurance. As we saw above, in Canada, the United States, and some European countries, there is a tax-expenditure subsidy for private insurance that is purchased by employers on behalf of workers. The size of this subsidy for any individual worker is equal to the total amount paid by the employer multiplied by the marginal income tax rate of the employee. But the latter, and typically the former as well, increase with rising incomes. Accordingly, the subsidy is much larger, in absolute terms, for those with higher incomes. Smythe (2001) estimates that in 1994 the subsidy from federal and provincial governments in Canada amounted to about fifty cents for households with an annual income under $5,000 and rose to $250 for those earning over $100,000. In the United States, Sheils and Hogan (1999) estimated a monotonically rising value of the subsidy in 1998, from an average of $71 for family incomes under $15,000 to $2,357 for those over $100,000. Thus the inherently regressive nature of private insurance financing increases markedly when tax exemptions subsidize private coverage. Not only are private premiums a smaller share of rising incomes; for those eligible for the tax-expenditure subsidy, the net cost is actually lower in absolute value.

Outside North America, however, private insurance is somewhat more complex. Where mostly people with higher incomes purchase private insurance, as a way of gaining preferred access to more timely, convenient, or perceived higher quality care – as in Germany, the Netherlands, Italy, Portugal, and the United Kingdom – private insurance premiums are correspondingly distributed progressively and take up a larger share of the incomes of wealthier people. But if private coverage enables the better-off to opt out of the general public insurance programs, as in Germany and the Netherlands, the overall financing system become much more regressive (Wagstaff et al. 1999; van Doorslaer et al. 1993, 42–4).

The range of possible outcomes appears in Figure 5.6, drawn from Wagstaff et al. (1999) and showing for a number of European countries (and the United States) the relationship between the proportion of health-care financing coming from taxation and an index of the overall progressivity or regressivity of health-system financing. Generally there is a clear relationship between tax finance and greater progressivity – or lesser regressivity. (Since health expenditures follow needs in being distributed highly regressively across the population, a mildly regressive financing system can still bring about a substantial net shift of resources down the income distribution. Even if lower-income

Figure 5.6
Relation between tax financing and progressivity of total health expenditures, selected OECD countries and years

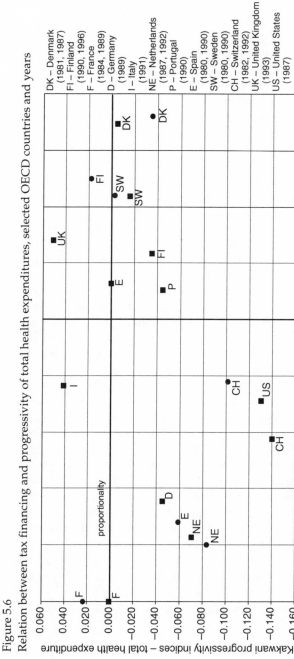

Sources: Wagstaff et al. (1999) and calculations by Hakkinen for Finland.

people are paying a larger share of their incomes to finance health care, the cost of the care that they receive may substantially exceed, on average, what they contribute to pay for it, and the converse holds for those with higher incomes.) But focusing on this relationship alone would ignore a lot of relevant detail.

The United States and Switzerland, the countries relying most heavily on private finance, have correspondingly the most regressive financing systems. But among those with primarily social-insurance systems – France, Germany, and the Netherlands – the former is close to proportionate while the latter two are also highly regressive. The key difference: France has no income ceiling for contributions and no opting out into private insurance for the very well-off. Social-insurance systems can thus have very different distributional effects, depending on the structure of the contribution system.

The most progressive financing systems, however, are tax-based, with no provision for opting out. Purchasers of private coverage must pay for it in addition to their public contributions. But the Nordic countries, where tax finance is most heavily used, appeared at the time of the study to have had *less* progressive tax systems than, for example, the United States, Germany, or Switzerland. (Or Canada, where there is overall a relatively low level of public finance for health care.) These data suggest a possible political trade-off between the progressivity of the tax system and the extent of reliance on tax finance for health care – perhaps reflecting the effect of political resistance from the better-off to too much income redistribution (Evans 2000, 2002a).

The overall distributive effect of choices among modes of financing health care obviously depends on the progressivity or regressivity of the tax system as a whole. Historically, Canadian tax systems have been estimated to be roughly proportionate to income, or mildly progressive, with the progressivity of the income tax offsetting the regressivity of other sources such as consumption taxes. However, income-tax cuts since 1997 focused primarily at the upper end of the income distribution and probably reduced both the progressivity of the income tax and its share in the overall tax mix. This would tend to reduce the redistributional effect of the tax-financed health-care system.

The most obvious examples of this form of regressive shifting in the tax mix have been provided by British Columbia and Alberta, both of which have reduced their income taxes and made up part of the lost revenue with increases in the provincial poll taxes known as health-care 'premiums.' Such a change in tax mix can lead to a considerable transfer of income from the lower and middle ranges of the income distribution to the upper and especially the very high end (Evans 2002b), and that indeed seems to be the intention (Fuller and Stephens 2002). But the federal government also introduced, in 2001, a five-year program of income-tax reduction, with the principal beneficiaries at the upper end of the income distribution.

Who Gets (How Much Care, from Whom, When)?

As noted above there is no logical connection between changes in the tax mix – however they may be labelled – and patterns of individual use of health care. This may, however, be too simplistic. Legally, the position is quite clear. Failure to pay provincial 'premiums' has no more effect on entitlement to medicare services than failure to pay income or any other tax. To qualify for federal transfers, provinces must cover 100 per cent of their eligible residents regardless of whether they have paid premiums. But almost no one in the public knows this. Most people assume that their coverage depends on their payment of premiums – a belief that may well inhibit some from seeking care. There is no hard evidence on the strength of this effect, but it is worth keeping in mind as both Alberta and British Columbia raise their premiums.

More generally, however, the pattern of revenue sources used may considerably affect the distribution of use across the population, and possibly its overall level and cost. Here, there are two distinct and diametrically opposed schools of thought, one rooted in standard economic theory and one in the perceptions of providers of health care.

The standard economic theory is familiar from first-year courses and from the business press. If people have to pay more for care from their own pockets, they will tend on average to use less of it. A shift to less third-party payment, public or private, and more user pay is thus predicted to lower total system costs. They will fall still further if people begin to act as 'prudent purchasers,' seeking out the lowest-cost providers and thus placing competitive pressure on providers to hold down prices. In terms of the identity above, raising C and lowering T and/or R causes a drop in Q, and perhaps in P as well. The result is a fall in W and/or Z; providers' incomes decrease, and some resources – particularly people – leave the industry.

Whether this highly simplified theory of human and institutional behaviour has any practical relevance has been quite controversial, dividing economists into distinct schools along national and ideological lines. But it is fundamentally an *empirical* question. Does the prediction hold, or does it not? More generally, under what circumstances might it hold? This empirical issue must be sharply distinguished from the *normative* question. If the prediction is valid, is that an argument for or against user fees? Traditionally, advocates of public insurance or provision – and advocates of public subsidization of private insurance – have assumed that removing financial barriers to care was in fact a *good* thing, enabling people to get the care that they need and thus improving the population's health overall. Larger values of Q – and consequent higher expenditures – meant meeting more needs and improving health.

A number of economists, however, advocate user fees on the ground that *reducing* general use of care increases the 'allocative efficiency' of the economy and is therefore necessarily a good thing. Unfortunately that evaluative judgment rests on a theoretical mistake, rooted in an incomplete grasp of theoretical welfare economics. It is crucial to understand the nature of this mistake in order to appreciate why a number of economists reach conclusions so different from those of most other participants in the health-policy debate.

In economic theory 'efficiency' has a very special, technical meaning that bears no necessary relation to any judgment about better or worse. 'Efficient' patterns of resource allocation can be, in A.K. Sen's words, 'perfectly disgusting' from the point of view of any ethical observer. Non-economists, however, will typically assume, from general usage, that efficiency is somehow necessarily a good thing (Barer and Evans 1992; Reinhardt 1992; Culyer and Evans 1996).

This technical meaning of 'efficiency' renders use of health care (or any other commodity) by people who are 'unwilling' – which includes unable – to pay for it as 'inefficient' regardless of need or the effectiveness of the care. Conversely, it makes use of care that is ineffective or even harmful by persons who are willing to pay for it (strikingly, even if they do not actually pay!) efficient. The finding that, for example, mental-health services in Ontario are used primarily by lower-income people with the most severe problems, while in the United States they are used more heavily by those at the higher end and for much less severe problems (Katz et al., 1997), indicates more 'efficient' allocation of psychiatric care in the United States.

But this judgment would not be widely shared in Canada or even, one suspects, in the United States. (Or even among economists as citizens, once they remove their theoretical hats.) Most people seem to regard health-care systems as social mechanisms to improve or maintain health and relieve suffering, at reasonable cost, equitably distributed over the population. We may not employ such terms precisely and may disagree on their interpretation. But there is no evidence that citizens in general accept the normative position that people should get only the care for which they are willing and able to pay. If citizens do not, then the normative foundation of the standard economic argument disappears. 'Allocative efficiency,' in the conventional meaning of the term in economics, is simply irrelevant.

What remains relevant, however, is a very different sort of argument often conflated with the former. It is often claimed in public debates in Canada that a shift from third-party to 'direct patient payment' will increase the overall effectiveness of the health-care system by discouraging 'frivolous' use of care and freeing up resources to provide more effective care that is now being unduly delayed or denied – rationed – for people with real needs. This argument slides into another related claim – that the system is 'underfunded,' in that needs are going unmet and effective care is unprovided because the public system cannot or will not meet all those needs.

While the simple-minded economic argument held (empirically) that a shift to more direct payment by patients would lower overall use and costs and (normatively) that this would be a good thing, this latter argument asserts that a greater flow of finance through private channels (user pay and/or private insurance) would increase overall use and cost, and *this* would be a good thing. The criterion for 'goodness' is the putative impact of more care on health, as it is for the claim that direct payment would free up resources by discouraging patients' 'abuse' of the system through 'frivolous' care-seeking that does not reflect real needs. The simple economic theory, in contrast, is totally silent on any relation between health care and health. The normative judgment – which cannot be derived from economic theory itself but must be imposed on it – is simply that people should get only what they are willing/able to pay for.[19] Health per se is irrelevant.

The empirical evidence on the impact of user fees on overall access to or use of health care is mixed, and its interpretation, as always, is controversial (Barer et al., 1998; Robinson 2002). Logically, it seems that user fees, if they are high enough (and enforced), *must* constrain some forms of use, at least for some people. And there is good evidence that, within observed ranges, they do – at least for physicians' services and for drugs. But the evidence is equally clear that they do not selectively discourage only unnecessary or 'frivolous' services. The principal impact of user fees, as one might expect, is to reduce use by those with lower incomes. And at least for drugs, there is evidence of a negative effect on health among some of those whose use has been curtailed (Kozyrskyj et al., 2001; Tamblyn et al. 2001). Thus the economist's objective of allocative efficiency hurts health status, particularly among the unhealthy and unwealthy.

But the fact that user fees may restrain some individual use does not in fact demonstrate that it reduces overall use and cost. Such a presumption is known as the logical 'fallacy of composition.' To the extent that the overall level of use is determined by system capacity, or more generally by the decisions and behaviour of providers, it is quite conceivable that reduced use by some may be made up by increased use by others. That is in fact what the Canadian evidence seems to show. In particular, a careful 'before-and-after' study of the introduction of medicare in Quebec produced precisely this result – a rise in use by lower-income people, a fall among higher-income people, and, overall, no change in total service provision (Enterline et al., 1973a, b; McDonald et al., 1974; Siemiatycki, Richardson, and Pless 1980; see also Barer et al., 1998).

Whether or not user fees tend to constrain total expenditures depends, however, on their effect on prices as well as on the use of care. The putative negative connection from C to Q is typically assumed to have no, or even a negative, implication for prices or fees. Yet physicians' organizations in Canada have consistently argued for the right to extra-bill their patients on the ground that this would provide a 'safety valve' if provincial governments too aggressively constrained their fees. They have argued that physicians would extra-bill in such a way as not to place an undue burden on their patients or restrict access to care. This implies that the rise in C would lead not to a fall in Q, but only to a rise in P – overall higher costs for care and incomes for physicians.

This argument seems convincing. It is hard to understand why physicians would so consistently argue for a policy that would lower their incomes by reducing their workload with no corresponding adjustment in fees. Their argument, however, fits more appropriately under the heading 'who gets paid,' since it rests on a claim for higher relative incomes rather than on concern for patterns of health-care use. It does,

Figure 5.7
Provincial government spending on medicare and on all health, as a share of
tax and of total revenue, 1980–81 to 2000–01

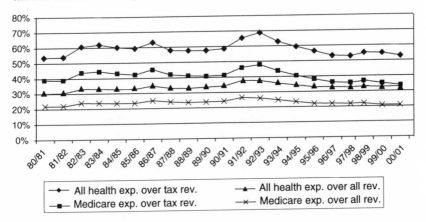

however, lead to the more general question of why one might advocate private financing – user fees or private insurance – in order to increase the use and/or costs of health care.

The argument is at root very simple. The costs of meeting patients' needs are allegedly increasing rapidly, as the population ages, technology advances, and public expectations grow. But governments cannot raise sufficient money from an already overtaxed public to meet those needs. Therefore private financing is needed, coming from 'those who can afford it,' to supplement public resources. Without private financing, patients' health will suffer. Q.E.D.

But such arguments contain both errors of fact and gaps of logic. In the first place the claim that public spending on health is absorbing a rising share of national income, or of public tax revenue, is simply false. Spending on medicare programs – physicians and hospitals – took up almost exactly the same percentage of gross domestic product (GDP) in 2001 (4.22 per cent) as in 1981 (4.11 per cent). This ratio has been virtually constant for the last five years, a full percentage point below its 1992 peak of 5.28 per cent and lower than in any year from 1982 to 1996 (CIHI 2001).

Figure 5.7 shows provincial government spending on these programs and on all health care, averaged across Canada, relative to total provincial revenues and to provincial tax revenue alone, between

1980–81 and 2000–01. Medicare spending absorbed 34 per cent of provincial tax revenue in 2000/01, well *down* from its 1980/81 level of 38.9 per cent (Canada, Department of Finance, 2002; CIHI 2002). That ratio reached a peak of 48 per cent in 1992/93, in the wake of the recession of 1989–91, but fell rapidly through the 1990s. All the ratios in Figure 5.7 show the same pattern: general economic conditions, not 'exploding' health-care costs, have generated the fiscal strains of the past decade. Relative to provincial revenues, both medicare and total provincial health spending are now at or below their levels of the early 1980s.

It is quite true that provincial health spending has been rising as a share of total program expenditures, and this has given rise to the argument that rising health-care costs are 'crowding out' other public programs. But this 'crowding out' reflects not rapid escalation in health spending but a relative decline in spending on non-health programs. Provincial governments have been working to restore their fiscal balance and eliminate deficits built up during the 1980s and the recession of the early 1990s. But this process is now complete and, on average, provincial governments are now in surplus. Several provinces have made substantial cuts to their income tax rates.[20]

If health spending is not currently outrunning public fiscal capacity, then it may be claimed that it will do so in the near future. But it has been repeatedly demonstrated that the common 'ageing population' argument does not stand up to quantitative analysis (see, for example, Barer, Evans and Hertzman 1995, 1998; Evans et al., 2001), while arguments based on technological advance and/or public expectations involve assumptions about political choices, not projections of historical inevitability (Evans 2002c).

Thus, it is never made clear exactly why Canadian governments cannot or will not make available sufficient public resources to meet the health needs of the population. The level of public financing is a political choice, and, despite claims to the contrary, there is no convincing evidence that Canadians are 'overtaxed' in the sense that some damage to economic performance is resulting. Surveys suggest that Canadians are actually willing to support higher levels of taxation in order to maintain and expand public health care. Contrasts are often drawn with tax burdens in the United States, but these neglect the fact that the level of tax finance for health care, as a share of national income, is actually substantially higher in the United States than in Canada.

The argument that governments cannot afford to meet growing health-care needs is often presented under the label of 'relieving the pressure on the public system,' but the extent to which private financing could do so depends on the assumed source of that pressure. If the public system is constrained by shortages of personnel, it is unclear how increased private financing could relieve this pressure. A 'parallel' private system would just draw personnel away from the public system by offering higher incomes, paid for from higher prices charged to private patients, and reducing the capacity of the public system. As in any private market, 'who gets' are those most able and willing to pay.

Yet a number of surgeons claim that they are working well below their capacity, constrained by limited access to operating facilities. Diagnostic specialists make similar claims about shortages of equipment. These limitations could be overcome with more private money, and indeed that seems to be happening as private clinics expand. (These developments raise a number of issues, but the focus of this paper is on the implications of alternative modes of financing, not on modes of delivery.)

What we can, however, state with some confidence is that 'separate but equal' public and private facilities will be neither separate nor equal, for perfectly straightforward economic reasons. If a separate, private tier of care were to 'take the pressure off the public system' to the extent that access and perceived quality were the same in both settings, no rational person would pay out of pocket to use the private system. The differences between the two, perceived or real, must be sufficient to maintain a price differential.

Nor will those distinctions be difficult to maintain, if, as is common in two-tiered systems, the same practitioners are permitted to work in both the public sector and the private sector. The economic incentives are obvious: to manipulate access to the public system so as to steer patients towards the more remunerative private care and to limit the time and effort put into the public system. Whether it is the Medicaid system for the poor in the United States, or the National Health Service in Britain, or Australia, or Israel, or Greece, or wherever, the same stories emerge. If practitioners can earn more in one setting than in another, the higher-priced venue draws their effort and commitment and their patients. The degree of distortion seems to depend, as one might expect, on the extent of the remuneration differential as well as on the prevailing medical culture.

No such distortion emerges if patients can 'go private' in a totally separate system, as when Canadians seek care at their own expense in the United States. But contrary to the prevailing rhetoric, very few actually do so – certainly not enough to sustain any sort of independent private market (Katz et al., 2002). Thus the survival of a two-tier system seems to depend on the maintenance of a significant differential of access and/or perceived quality between the two tiers. But this differential need not emerge solely from manipulation by care providers. A government committed to the expansion of private payment as well as of private care could also maintain such a differential by the simple expedient of underproviding facilities in the public sector and permitting private investors to offer and charge privately for such services. Private financing would then indeed expand the range of 'who gets,' but public and private patients will not get the same thing.

Who Gets Paid (How Much, for Doing What)?

Alternative modes of financing could affect both the total amount of income drawn from the health-care sector – equal to total health-care expenditures – and total revenue. But they will also influence who gets paid, and how much, for what kinds of activities.

As we saw in Figure 5.3, people receive payment for supplying various types of resources to the firms that provide health-care goods and services. But they are also paid for supplying associated administrative and other 'overhead' services, without which provision of care services on a large scale and in a co-ordinated fashion would be impossible. Administrative overhead is an essential part of a modern health-care system. But the level of such overhead costs varies considerably, depending on differences in both the way in which the delivery system is organized and in the financing channels employed.

These differences take two forms. One class of overhead – 'prepayment and administration expense' – refers to the costs of running the organizations, public or private, that actually assemble funds and disburse them to providers. The second class is incurred within provider organizations – clinics, hospitals, and other such agencies – to manage their internal affairs and deal with external funding organizations. Comparative analysis of health-care systems has demonstrated conclusively that private insurance requires much higher administrative overheads, for both reimbursing agencies and providers, than do public systems. Nor are these discrepancies difficult to understand.

The primary function of private insurance firms is underwriting, assessing the relative risk status of potential insurees, and setting premiums for groups according to their risk. Attached to this core function are billing and claims administration and marketing. Profitability depends crucially on the ability to identify risks accurately. If the risk associated with a policy is underestimated, and the premium set too low, underwriting losses result; if the estimate and the premium are too high, a competitor may take away the business.

But if a political decision has been made to levy contributions according to ability to pay rather than risk status, neither underwriting nor marketing is needed. In a universal, tax-based system, therefore, no one needs to be paid for these activities, and the corresponding costs disappear. Not surprisingly, private insurance firms tend to oppose bitterly the loss of their markets, and in the United States they have successfully campaigned against national health insurance. But public systems can raise financing, administer claims, and spread risk over the population more efficiently than private firms can. The unique product that private firms offer – at considerable extra cost – is the differentiation of premiums according to risk status, identifying and charging more to the least healthy. If that is how citizens collectively want to finance health care, then the services in which private insurers specialize may be worth paying for. But if not, not.

In Canada, the estimated cost of prepayment and administration amounted in 1999 to 13.6 per cent of total payments to private insurers. By contrast, the total reported outlays for prepayment and administration in the public sector were only one percent of outlays for hospitals and physicians' services. U.S. data show a similar pattern: out of $80.9 billion for prepayment and administration in 2000, $53.1 billion was spent by private insurers, and $21.5 billion by the public Medicare and Medicaid programs. These sums represented 19.6 per cent and 6.3 per cent, respectively, of total outlays through these channels (Levit et al., 2002). For the federal Medicare program alone, which more closely parallels Canada's medicare, overhead represented 3.3 per cent. The complexities of financing in the much more fragmented U.S. health-care environment add significantly to both public and private administrative costs, but the differential remains very large.

But the administrative cost differential can in fact be much larger than is reflected in the payment system alone. Complex financing systems require correspondingly complex administrative systems in the provider institutions themselves. A pair of U.S. researchers have produced a series of studies identifying the differentials in administrative costs between Canada and the United States (Himmelstein and Wool-handler 1986; Woolhandler and Himmelstein 1991; Woolhandler, Himmelstein, and Lewontin 1993; Himmelstein, Lewontin, and

Woolhandler, 1996); Woolhandler, Campbell, and Himmelstein (2003). They estimate comparative costs both in the payment agencies themselves and in the hospitals and other provider organizations that must deal with a wide variety of constantly changing forms and levels of coverage. Simply determining whether a patient is insured, and if so for what, is a major administrative task in a highly competitive and fluid market environment.

Combining both forms of overhead, provider and payer, Woolhandler, Campbell, and Himmelstein (2003) estimate the total expense in 1999 as $284.3 billion or $1059 per capita in the United States, compared with $307 (U.S.) in Canada. The excess administrative cost, relative to Canada's universal, public single-payer system, is $752 per capita, or 17 per cent of the total of $4392 (Levit et al., 2002). Americans spent 13.2 per cent of their national income on health care in 1999, compared with 9.2 per cent in Canada (CIHI, 2001); if one could remove the excess cost of the private insurance system the American ratio would fall to 10.9 per cent. Differences in the overhead costs generated by the payment system thus account for over half of the total difference between the two countries in that year. If these funds could be transferred from administrative activities to clinical care, they would be sufficient to provide full coverage for all Americans (over forty million) who currently have no insurance coverage at all.

Such a transfer, however, would be a direct attack on very powerful economic interests. These excess administrative expenditures simultaneously provide income for administrators, accountants, actuaries, benefits managers, lawyers, salesmen of all kinds, specialists in private capital markets, and private investors. Their services may contribute little or nothing to running an efficient health care system, let alone to anyone's health, but they are paid for, and often very well. Collectively they have always been able to mobilize decisive political influence to block attempts to rationalize the American health insurance system – i.e., to eliminate their incomes. The enormous overhead costs of the American payment system have been known for nearly twenty years; Woolhandler, Campbell, and Himmelstein (2003) merely provide a reminder and a confirmation that despite advances in information-handling technology the burden is growing over time. The choice of financing channel determines 'who gets paid,' and those who are paid do not easily surrender their incomes.

The evidence on administrative costs of private insurance is relatively clear and rarely contested by students of health-care systems.

The effects on 'who gets paid' of the mix between out-of-pocket and other forms of finance are themselves more mixed, and contingent on just how the payment process is organized. As noted above, physicians' representatives have for many years pressed for the right to extra-bill patients, over and above provincial reimbursement schedules, on the explicit ground that this would yield them higher fees and incomes. In the identity above, P would rise without any (significant) reduction in Q, and total health expenditures would increase.

It seems likely that any form of user fee that was to be collected by physicians would (re)open the door to such extra-billing – once patients are being charged for care, it may be difficult for them to keep track of how much they are being charged and of whether the practitioner is adding in an extra fee of his or her own. On the other hand, if medicare payments are added in whole or in part to taxable income, a ban on extra-billing could easily be maintained administratively. Whether it could be maintained politically is another question.

User charges for hospital services would not appear to raise this issue; the amount of such charges could simply be deducted from the hospital's global budget allocated by the province. There would, of course, be extra administrative costs for the hospital, to keep track of and collect such charges. These could become significant – in the United States, hospital finance departments add at least 10 per cent extra to hospital budgets – if a large competitive market were to develop for private insurance. In the identity above, this amounts to an increase in Z and P along with C – more people employed in the hospital, at greater cost, for no increase in care output. This is exactly what has happened in the U.S. system over the last two decades – 'cost without benefit,' as Himmelstein and Woolhandler (1986) put it succinctly – but it would seem unlikely in Canada in the near term unless private coverage expands dramatically.

This point is quite separate from the debate over the impact of private *delivery* of hospital services. Advocates argue that this would lead to greater efficiency of provision – represented as raising productivity, or the ratio of Q to Z in the basic identity. This would lower unit costs – a fall in P – permitting either lower expenditures or greater output, or both. Opponents argue that there is no evidence to support this assumption and that the real objective is 'union-busting' – lowering wages and transferring incomes to private-sector managers and investors without generating any net savings. They also point to evidence of systematic differences in quality of care between public and private facilities (for example, Devereaux et al., 2002), presumably a result of cutting costs to increase profits. This paper addresses only choice of financing mechanisms, taking no position on delivery.

The experience with mixed public–private financing for pharmaceuticals, however, illustrates what may be the most important issue under the heading 'Who Gets Paid? Experience with universal, comprehensive tax-financed programs, in Canada and elsewhere, has shown that governments – when they want to be – are much more effective at cost control than any known private-sector institutions. Whether such control is a good or a bad thing – opinions tend to differ between payers and paid – there is no doubt that public finance restricts income opportunities in the provision of health care. This would explain the otherwise anomalous and fierce opposition of the pharmaceutical industry to universal 'Pharmacare' in Canada.

The industry appears to share the view taken by the National Forum on Health (1997) that a Pharmacare program, with provincial and federal governments sharing costs, would change the incentives faced by those governments in favour of stronger control measures. In a multipayer system, it appears politically less costly not to take on the industry but to react to cost escalation by transferring a larger share of costs to users. From the industry's point of view, this is the best of all worlds, with governments accepting responsibility for those who cannot afford the product, but unable or unwilling to control overall costs/sales. A national Pharmacare program analogous to medicare might 'hold their feet to the fire,' and the result could be lower incomes and profits for drug makers and lower rates of cost escalation.[21]

A Triple Threat: Medical Savings Accounts

The hybrid financing approaches under the general label of medical savings accounts (MSAs) are more difficult to categorize because they would probably have significant effects on who pays, who gets, and who gets paid.

Advocates argue that MSAs would both reduce total health-care costs and open up more choice, in that people could decide how to spend the accounts under their own control. Since they involve increased user fees for the heaviest users of care, and allegedly lower total costs, they would shift the financing mix from taxation to user pay. The answer to 'who pays?' becomes more regressive. But by opening up choices for users, and billing opportunities for providers, MSAs would also change the pattern of 'who gets paid.' Further, since these schemes place more public resources in the hands of the lowest users of care and take them away from the highest users, they might be expected to shift the balance of who gets' in favour of the healthiest.

Critics, however, have emphasized the very high concentration of health expenses on relatively few, very ill individuals, a concentration that persists over time. As Forget, Deber, and Roos (2002) point out, on the basis of a simulation of a typical MSA specification with actual use and corresponding expenditure data from Manitoba, the majority of the population would not reach their account limits – unless they greatly increased their spending on health-related commodities. Those few who generate very high expenses would move into the 'catastrophic,' range where expenses (at the margin) would be fully covered. For them the MSA would in effect impose a tax equal to the difference between the account allowance and the catastrophic limit – a poll tax on the very ill. Only those few whose annual expenditure fell into the gap between the account balance and the catastrophic limit would have any financial incentive to limit their use.

Yet the majority of the population who are basically healthy would now both have opportunities to spend public money on a much broader range of designated health services and face higher prices charged by providers freed from the constraints of public bargaining. As Forget et al. show, an increase in covered outlays among this large group could easily wipe out, and indeed greatly exceed, any reduction in costs resulting from price-responsiveness among those in the gap between the account level and the catastrophic limit. Their analysis suggests that MSAs would probably increase both public and total spending on health care (and thus providers' incomes).[22] But they would certainly increase the financial burden on the relatively ill and the very ill while expanding spending opportunities for the healthy.

Forget et al. provide the most recent and thorough empirically grounded critique of MSA proposals, though by no means the first (Deber 1999; Hurley 2000; Schaafsma 2002). Advocates, by contrast, have brought forward no credible empirical analysis to support their claims. Their figures simply do not add up, leading to justifiable suspicion as to their real motivations.[23] 'MSAs will not save money but will instead, under most formulations, lead to an increase in spending on the healthiest members of the population ... with little attention to the appropriateness or health benefits ... When one adds ... concerns about equity ... MSAs have very little to recommend them. It is past time that they be buried' (Forget, Deber, and Ross 2002, 146–7).

Shifting Financial Sources: What Are the Objectives?

'Would you tell me, please, which way I ought to go from here?' said Alice.
'That depends a good deal on where you want to get to,' replied the
Cheshire Cat.

As noted at the outset, it appears unlikely that a modern system of health
care can function without a predominant role for public financing. Certainly no such system now exists. But it is certainly possible to alter the
mix of sources while maintaining the predominance of public finance;
one observes considerable variation both between countries and to a
lesser extent within countries over time. What scope might there be for
altering the mix in Canada, and what might the consequences be?

The discussion focuses on potential shifts to more private financing
for the services of physicians and hospitals, because those possibilities
appear to dominate public discussion. A move towards more public
financing, particularly for prescription drugs, would raise some very
interesting issues. But a national Pharmacare program seems to have
drifted off the public agenda for the moment.

As Figure 5.2 shows, Canada is already towards the top of the range
among OECD countries in terms of the private share of financing for
all health care.[24] Private financing for the services of physicians and
hospitals is, however, relatively low – about 1.2 per cent for physicians
in 2001 and 7.4 per cent (mostly charges for extended care) for hospitals (CIHI 2001). Would an increase in these percentages take Canadians closer to where they wish to go?

This is a question about policy *choices* and public priorities. If instead
one takes it as axiomatic that the current medicare system is (or soon
will be) 'underfunded' and that no more money can be raised from
public sources, then very little further analysis is needed. The answer
must be increased user fees, in some form or other, and possibly an
extension of private insurance to permit those who can buy it to cover
those charges. This is an example of the logical fallacy known as 'petitio
principii,' or begging the question, in which the desired conclusion is in
effect taken as given in the initial assumptions.[25] We can bypass this
logical trap and consider alternative funding sources on their merits.

There exist a myriad of possibilities and proposals for shifting medicare costs from public to individual budgets, and a detailed analysis of
any one of them would be a significant research project in itself. Here,
we consider two 'pure types' of user fees – a 20 per cent coinsurance
rate applied to all public expenditures for hospital care and physicians'

services and an annual per-person 'deductible' of $300 applying to the same expenditures.[26] The various hybridizations discussed above are essentially similar to these in their effects.

For simplicity, we assume that these amounts are billed directly to individuals by the government (parents would be responsible for their children's use), maintaining the current single-payer system of direct reimbursement. A shift to a model similar to private insurance, in which individuals paid their own bills and then sought reimbursement from government, would probably trigger major changes – and major cost inflation – in the whole system.

In round figures, averaged across Canada, the public sector paid out about $1,000 per capita for hospital care and $450 for physicians' services in 2001. if there were no other changes, a 20 per cent coinsurance charge would raise an average of about $300 per person per year, or $1,200 for a family of four, and would add about $9 billion to total provincial revenue – a substantial sum. A deductible, requiring each person to reimburse the public treasury for expenditures up to $300 in each year, would (if everyone exceeded this limit) generate roughly the same amount from the Canadian population of about 31 million. For comparison, however, the federal Department of Finance estimates that provincial income tax cuts since 1996/97 have reduced annual revenue by about $20 billion.

The share of total Canadian health-care costs raised from out-of-pocket charges would increase by over 50 per cent, from 16 per cent to 26 per cent, or higher than in any other country shown in Figure 5.1. The privately financed share would rise from about 30 per cent to nearly 40 per cent, almost equal to that in the United States (adjusted for tax-expenditure subsidies) and well above all other OECD countries shown in Figure 5.2. But are these serious options?

In a word, no. Neither form of user charge will actually yield these amounts, and for the same reason – the very high proportion of service use and costs accounted for by a small proportion of the population.[27] The 'average' level of expenditure is made up of relatively few heavy users and a large number whose use is well below average – some, nothing at all.

Consider first the deductible. Forget, Deber, and Roos (2002) find that the lowest-using half of the Manitoba population accounts for only 4 per cent of hospital and physician expenditures. If the overall average is $1,500, then the average for the bottom half is $120 and that for the top half is $2,880. If none of those in the bottom half reaches the deductible (Forget et al. do not report the median level of expenditure), then the low-using half will contribute only 40 per cent of the expected amount, lowering the estimated revenue from $9 billion to $7.2 billion. (About 15 per cent will contribute nothing.) But within the high-using half of the population, the top decile accounts for the lion's share of spending, with an average per capita of about $8,100. The next decile contributes about $1,600, and the next three – from 80 per cent to 50 per cent – average only $520 each. If no one in the bottom half reaches the deductible level, then it is virtually certain that some in the top half do not either – further reducing the revenue raised.

Still another consideration is the evidence from Figure 5.4 – not particularly surprising – that people with low incomes tend to use, on average, more services. It seems likely that people below some income level will be exempt from paying the deductible. If the bottom decile of the income distribution is excused, and if we assume, conservatively, that the incidence of high use is not greater among this group, then the revenue potential falls another 10 per cent, to about $6.5 billion. If, however, high users – who would otherwise have to pay the full deductible – are more prevalent among this bottom income group, then the extent of revenue loss will be greater.

Allowing for low and non-users and for the very poorest still leaves a respectable amount of additional revenue potential. But the deductible requirement begins to look rather like a poll tax with full or partial exemption for the healthy and the poor. If the objective of the deductible is simply to bring in money, why not just impose a poll tax on the whole population (again exempting the poorest) – as Alberta and British Columbia do with the health insurance 'premium'? This will bring in substantially more money without raising the questionable ethics of exempting the healthy and imposing the full charge only on the most ill. Unless one has some clear reason for *wanting* to 'tax the sick,' a poll tax seems a superior vehicle for raising additional revenue without unduly burdening the wealthy.

The same issues arise in more extreme form with the 20 per cent coinsurance charge. That mechanism also exempts non-users and bears relatively lightly on the low-using majority. But this would not erode its revenue-raising potential, *if* in fact the coinsurance were paid on all services used. The level of contribution would rise proportionate to use, with the heaviest users making up the amounts not contributed by the light or non-users. In reality, of course, this will not happen.

The very heavy users are not only disproportionately elderly, female, and in poor health. They are also much more likely to be poor.

In Figure 5.4, the permanently institutionalized population – about eighteen thousand persons out of over one million – had virtually no income at all yet were estimated to account for over 20 per cent of public outlays on health care in 1994.[28] Together with the bottom two deciles, they were responsible for nearly half of the total. Even for those who 'can afford it,' however, the coinsurance charge will bear very heavily on that small proportion of the population that has the misfortune to be very ill. But for many of the heaviest users, the money simply is not there. They will either be unable to obtain the services that they need, or they will be exempt from the coinsurance charge. Either way, they will not pay. Exempting only the bottom income decile and the permanently institutionalized lowers the revenue estimate by about 30 per cent, from $9 billion to $6.3 billion.

But there will remain a considerable number of high and very high users in the rest of the population, some of whom will have incomes just above the bottom income decile. 'Those who can afford it' may seek private insurance coverage against the risk of these large outlays – that is, after all, what insurance is for. But private for-profit insurers in a competitive marketplace cannot afford to sell coverage to high-risk individuals. What they can sell are contracts covering employee groups – pre-selected as relatively healthy by virtue of being employed – from which individuals are not permitted to opt out. And even on these contracts they receive a large public subsidy. Private insurers would probably offer to extend this coverage to include large medicare coinsurance charges for this subsidized and relatively healthy employed population. But they will not cover the elderly and chronically ill, who account for most of the high use.

Conceivably, such private coverage might be mandated, but that would require both further public subsidies and a considerable regulatory effort to prevent insurers from behaving as their profit motivation leads them to behave – avoiding the high risks, or simply pricing them out of the market. And there will be substantial overhead costs, for both insurers and government, to run such a system. Australia provides perhaps the best example of the problems raised by this sort of 'swimming upstream' – trying to use a financing mechanism for what it was never designed to do (Hurley 2001).

The simplest way of mitigating the impact of a coinsurance requirement would be to place a ceiling on the level of expenditure for which coinsurance must be paid.[29] If this limit were set at, say, the average level of medicare expenditure – about $1,500 – then no one would have to pay more than $300 out of pocket in any one year. At this point, however, the coinsurance requirement begins to look rather like the deductible. Those with heavy expenses pay $300, those with no use (or little income) pay none, and the majority of the population contribute somewhere between zero and $300.

The difference is that the coinsurance requirement with these parameters yields much less revenue than the $300 deductible, because fewer than one quarter of the population will reach the 'average' level of expenditure and pay the full $300. For an equivalent amount of money to be raised, the ceiling expenditure level would have to be substantially higher than $1,500, implying a substantially greater financial burden for the heaviest users. The arithmetic is straightforward; for any given amount of revenue raised, the coinsurance requirement with a ceiling must place a heavier burden on the highest users of care and a correspondingly lighter burden on low users – and of course no burden on non-users. Again, the poll tax looks like the superior alternative.

Why then is there such energetic advocacy of alternative, private financing mechanisms, if regressive income redistribution can be achieved more simply just by modifying the tax mix? In fact, however, advocates for changing the financing mix in the direction of less taxation and more private financing do *not* highlight the regressive transfer of income from the unhealthy and unwealthy to the healthy and (especially) the wealthy that are their primary and inevitable effect. They argue instead that linking financial liability to the use of care will bring other benefits, leading to a more efficient and more effective health-care system. Some even claim that it will be less costly, although, as we saw above, the preponderance of advocacy seems to hold that the Canadian health-care system needs more money, not less. So do we deplore on equity grounds the fact that private financing alternatives will face (some) users with personal financial consequences from the use of care and present the heaviest users with the heaviest consequences, or do we celebrate and embrace that fact for its supposed beneficial effects? What might those beneficial effects be? To put the matter in another way, why might one support 'taxing the sick'?

Advocates tend to refer, in general terms, to 'limiting demand' for health care and encouraging patients to be more discriminating in identifying appropriate and inappropriate care. Such emphasis would seem inconsistent with the view that the Canadian health-care system is 'underfunded' and therefore requires *more* money to meet currently unmet needs. Which is it to be, do Canadians need to spend more, or less? One cannot have it both ways.

A reconciliation might be that there is a good deal of inappropriate use in the present system crowding out genuine needs, and that charges to users – small ones, so as not to restrict access for real needs – would selectively deter inappropriate care. More money is still needed, but not as much more.

This view has been remarkably resilient in the face of consistent evidence that selective deterrence is exactly what user charges do *not* achieve. To the extent that they influence patients' care-seeking, they discourage appropriate and inappropriate care alike. Nor is this surprising, given the implausibility of the proposition that patients deliberately seek out care – especially in hospital! – they know to be inappropriate, simply because it is free. There are in fact some very odd patterns of care-seeking to be found in the Canadian data, but they are mostly associated with mental illness and/or serious problems of substance abuse, and they are neither quantitatively significant nor growing.

The major pressures for cost escalation arise not from individuals' decisions to seek care, but from the therapies offered in the doctor's office – from recommendations for various diagnostic and therapeutic procedures to prescription drugs – are under physicians' control. If inappropriate care is a concern – and it should be – then focusing on patients' behaviour amounts to looking (perhaps deliberately) in exactly the wrong direction.

Insofar as a general policy of user charges may provide a less politically contentious alternative to a serious examination and modification of care patterns, it may actually inhibit efforts to discourage inappropriate care. This has certainly happened in Canada in the case of prescription drugs. And the reason is clear from Figure 5.3. Whether or not care is appropriate, people are paid for providing it. Effective policies to discourage it threaten those incomes and generate strong opposition. Ineffective policies, which merely transfer costs rather than reducing them, do not.

What, then, do user charges do? Again, the evidence is very clear. They selectively deter access by those with lower incomes, thereby increasing access for those with greater ability to pay.[30] Some advocates seem to confuse the two, implicitly assuming that the health problems of the better-off are more serious, or at least more deserving of attention.[31] User charges help them to get it.

If that is considered a proper objective for Canadian health policy, then private financing will be necessary. Simply making the tax system more regressive will not do the job. Yet the fact that advocates base their claims not on this point, but rather on the spurious claim of selectively discouraging inappropriate care, suggests that they fear their real objective may not receive sufficient weight in the political process.

Insofar as they improve access for those better able to pay, because of private resources or private insurance, user charges do not necessarily reduce the overall use of health care. Their effect on total expenditures is even more doubtful insofar as they create opportunities for providers to increase their fees. There is in fact no evidence that private financing assists in global cost containment – the United States is a glaring counter-example. Cross-national comparisons show considerable variation in the costliness of various national systems, reflecting different policy choices. The financing system appears to be a factor, but it is public, not private financing, that conduces to global cost control.

There are circumstances in which user payments may be used either to steer patients in the direction of more appropriate care or to ration access to services that are not considered therapeutically necessary (Evans et al., 1994b). The reference pricing system for pharmaceuticals in British Columbia, for example (note 21 above), relies on expert clinical and pharmacological judgment, based on the scientific literature, to identify drugs that are therapeutically equivalent, though chemically different. When two drugs are judged equivalent, the public Pharmacare program will reimburse only the price of the lower-cost drug. Patients may, if they wish, pay the difference to purchase the more expensive drug, and some do. The program has been quite successful in reducing costs for those drugs that have been reference-priced, without any evidence of harm to patients. The higher-cost drug is 'not medically necessary.'

There are obvious risks, however, and the program requires not only a high level of guiding expertise but also a readily accessible system for exempting patients who either cannot tolerate the cheaper drug or do not find it effective. In such cases, the higher-cost drug is 'medically necessary,' and a public agency that withheld reimbursement, or simply placed obstacles in the way of those seeking therapeutically justified exemptions, would not be meeting its obligations.

The same argument has been accepted for years as a basis for preferred-accommodation differentials in hospitals – charges to patients for private or semi-private rooms that are not judged necessary on the basis of the patient's medical condition. And user charges in long-term care facilities have an equally lengthy history as a way of 'clawing back' public pensions for those with very low incomes, on the ground that room and board are being provided in the institution and should not be subsidized twice. More recently, some provinces have begun to try to recapture the whole of the room-and-board costs in long-term care, but it is unclear how many patients could afford this. In any case, such charges are grounded on the distinction between general maintenance and 'medically necessary' care.

But the issue of medical necessity can be slippery; it is apparently being used by private medical resonance imaging (MRI) clinics – perhaps with the encouragement of some provincial governments – to exploit waiting times at public facilities. The argument is made that while an MRI procedure is needed, it is not needed immediately, and therefore the private clinic charging patients for more timely service is in fact selling a service that is not medically necessary. It is not clear, however, if patients understand that they are paying for an 'unnecessary' service. Certainly, it is not in the interest of clinic staff to tell them. A provincial government seeking ways to evade the provisions of the Canada Health Act might simply fail to fund adequate MRI capacity, thus saving taxpayers' money at the expense of patients.

Thus, while the use of financial incentives to encourage patients to make the most cost-effective choices among therapeutically equivalent alternatives has a certain appeal, that appeal rests on the assumption that patients have genuine choices to make and sufficient information to make them. The economic incentives to market 'value-added services' do not encourage the provision of unbiased information. Governments looking for ways to contain public expenditures (and not strongly committed – in fact, perhaps opposed – to the underlying principles of medicare) have little incentive to remedy this imbalance. The offloading of costs onto patient, and the expansion of private profit opportunities, can then masquerade as a policy of encouraging patients to make appropriate choices of therapy.

So how to reply to the Cheshire cat? If the objective is simply to reduce the extent to which Canadian governments redistribute income from the more to the less wealthy – from those who earned it to those who did not, as Conrad Black (2000) put it with such charming directness – then there is no good reason to change the financing mix away from taxation. Reducing the income tax and introducing or raising poll taxes will do the job more simply, with less administrative expense, and will shift more money than will user fees because it will not exempt (wholly or partially) such a large proportion of the population. The regressive potential of such a shift in mix is considerable, moving thousands of dollars a year into the hands of upper-income groups (tens of thousands for the very wealthy) at the expense of those in the middle- and lower-income brackets (Evans 2002c). Moreover, it cannot be interpreted as being in violation of the Canada Health Act so long as those in default are not explicitly denied care. (If they are deterred by the erroneous belief that they are not covered, well, that is not the fault of the provincial government. They should read the legislation.)

But if the objective of reform is also to improve access to care for the better-off, then some form of private payment is essential. A straight-forward coinsurance charge might seem the best option, even though a deductible might bring in more money, because it would bear more on the heaviest users and thus have the greatest potential for freeing up resources by discouraging use by this group. But if one accepts the argument that these people, being in the main very ill, have little choice as to the use of care, and if denying care to the very ill who simply cannot pay seems politically unacceptable, then that would suggest the deductible as a way of deterring unnecessary use by low-income people who are not very ill – relatively low users – so as to increase access for 'those who can afford it.'

It will, however, be hard to avoid interpreting either of these policies as violating the access provisions of the Canada Health Act. That is, after all, their purpose. Thus, while the various hybridizations of alter-native funding sources have little to recommend them on economic grounds, they may serve to make that violation less transparent. (The public subsidy to private insurance, of course, also serves to make the fiscal system more regressive, thus furthering the objective so clearly expressed by Lord Black.) This lack of transparency may be advanta-geous as a basis for legal as well as political challenges, if the federal government should attempt to enforce the act against a province intro-ducing such policies.

If, however, one takes as an objective the reform of the system of health-care delivery itself – the demanding (and politically dangerous) task of improving the effectiveness of the care delivered and the effi-ciency with which it is produced – then expanding private financing has nothing to offer. The focus must be on changing the information available to and the incentives bearing on those who deliver the care – the funding structure, not the financing mix (upper right of Figure 5.3, not upper left). This is a huge topic and task, challenging every nation in the developed world; further privatizing the financing mix will not make it easier and is likely to make it more difficult.[32]

But if neither transferring income from the less to the more wealthy, nor increasing their access at the expense of the less wealthy, is considered a major priority for Canadian public policy, and if potential improvements in the cost-effectiveness of the health care system (for which there is considerable evidence) are believed politically infeasible or insufficient to permit it to meet present or emerging needs, then the clear implication is that more funding should be made available from tax revenue. This could, but need not, require higher tax rates; it depends on the general fiscal situation.

But that situation is vastly improved from five years ago, for both the federal and the provincial governments.[33] Those who claim that public health-insurance programs are taking up an increasing and unsustainable share of national income and/or public revenues have simply failed to check the fiscal facts. Nor is there any basis for the claim that Canada has reached some absolute limit, for political or economic reasons, in the amount of public money available for health care. The real motive underlying proposals for more private financing is very simple. 'The more private funding we have, the more those with high incomes can assure themselves of first class care without having to pay taxes to help support a similar standard of care for everyone else' (Roos and Frohlich 2002).

NOTES

1 Here and subsequently, references to OECD data are drawn from OECD 2001.
2 The widespread impression that U.S. health-care is financed primarily from private sources is in fact incorrect for reasons discussed below (Fox and Fronstin 2000; Woolhandler and Himmelstein 2002).
3 In the abstract, it can be argued that some changes generate sufficient benefits for the gainers that they could compensate all the losers and still come out ahead. But unless the compensation is actually paid – which is never part of real-world proposals – then the possibility is irrelevant. The argument that a policy change meeting this criterion represents a general social benefit *even if the compensation is not paid* is logically unsound and simply fraudulent, as Reinhardt 1992 shows.
4 The underlying algebra and the disaggregation of these identities to the

individual transactor level are discussed in Evans and Stoddart 1994a, along with the imputations, taken from the national income accounting framework, necessary to ensure identity.

5 The dimensions of 'privateness' are discussed in more detail in Evans et al. 2000.

6 They have also led to criminal fraud charges being laid against a number of the largest for-profit health-care corporations in the United States (Evans et al. 2000).

7 Patients were reportedly charged as much as $750; at other hospitals in Alberta, the flexible implants were included as part of the standard, publicly reimbursed cataract procedure. Bought in bulk, the implants might cost $25.

8 The government of Quebec, however, removed this subsidy from its provincial income-tax system in 1993 and now taxes employer-paid premiums as personal income (Smythe 2001).

9 The government of Quebec, however, removed this subsidy from its provincial income-tax system in 1993.

10 CIHI 1999, 14, reports private insurance expenditures in Canada in 1997 at $8.5 billion; if one assumes that this amount had grown since 1994 at the same rate as total health spending, the figure for 1994 would be about $7.9 billion.

11 This advantage is partly offset by the medical-expense deduction for out-of-pocket payments, but as noted below this is of much more limited value.

12 There is widespread agreement among economists that this subsidy is bad policy, although their reasons differ radically. Some, such as Martin Feldstein, believe that it encourages overinsurance, leading to overuse of health care, although he and many other economists define 'overuse' in a way that bears no relation to the ordinary-language meaning of the term and would probably be rejected by most people (see below). Others, including this author, believe that, in the absence of the subsidy, private coverage would shrink so much as to increase greatly the public pressure for expanded public coverage – of drugs in Canada and of health care generally in the United States. Still others may simply regard the distribution of the benefits of the subsidy as unfair.

13 An individual seeking to purchase health insurance may know that he or she is at higher-than-average risk of making a claim; insurers cannot easily monitor individual health status.

14 Canada, Department of Finance (2000, Table 1), estimates the federal component of the subsidy to private insurance as being about five times as large as the medical-expense deduction.

15 The Australian government has, for a number of years, been trying to use regulatory authority and financial incentives to preserve a major role for private insurance alongside a public system. The ostensible purpose is to transfer costs from public to private budgets; in fact it appears that the costs to the government of trying to maintain both systems outweigh any hoped-for savings. The government is actually incurring substantial extra public costs to pay for its ideological predilections (Hurley 2001).

16 A regressive financing system, like a regressive tax, takes a larger proportion (on average) of the incomes of people with lower incomes – though not necessarily a larger absolute amount. A progressive system takes a larger share of the incomes of higher-income people, and a proportionate one takes, on average, a more or less equal share at all income levels.

17 This figure is well below the $1,500 used above for illustrating the regressive effect of taxing health-care expenditures. Part of the difference is accounted for by the increase from 1997–99 to 2001, but most reflects the fact that a significant proportion of hospital costs cannot be attributed to individuals. This represents a limitation on the scope of any such user fees, unless an arbitrary attribution is made for billing purposes.

18 These calculations apply the relative variations in use patterns found by Forget, Deber, and Roos 2002 to the average level of expenditure reported by CIHI 2001. If it were not feasible to identify or attribute the full amount of provincial spending on physicians and hospitals to individuals, the increased tax liabilities would have to be scaled down accordingly – as would the revenue potential. But the proportionate impact on differently situated individuals would remain the same. Also, these calculations assume that the distribution of utilization is the same in each income class; in fact, heavier users are disproportionately represented in the lower income brackets. Thus, these calculations understate, to some degree, the additional liability of the 'average' individual in the lower-income brackets and overstate liabilities higher up the scale.

19 David Hume is credited with pointing out the logical fallacy of imagining that one can derive normative propositions such as 'What ought to be done?' from positive propositions such as 'If A holds, then B follows.' The fallacy is committed with depressing frequency by economists making policy recommendations based – they think – on 'value-free' economic analysis.

20 This fiscal history is described in more detail in Evans 2002c.

21 The Pharmacare program in British Columbia has had some success in controlling prescription-drug expenditures through its reference pricing system (Marshall et al. 2002; Schneeweiss et al. 2002;). But it has not pursued

this approach aggressively. A nation-wide system backed by both federal and provincial governments might significantly moderate the escalation of drug costs but by the same motion would restrain the escalation of industry sales and profits.

22 The net effect depends on the behaviour of the large majority of the population whose allocated spending accounts will exceed their actual outlays. Will they use the excess to pay for health-related commodities that they were previously paying for privately, or will they increase their overall spending on such commodities – buying more and/or paying higher prices for services previously reimbursed by governments? In the former case, public spending will go up but total spending will not; in the latter case, total spending will go up as well. If, as seems likely, the increase in public spending exceeds the extra revenue from user charges on those who exceed their allocated accounts, then the requirement for tax finance will increase as well. Rather than shifting the burden of payment from taxpayers to users of care, the MSA scheme is likely to increase it for both.

23 See, for example, the review by Roos and Frohlich 2002 of a book edited by one of the leading advocates of MSAs.

24 An adjustment for the tax-expenditure subsidy to private insurance, however, would lower Canada's private share by about three percentage points, bringing it closer to the middle of the pack.

25 The common interpretation of 'begging the question' as referring to an observation or argument that strongly suggests a further question is incorrect.

26 Individuals would be liable either for 20 per cent of all expenses billed (physicians' fees) or estimated to have been incurred (hospitals) on their behalf or for all such expenses up to an annual ceiling of $300.

27 There is still another reason: the proportion of costs that cannot be attributed to individuals. In what follows, we continue to use the CIHI estimate for 2001 of about $1,500 per-capita expenditure on physicians and hospitals. But as noted above, Forget et al. were able to attribute only about 62 per cent of the CIHI estimate for Manitoba in their study years. If nearly 40 per cent of costs cannot be attributed to individuals, the scope for raising revenue through private financing declines significantly.

28 This group is too small to matter much with respect to the revenue-raising potential of a deductible, which is proportionate to numbers of people. But it matters a lot when contributions are linked to the level of expenditure.

29 That limit could be based on individual incomes, as for that matter could be the deductible level; it would mitigate somewhat the regressivity of this form of financing. But this creates another problem. The degree of inequal-

ity of income is such that if the limit were directly proportionate to income, most of those in the highest income groups would effectively be uninsured by the public system, creating an obvious pressure for a two-tier system of both insurance and provision. Yet if the limit varies over a narrower range than income does, then the financing system remains regressive.

30 There are two major sources for this evidence. Several papers from the RAND Health Insurance Study in the 1980s are referenced in Barer et al. 1998, but their conclusions were foreshadowed in the papers from the Montreal study of the early 1970s, referenced above (Enterline et al., 1973a, b; McDonald et al., 1974; Siemiatycki, Richardson, and Pless 1980).

31 The confusion is significant, because most of those who advocate user fees on the basis of economic theory have adopted precisely this normative view – that 'efficient allocation' of health-care resources means providing care to those, and only those, who are able and willing to pay for it. (While this value judgment is not widely shared, at least openly, it may have more adherents than are willing to admit it – or are even clearly aware of it.) There remains continuing controversy in the economic literature over whether user fees do or do not serve to limit overall expenditures. It appears that they have little or no effect on hospital use but do affect individuals' decisions in the anticipated direction, discouraging use. The controversy arises over whether these effects on individuals can be added up to an aggregate effect. Insofar as they discourage needed care, one might find harm to health and greater costs later. Some evidence of harm has emerged for pharmaceutical user charges, but the net financial costs are not clear. More important (in this author's judgment), use of both hospitals and physicians is largely determined by physicians' judgments as constrained by the availability of supply. What one patient does not use another will.

32 The U.S. experience does show that a greater share of private financing is conducive to greater flexibility and change in the delivery system, but unfortunately not to improvement (Oberlander 2002).

33 Granted, the economic outlook at mid-2002 seems distinctly worrying. But the news is bad for the public and the private sectors alike. A severe recession that strains public resources will not make health care any more affordable through private channels.

REFERENCES

Armstrong, W. 2000. *The Consumer Experience with Cataract Surgery and Private Clinics in Alberta*. Consumers' Association of Calgary, Alberta Chapter, Jan.

Barer, M.L., and R.G. Evans. 1992. 'Interpreting Canada: Models, Mind-Sets and Myths.' *Health Affairs* 11, no. 1: 44–61.

Barer, M.L., R.G. Evans, and C. Hertzman. 1995. 'Avalanche or Glacier? Health Care and the Demographic Rhetoric.' *Canadian Journal on Aging* 14, no. 2: 193–225.

Barer, M.L., R.G. Evans, C. Hertzman, and M. Johri. 1998. 'Lies, Damned Lies, and Health Care Zombies: Discredited Ideas That Will Not Die.' HPI Discussion Paper No. 10, University of Texas–Houston Health Policy Institute, Houston, Texas. www.chspr.ubc.ca

Black, C. 2000. 'The Most Boring Election in History.' *National Post*, 1 Dec. 2000.

Canada, Department of Finance. 2000. *Canada Federal Tax Expenditures.* Ottawa: Department of Finance.

– 2002. 'Fiscal Reference Tables September 2001.' Ottawa: Department of Finance. www.fin.gc.ca/toce/2002/frt_e.html

CIHI. 1999. *National Health Expenditure Trends: 1975–1999.* Ottawa: Canadian Institute for Health Information, Dec.

– 2001. *National Health Expenditure Trends: 1975–2001.* Ottawa: Canadian Institute for Health Information, Dec.

Culyer, A.J., and R.G. Evans. 1996. 'Normative Rabbits from Positive Hats: Mark Pauly on Welfare Economics.' *Journal of Health Economics* 15, no. 2: 243–51.

Deber, R.B. 1999. 'Medical Savings Accounts: A Fine Idea Unless You're Sick.' *Health Policy Forum* 2, no. 1: 4–5.

Devereaux, P.J., P.T.L. Choi, C. Lacchetti, B. Weaver, H.J. Schünemann, T. Haines, J.N. Lavis, B.J.B. Grant, D.R.S. Haslam, M. Bhandari, T. Sullivan, D.J. Cook, S.D. Walter, M. Meade, H. Khan, N. Bhatnagar, and G.H. Guyatt. 2002. 'A Systematic Review and Meta-analysis of Studies Comparing Mortality Rates of Private For-profit and Private Not-for-profit Hospitals.' *CMAJ* 166, no. 11: 1399–1406.

Enterline. P.E., et al. 1973a. 'Effects of Free Medical Care on Medical Practice: The Quebec Experience.' *New England Journal of Medicine* 288: 1152–5.

– 1973b. 'The Distribution of Medical Services before and after "Free" Medical Care: The Quebec Experience.' *New England Journal of Medicine* 289: 1174–8.

Evans, R.G. 2000. 'Financing Health Care: Taxation and the Alternatives.' HPRU Discussion Paper No. 2000: 15D, Centre for Health Services and Policy Research, University of British Columbia, Vancouver. www.chspr.ubc.ca

– 2002a. 'Financing Health Care: Taxation and the Alternatives.' In E. Mossialos, A. Dixon, J. Figueras, and J. Kutzin, eds., *Financing Health Care: Options for Europe* Buckingham: Open University Press, 39–58. (An edited version of Evans 2000). www.euro.who.int/document/e74485.pdf

– 2002b. 'Getting to the Roots: Health Care Financing and the Inegalitarian Agenda in Canada' Presentation to the Senate Standing Committee on Social Affairs, Science and Technology, Ottawa, 3 June. HPRU Discussion Paper No. 2002: 7D, Centre for Health Services and Policy Research, University of British Columbia, Vancouver. www.chspr.ubc.ca

– 2002c. Financing the Canadian Health Care System: Experience, Challenges, Options and Traps.' Paper prepared for the Commission on the Future of Health Care in Canada (Romanow Commission), July.

Evans R.G., M.L. Barer, S. Lewis, M. Rachlis, and G.L. Stoddart. 2000. 'Private Highway, One-Way Street: The De-Klein and Fall of Canadian Medicare?' HPRU No. 2000:3D, UBC Centre for Health Services and Policy Analysis, Vancouver. www.chspr.ubc.ca

Evans, R.G., M.L. Barer, and G.L. Stoddart. 1994a. *Charging Peter to Pay Paul: Accounting for the Financial Effects of User Charges.* Toronto: Premier's Council on Health, Well-being and Social Justice, June. www.chspr.ubc.ca

Evans, R.G., M.L. Barer, G.L. Stoddart, and V. Bhatia. 1994b. *It's Not the Money, It's the Principle: Why User Charges for Some Services and Not Others?* Toronto: Premier's Council on Health, Well-being and Social Justice, June. www.chspr.ubc.ca

Evans, R.G., K. McGrail, S. Morgan, M.L. Barer, and C. Hertzman 2001. 'Apocalypse No: Population Aging and the Future of the Health Care System.' *Canadian Journal on Aging* 20, Suppl 1: 160–91. www.chspr.ubc.ca

Feldstein, M.S. 1971. 'A New Approach to National Health Insurance.' *Public Interest* (spring): 93–105.

Finkelstein, M.M. 2001. 'Do Factors Other Than Need Determine Utilization of Physicians' Services in Ontario? *CMAJ* 165, no. 5: 565–70.

Forget, E.L., R. Deber, and L.L. Roos. 2002. 'Medical Savings Accounts: Will They Reduce Costs?' *CMAJ* 167, no. 2 (23 July: 143–7).

Fox, D.M., and P. Fronstin. 2000. 'Public Spending for Health Care Approaches 60 Percent' (Letter). *Health Affairs* 19, no. 2 (March–April): 271–4.

Fuller, S., and L. Stephens. 2002. *Cost Shift: How British Columbians Are Paying for Their Tax Cut.* Vancouver: Canadian Centre for Policy Alternatives.

Gordon, M., J. Mintz, and D. Chen. 1998. 'Funding Canada's Health Care System: A Tax-based Alternative to Privatization.' *CMAJ* 159: 493–6.

Himmelstein, D.U., J. Lewontin, and S. Woolhandler. 1996. 'Who Administers, Who Cares? Medical Administrative and Clinical Employment in the United States and Canada.' *American Journal of Public Health* 86, no. 2: 172–8.

Himmelstein, D.U., and S. Woolhandler. 1986. 'Cost without Benefit: Administrative Waste in U.S. Health Care.' *New England Journal of Medicine.* 314: 441–5.

Hurley, J. 2000. 'Medical Savings Accounts: Approach with Caution. *Journal of Health Services Research and Policy* 5, no. 2: 30–2.

– 2001. 'Parallel Private Health Insurance in Australia: A Cautionary Tale and Lessons for Canada.' Working Paper No. 01: 12, Centre for Health Economics and Policy Analysis, McMaster University, Hamilton, Ont. www.chepa.org

Katz, S.J., K. Cardiff, M. Pascali, M.L. Barer, and R.G. Evans. 2002. 'Phantoms in the Snow: Canadians' Use of Health Care Services in the United States.' *Health Affairs* 21, no. 3: 19–31.

Katz, S.J., R.C. Kessler, R.G. Frank, P. Leaf, and E. Lin. 1997. 'Mental Health Care Use, Morbidity, and Socioeconomic Status in the United States and Ontario.' *Inquiry* 34, no. 1: 38–49.

Kozyrskyj, A., C. Mustard, M. Cheang, and F. Simons. 2001. 'Income-based Drug Benefit Policy: Impact on Receipt of Inhaled Corticosteroid Drugs by Manitoba Children with Asthma.' *CMAJ* 165, no. 7: 1–7.

Levit, K.R., C. Smith, C. Cowan, H. Lazenby, and A. Martin. 2002. 'Inflation Spurs Health Spending.' *Health Affairs* 21, no. 1: 172–87.

Lewis, S.J. 1998. 'Still Here, Still Flawed, Still Wrong: The Case Against the Case for Taxing the Sick.' *CMAJ* 159: 497–9.

Marshall, J.K., P.V. Grootendorst, B.J. O'Brien, L.R. Dolovich, A.M. Holbrook, and A.R. Levy. 2002. 'Impact of Reference-based Pricing for Histamine-2 Receptor Antagonists and Restricted Access for Proton Pump Inhibitors in British Columbia.' *CMAJ* 166, no. 13 (25 June): 1655–62.

McDonald, A.D., J.C. McDonald, V. Salter, and P.E. Enterline. 1974. 'Effects of Quebec Medicare on Physician Consultation for Selected Symptoms.' *New England Journal of Medicine* 291, no. 13: 649–52.

Morgan, S. 1998. 'Quebec's Drug Insurance Plan: A Prescription for Canada?' HPRU Discussion Paper No. 1998: 2D, Centre for Health Services and Policy Research, University of British Columbia, Vancouver. www.chspr.ubc.ca

Mustard, C.A., M.L. Barer, R.G. Evans, J. Horne, T. Mayer, and S. Derksen. 1998b. 'Paying Taxes and Using Health Care Services: The Distributional Consequences of Tax Financed Universal Health Insurance in a Canadian Province.' Presented at the Centre for the Study of Living Standards Conference on the State of Living Standards and the Quality of Life in Canada, Ottawa, 20–31 Oct. www.csls.ca/oct/must1.pdf

Mustard, C.A., M. Shanahan, S. Derksen, et al. 1998a. 'Use of Insured Health Care Services in Relation to Income in a Canadian Province.' In M.L. Barer, T.E. Getzen and G.L. Stoddart, eds., *Health, Health Care and Health Economics: Perspectives on Distribution*, Chichester: John Wiley, 1998, 157–78.

National Forum on Health. 1997. *Canada Health Action: Building on the Legacy: Volume 1*, Final Report of the National Forum on Health. Ottawa.

Oberlander, J. 2002. 'The U.S. Health Care System: On a Road to Nowhere?' *CMAJ* 167, no. 2: 163–8.

OEC (Ontario Economic Council) 1976. *Issues and Alternatives – 1976 Health.* Toronto: Ontario Economic Council.

OECD. 2001. *Health Data 2001* (CD-ROM). Paris: Organization for Economic Co-operation and Development.

Pauly, M.V., P. Danzon, P. Feldstein, and J. Hoff. 1991. 'A Plan for "Responsible National Health Insurance."' *Health Affairs* 10, no. 1: 5–25.

PMPRB. 2002. *Patented Medicine Prices Review Board: Annual Report 2001.* Ottawa: Patented Medicine Prices Review Board.

Rasell, E., J. Bernstein, and K. Tang. 1993. 'The Impact of Health Care Financing on Family Budgets.' Economic Policy Institute Briefing Paper, April. Washington, DC: EPI.

– 1994. 'The Impact of Health Care Financing on Family Budgets.' *International Journal of Health Services* 24, no. 4: 691–714.

Reid, R., R.G. Evans, M.L. Barer, S. Sheps, K. Kerluke, K. McGrail, C. Hertzman, and N. Pagliaccia. 2003. Conspicuous Consumption: Characterizing High Users of Physicians' Services in One Canadian Province.' *Journal of Health Services Research and Policy.*

Reinhardt, U.E. 1992. 'Reflections on the Meaning of Efficiency: Can Efficiency Be Separated from Equity?' *Yale Law and Policy Review* 10, no. 2: 302–15.

Robinson, R. 2002. 'User Charges for Health Care.' In E. Mossialos, A. Dixon, J. Figueras, and J. Kutzin, eds. *Financing Health Care: Options for Europe.* Buckingham: Open University Press, 161–83. www.euro.who.int/document/e74485.pd

Roos, N.P., and N. Frohlich. 2002. Review of D. Gratzer, ed., *Better Medicine: Reforming Canadian Health Care*, Toronto: ECW Press, in *Winnipeg Free Press,* 23 June, D2.

Schaafsma, J. 2002. 'Medical Savings Accounts Costly to Government.' Department of Economics, University of Victoria, Victoria.

Schneeweiss, S., A.M. Walker, R.J. Glynn, M. Maclure, C. Dormuth, and S.B. Soumerai. 2002. 'Outcomes of Reference Pricing for Angiotensin-Converting Enzyme Inhibitors.' *New England Journal of Medicine* 346, no. 11 (14 March): 822–9.

Shiels, J. and P. Hogan. 1999. 'Cost of Tax-exempt Health Benefits in 1998.' *Health Affairs* 18, no. 2: 176–81.

Siemiatycki, J., L. Richardson, and I.B. Pless. 1980. 'Equality in Medical Care under National Health Insurance in Montreal.' *New England Journal of Medicine* 303; no. 1: 10–15.

Smythe, J.G. 2001. 'Tax Subsidization of Employer-Provided Health Care

Insurance in Canada: Incidence Analysis.' Working paper, Department of Economics, University of Alberta, Edmonton, 19 Aug.

Tamblyn, R., R. Laprise, J.A. Hanley, M. Abrahamowicz, S. Scott, N. Mayo, J. Hurley, R. Grad, E. Latimer, R. Perreault, P. McLeod, A. Huang, P. Larochelle, and L. Mallet. 2001. 'Adverse Events Associated with Prescription Drug Cost-Sharing among Poor and Elderly Persons.' *JAMA* 285, no. 4: 421–9.

van Doorslaer, E., A. Wagstaff, and F. Rutten, eds. 1993. *Equity in the Finance and Delivery of Health Care: An International Perspective.* New York: Oxford University Press.

van Doorslaer, E., A. Wagstaff, H. van der Burg, et al. 1999. 'The Redistributive Effect of Health Care: Some Further International Comparisons.' *Journal of Health Economics* 18, no. 3:, 263–90.

Wagstaff, A., E. van Doorslaer, H. van der Burg, et al. 1999. 'Equity in the Finance of Health Care in Twelve OECD Countries.' *Journal of Health Economics* 18, no. 3: 291–14.

Woolhandler, S., and D.U. Himmelstein. 1991. 'The Deteriorating Administrative Efficiency of the U.S. Health Care System.' *New England Journal of Medicine* 324, no. 18: 1253–8.

– 2002. 'Paying for National Health Insurance – and Not Getting It.' *Health Affairs* 21, no. 4 (July–Aug.): 88–98.

Woolhandler, S., D.U. Himmelstein, and J.P. Lewontin. 1993. 'Administrative Costs in U.S. Hospitals.' *New England Journal of Medicine* 329, no. 6 (5 Aug.): 400–4.

Woohandler, S., T. Campbell, and D.U. Himmelstein. 2003. 'Costs of Health Care Administration in the United States and Canada.' *New England Journal of Medicine* 349, no. 8 (21 August): 768–75.

6 Determining the Extent of Public Financing of Programs and Services

CYNTHIA RAMSAY

Public-sector spending accounts for almost 73 per cent of total spending on health and represents about 30 per cent of governments' total revenues in Canada (Canadian Institute for Health Information [CIHI] 2001; Conference Board of Canada 2001). The Conference Board of Canada (2001) projects that public-health expenditures will rise from 31.1 per cent in 2000 to 42.0 per cent by 2020 as a share of total provincial and territorial government revenues, reducing the funding available for other social programs and government initiatives. As well, several other analysts and research organizations are concerned about the financial pressures on the current health-care system: advances in technology, new pharmaceuticals, population ageing, and so on (Baxter 2002; Standing Senate Committee 2002; Baxter and Ramlo 1998; Canadian Institute of Actuaries 1995; 2001). In this context, the goal of the Commission on the Future of Health Care in Canada – a sustainable, high-quality and universal health-care system – must involve an examination of how public health-care funding is allocated and whether the money is 'well spent.'

In general, hospital and physicians' services are government funded, as required by the Canada Health Act (CHA). However, the central concept of the CHA – medical necessity – has not been officially defined, and what is publicly insured varies from province to province, even for services provided in-hospital, such as certain prosthetic devices and crutches (Prince Edward Island Department of Health and Social Services 2001). This may not be problematic in and of itself, but

it begs the question of whether Canada needs a more structured framework for making decisions about financing health care.

This paper examines this question from a macro-level perspective.
The first section provides an overview of health-care services currently
paid for by the public and private sectors in Canada, outlines two
models for setting priorities, and describes how five other countries –
Australia, New Zealand, Singapore, the United Kingdom, and the
United States – deal with financing issues and considers the lessons for
Canada. The second section discusses how public funding of services
is related to the quality, accessibility, and cost of services and to population health. The final section proposes four principles for decisions
on public funding.

Government Funding of Health-Care Services

Current Arrangements

Total health-care spending in Canada is projected to have been almost
$96 billion in 2000 and more than $102 billion in 2001. The public-
sector share of health spending has risen from 70.2 per cent in 1997 to
72.6 per cent in 2001 (CIHI 2001). Table 6.1 outlines the basic structure
of health-care financing in Canada.

Most provinces cover only a portion of the fees charged by chiropractors and other non-physician health-care providers. Only some
pay for hearing aids for certain age groups and coverage of prescription drugs varies. Most provincial insurance plans do not cover acu-
puncture, naturopathy, cosmetic surgery, physical examinations for
employment or insurance purposes, and sterilization reversals. With
respect to these differences, a paper by the National Forum on Health
asked two questions: What is the proper way for provincial insurance
plans to define 'medically necessary'? What standards of evidence
should govern decisions about insuring or not insuring services
(National Forum on Health 1995)?

Since the National Forum on Health, there has not been much movement towards answering these questions and building a framework
for determining core services. However, there have been many methods proposed, and a few provinces have said that they are now going
to be examining this issue seriously.

Most recently, Alberta accepted all the recommendations for reform
proposed by an advisory council. The council states that the CHA was
never designed to cover the full range of health-care services now

Table 6.1
The financing of health-care services in Canada

Service	Method(s) of financing
Hospitals	100 per cent public financing for medically necessary services; private payment for upgraded accommodation or non-medically necessary services provided in hospitals
Private clinics	Privately funded for services not considered medically necessary
Long-term care	Mixed
Home care	Partial public coverage provided in most provinces
Physicians	100 per cent public payment for medically necessary services; majority is paid fee-for-service, with some salary and capitation payments; private payment for non-medically necessary services
Other health-care professionals	Mainly private (insurance and out-of-pocket); some services covered by provincial plans for long-term care or home care
Prescription drugs	Mixed: drugs within hospitals covered by government-allocated hospital budgets; provincial plans pay for a large percentage of drugs dispensed outside hospitals; coverage is typically limited to target populations; balance funded privately
Non-prescription drugs	Private
Dental/optometry care	Mainly private; some provincial plans cover some services for children and seniors
Alternative medicine	Mainly private; limited coverage by some provincial plans
Ambulance services	Partial public coverage in some provinces; special programs for residents in remote areas
Public health programs	Public
First Nations health	Public directly delivers some services

Sources: El Feki 1998, 38; National Forum on Health 1995; Newfoundland Department of Health and Community Services 1999; Prince Edward Island Department of Health and Social Services 2001; Government of New Brunswick 2002; Nova Scotia Department of Health 2001; Government of Quebec 2001; Ontario Ministry of Health and Long-Term Care 2000; Manitoba Health 2002; Saskatchewan Health 2000; Alberta Health and Wellness 2002; British Columbia Ministry of Health 2002.

available; over the years, many new treatments and technologies have been added to the list of insured services. Generally, decisions involve assessment of the technology, analysis of the impact, expert consultations, government review, development of legislation if necessary, review by the legislature or government and implementation. Ultimately, the funding decision is made by the health minister or by the government collectively (Premier's Advisory Council 2001).

As there will probably be continued pressure to add more treatments, programs, and drugs to Alberta's list of insured services, the government needs to reconsider what gets insured and what does not and decide what services could be funded in other ways. One of the council's proposals was for a permanent expert panel to review and make decisions on which health services and treatments should be publicly funded. The panel will start by reviewing the broad categories of services currently provided and deciding which ones should be 'grandfathered' for continued public funding (Premier's Advisory Council 2001).

In Quebec, the Clair Commission also recommended a permanent committee to review and decide which services to insure publicly (Standing Senate Committee 2002). Saskatchewan is also moving to formalize evidence-based funding of health care. Its 2001 action plan supports a new quality council to advise government, develop evidence-based approaches, and promote effective practices throughout the system (Saskatchewan Health 2001).

A rationalization of services is not easy to achieve. Ontario's deinsurance initiative of 1994 illustrates the variety of principles and interests involved in the process. The initiative was part of an agreement between the Ontario Medical Association (OMA) and the Ministry of Health to cut $20 million worth of services in order to keep within the budget allocated to the profession, which had been recently capped. The services for deinsurance were nominated by the OMA and the ministry and reviewed by an ad hoc commission. Because the CHA requires that provinces insure all medically necessary care, the candidates for deinsurance had to seem 'medically unnecessary' in some sense – cosmetic surgery, for example. Additionally, since deinsured services would be privatized, an existing or potential private market helped 'flag' certain choices. It was a difficult process, and there were attempts to include the public in the decision making. None the less, even the chair of the ad hoc commission described the final selection as 'bizarre' (Giacomini 1999, 728–30).

Setting Priorities: Two Models

John Williams and Michael Yeo (2000), ethicists at the Canadian Medical Association (CMA), make a few general suggestions about priority setting in Canada:

- Regional boards and the federal and provincial governments should clarify the values and principles that guide their priority-setting work, as regards both the goals of health and health care and the means for attaining them.
- Decision making at all levels should be 'transparent' and open to scrutiny.
- Public education programs should prepare people to participate in priority setting and to demand accountability from the decision makers. (132)

The CMA's Core and Comprehensiveness Project
The CMA has constructed a decision-making framework for core (publicly funded) health-care services. The association uses the terms *core*, *basic*, and *optional* services, rather than *medically necessary*. It recognizes three key factors to making decisions: quality of care (effectiveness, appropriateness, efficiency, patients' acceptance, and safety), ethics (fairness, age, lifestyle, the identifiable patient versus the statistical patient, and futility), and economics (cost-effectiveness analysis). The CMA states that an ethical process recognizes that decisions are made between patients and physicians, in the community or by society, and by governments. It advocates for public involvement in the decision-making process (Wilson, Rowan, and Henderson 1995; Walters and Morgan 1995; Sawyer and Williams 1995). The CMA first used its model to make recommendations on three clinical issues: prostate specific antigen (PSA) screening, gastroplasty, and the annual physical examination (Deber et al. 1995, part 2).

The Four-Screen Model
The Public/Private Mix in Health Care, by Deber et al. (1995), proposes a four-screen (Deber–Ross) model of prioritizing government financing decisions on health care. Decisions about coverage are made as a function of four screens, with only those interventions passing an earlier screen considered at the next stage, or screen. Screen 1 (effectiveness) examines whether the intervention works. Screen 2 (appropriateness)

incorporates information about the risks and benefits to particular individuals. Screen 3 (informed choice) incorporates the views of recipients of care, and screen 4 (public provision) asks whether a third party should pay for the intervention. This stage involves such factors as minimizing cost, social values, and advancement of knowledge (Deber et al. 1995, part 2).

The model begins at the level of the individual, but implementation is simplified if the model is then aggregated to determine a global budget. Rather than listing procedures covered, the budget is based on an estimation that, for a given population, there should be, for example, approximately X hip replacements, Y cases of diabetes, and Z people with high blood pressure. This model presupposes reform of health-care delivery in Canada (Deber et al. 1995, part 2).

Five Other Countries' Approaches

In all countries, the government plays a significant role in the financing of health care. The programs and services that they fund publicly vary, as does the method of determining financing arrangements. This section looks at publicly covered services in Australia, New Zealand, Singapore, the United Kingdom, and the United States, and how these coverage decisions are made.

Australia

The Commonwealth (national) and state and territorial governments account for about 70 per cent of health in Australia. The Commonwealth government is the primary public insurer of prescription drugs and physicians' services, and it pays for some 50 per cent of hospital expenditures (Standing Senate Committee 2002b, 8).

The Commonwealth's Medicare program provides 'free' treatment to Medicare patients in public hospitals and free or subsidized treatment to patients treated by doctors (and optometrists, or dentists, for some services). Patients may insure with private organizations for the gap between the Medicare benefit (subsidy) and the fees (Ramsay 2001).

Medicare pays benefits for services considered 'clinically relevant,' such as consultation fees for doctors, tests and exams by practitioners to treat illness, eye tests performed by optometrists, and most surgical and therapeutic procedures carried out by doctors. Medicare does not cover such things as dental exams and treatment, ambulance services, home nursing, physiotherapy, chiropractic, glasses and contact lenses, hearing aids, prostheses, medicines, and non–clinically necessary services (Health Insurance Commission 2001).

In what it calls an effort to ease the financial burden on the public health system, the national government has implemented reforms to make private health care more affordable and to increase choice for consumers. Specifically, it encourages the purchase of private health insurance with a 30 per cent refundable tax credit (Australian Department of Health and Aged Care 2000, 4). However, there is debate as to whether tax relief on the purchase of private insurance is an effective use of public funds, as it could cost governments more than it would save them (Standing Senate Committee 2002b, 11; Emmerson, Frayne, and Goodman 2000, 31–2). As well, some observers contend that private insurance or private hospitals result in longer queues in the public system (Standing Senate Committee 2002b, 11–12; Currie 2000).

The government's approach to Medicare is increasingly to fund interventions that are safe, clinically effective, and cost-effective. During 2000–1, it contracted the Quality and Safety Council and the National Institute of Clinical Studies to examine a 'whole of system' approach to quality and safety, focusing on best-practice models for acute care and on the treatment of a range of priority areas. Already, the advisory committees on pharmaceutical benefits and on medicare services have recommended funding for services and medicines proven to be appropriate and effective (Australian Department of Health and Aged Care 2000).

New Zealand

In 1998–9, publicly funded health and disability-support services accounted for around 77.5 per cent of total health expenditures in New Zealand. Individuals may also choose to use private health-care services; the proportion of health expenditure financed privately has risen from 12.0 to 22.5 per cent over the last two decades (New Zealand Ministry of Health 2001b, 12–13).

Most New Zealanders are eligible for publicly funded health and disability services, as they are either permanent or long-term residents. Eligible people may receive free inpatient and outpatient public-hospital services, subsidies on prescription items, and a range of support services to help with disabilities. There is a fee-for-service system for primary care, although visits to the doctor and prescription items are generally free for children under age 6 and basic dental care for children is usually free until age 16. Many people who have to visit doctors frequently or who require a lot of medication may receive a government subsidy (New Zealand Ministry of Health 2001a).

In 2000, the central government transferred decision making to community-focused district health boards (DHBs). It provides broad guidelines on what services the DHBs must provide, and national priorities have been identified in the New Zealand Health Strategy (New Zealand Ministry of Health 2001b).

The national Health Funding Authority is expected to reflect the needs of users and is obliged to consult communities about its plans for the purchase of services. As well, the National Health Committee (NHC), set up in 1992, advises the government on the types of health and disability services that should be publicly funded and their relative priorities, given available resources. Over the years, the NHC has engaged the public in its work, through town-hall meetings, focus groups, and calls for submissions. The NHC even runs a consumer-training program in guidelines development (Edgar 2000).

The NHC's rationing process considers the effectiveness of services, value for money, fairness in access and use, and consistency with communities' values (Edgar 2000). Four assumptions underlie its work:

• Rationing of services is inevitable.
• The processes for making rationing decisions must be 'transparent.'
• Communities must be involved – their values are essential when rationing decisions mean that not everyone will get all the health services they want.
• There are transparent tools – guidelines and priority criteria – that can help decision makers (Edgar 2000, 186).

While there have been few well-designed research studies on NHC initiatives, the committee plans to continue learning how to make difficult choices. Even if total spending on health care were to double, decisions would still be necessary on the margins of funding, and acceptance of such decisions is important (Edgar 2000).

Singapore
Health services in Singapore are provided by three different ministries and by the private sector. In 1999, Singapore spent about 3 per cent of gross domestic product (GDP) on health care; government health spending accounted for 0.8 per cent of GDP (Singapore Ministry of Health 2001, 10).

The Ministry of Health provides preventive, curative, and rehabilitative services; formulates national health policies; co-ordinates planning and development between the public and private health sectors; and regulates health standards (Singapore Ministry of Health 2001). It emphasizes the building of a healthy population through preventive care and the promotion of healthy living. Immunization, health education in schools, and dental services are free (Hsiao 1995).

Primary health care is delivered at government outpatient polyclinics and private medical practitioners' clinics. There is an outpatient consultation fee, which covers medication. At the government polyclinics, all services are subsidized (Hsiao 1995). However, copayments apply even to most heavily subsidized hospital wards and are designed to limit demand by making patients cost-conscious (Ham 1996).

To ensure that basic medical services are available to all Singaporeans, the government also subsidizes medical services at public hospitals and government clinics. The basic medical package is intended to reflect up-to-date medical practice that is cost-effective and of proven value. It excludes non-essential or cosmetic services, experimental drugs, and procedures of unproven value. The goal of the system is to allocate resources in such a manner as to do the most good for the largest number of people (Ham 1996).

Singaporeans are required by law to save for their medical expenses. Under the Medisave scheme, all working persons must set aside 6 to 8 per cent of their income for a personal Medisave account. Singaporeans use this account to help pay for any hospitalization costs for them or their immediate family. In addition, Medishield, a voluntary insurance plan, helps them meet any medical expenses arising from a major accident or prolonged illness. Medishield reimbursements are based on a system of deductibles and co-insurance, and there are claim limits per policy year and per lifetime. As well, Medifund, an endowment fund set up by the government, helps low-income citizens pay for medical care. The amount of help given to a patient depends on individual circumstances and is decided by a committee at the hospital level (Ramsay 2001).

The government has also introduced low-cost community hospitals for the convalescent sick and elderly not requiring the more expensive care of the acute general hospitals. Health-care services for the elderly are mostly in the hands of government-subsidized voluntary welfare organizations. Most support services to hospital and primary-health-care programs exist in both the public and private sectors (Singapore Ministry of Health 2001).

The United Kingdom

The National Health Service (NHS) is the main provider of health care in the United Kingdom. Its ideal is universal coverage for all citizens, paid for from general tax revenues. But initial cost estimates for the NHS were soon exceeded, and fees were added for such services as prescriptions and dental care. However, today, about 85 per cent of prescriptions are dispensed to people who are exempt from the charges (British Medical Association [BMA] 1999).

About 11 per cent of the population have private medical insurance (Ramsay 2001). Direct payment for elective surgery in the private sector accounts for about 19 per cent of private treatment, and the sector also provides the majority of places in residential and nursing homes (BMA 1999).

Despite cost pressures on the system, the NHS's 10-year modernization plan (*The NHS Plan*) rejects the suggestion that the NHS should cover only a defined set of individual conditions or treatments: 'First, advocates of this position usually have great difficulty specifying what they would rule out. The sorts of treatments that commonly feature include varicose veins, wisdom teeth extraction or cosmetic procedures. The problem is that these sorts of services account for less than 0.5 percent of the NHS budget, and are not major cost-drivers for the future. Instead, the vast majority of spending – and spending increases – go on childbirth, elderly care and major conditions such as cancer, heart disease and mental health problems' (United Kingdom Department of Health 2001, chap. 3). The other reason given for not restricting spending to a defined set of core services is that effectiveness is subjective: different patients under different circumstances can derive different benefits from the same treatment.

However, *The NHS Plan* acknowledges that priorities are necessary. The National Institute for Clinical Excellence, with the aid of a Citizens Council, provides guidance on the clinical and cost-effectiveness of new and existing health technologies, including medications (United Kingdom Department of Health 2001). While the context for ranking decisions is national, local health authorities make many choices, and, more often, individual physicians do the rationing implicitly by applying clinical judgment to individual cases (BMA 1999).

The United States
Medicare/Medicaid. The U.S. federal government runs two main health-care programs. Medicare covers the elderly (aged 65 and over) and the disabled; Medicaid provides health insurance and services for lower-income Americans. Medicare covers more than 39 million people, and Medicaid, 36 million (Health Care Financing Administration [HCFA] 2001a; c). In 1997, the public sector accounted for 46.4 per cent of total spending on health care (Ramsay 2001).

Medicare reimburses the elderly for their health-care expenses. Among seniors, 98.6 per cent are in Medicare, and most (70 per cent) have both Medicare and additional private insurance for other costs (Ramsay 2001). Medicare Part A is hospital insurance that pays for part of inpatient hospital care, critical-access hospitals, skilled nursing facilities, hospice care, and some home care. Part B is optional and covers medically necessary doctors' services, outpatient hospital care, and some services that Part A does not cover, such as the services of physical and occupational therapists. For both parts, there are premiums, deductibles, and copayments.

State governments contribute to Medicaid and also fund such items as public health services (for example, immunizations and Native health), community-based services (for example, mental-health and substance-abuse services), state university–based teaching hospitals, and state employees' health premiums. As Medicaid is a joint federal–state program, its benefits and eligibility requirements vary from state to state. Coverage is available not to all low-income people, but to those who are considered by the various state definitions to be 'categorically' or 'medically' needy; most states fund assistance programs for specified poor persons who do not qualify for Medicaid (Standing Senate Committee 2002a, 48). Nominal deductibles and cost sharing are in effect for some Medicaid recipients for certain services, but exemptions from cost sharing include pregnant women and children under 18 (HCFA 2001b).

In general, basic Medicaid coverage must include inpatient and outpatient hospital services, physicians' services, surgical dental services, nursing-facility services and home health care for some individuals, family-planning services and supplies, rural clinic and ambulance services, laboratory and X-ray services, and periodic screening. The most commonly covered optionals include clinic services, intermediate-care facility/mentally-ill services, optometrists' services and eyeglasses, prescribed drugs, prosthetic devices, and dental services (HCFA 2001b).

The HCFA, now renamed the Centers for Medicare and Medicaid Services, track emerging technologies and patterns of care to determine the need to change national coverage policies. In making these decisions, the HCFA considers whether an item or service demonstrates medical benefit and added value (in terms of either more health benefits or lower cost) to what is already covered for the Medicare population (HCFA 2001d). It uses the internet to inform people about how coverage decisions are made and the progress of each issue under coverage review (HCFA 2001e).

Oregon. The Oregon Health Plan (OHP) provides insurance coverage for some one million low-income residents, but an estimated 400,000 remain without health coverage (Oregon Health Services Commission 2001a).

The OHP is the only state Medicaid program that explicitly rations medical care, funding services using various measures of value. In broad terms, covered services include diagnosis, physicians' services, medical and dental check-ups, family-planning services, maternity, prenatal, and newborn care, prescriptions, hospital services, comfort care and hospices, dental services, alcohol and drug treatment, and mental-health services. It does not cover services for conditions that will get better on their own, conditions that have no useful treatment, treatments that are not generally effective, cosmetic surgeries, gender changes, treatment for infertility, and weight-loss programs (Office of Medical Assistance Programs 2001).

There is a priority list of 736 medical conditions and their related treatments. As of October 2001, government funding included 566 of these condition–treatment pairs. Table 6.2 indicates the complexity of the funding list.

The impetus to rank procedures came in 1987, when the state de-insured transplants for Medicaid patients. As a consequence, a boy needing a bone-marrow transplant died before his family could raise enough private money for the procedure. The incident led to public outrage and a more systematic and evidence-informed method of rationing.

The initial process involved ranking health services by their value to the community and their cost-effectiveness. Multiple rankings were required before the end result was achieved. In later stages, analysts

Table 6.2
Selected services covered by the Oregon Health Plan as of October 2001

Ranking	Diagnosis	Treatment
Government-funded services include:		
1	Severe/moderate head injury: hematoma/edema with loss of consciousness	Medical and surgical treatment
2	Type I diabetes mellitus	Medical therapy
565	Symptomatic urticaria	Medical therapy
566	Dysfunction of nasolacrimal system	Medical and surgical treatment
Government funding does not include:		
567	Chronic anal fissure, anal fistula	Sphincterectomy, fissurectomy, fistulectomy, medical therapy
568	Dental conditions (ex. broken appliances)	Periodontics and complex prosthetics
735	Spastic dysphonia	Medical therapy
736	Disorders of refraction and accommodation	Radial keratotomy

Source: Oregon Health Services Commission 2001b.

ranked finer categories (eventually diagnosis–treatment pairs) according to an algorithm that used criteria including cost-effectiveness, public opinions of service types and health states, and expert opinions of the ranks produced. Eventually, 17 categories were developed and then ranked by a state-appointed Health Services Commission. They covered more than 10,000 medical procedures, which were reduced to 709 diagnosis–treatment pairs.

Oregon's efforts to rationalize the Medicaid benefit package met with lobbying by providers and consumers who wanted to protect their own favoured services from rationing. Lobbyists proscribed or delayed the addition of particular services; for example, most psychiatric care stayed out of the ranking. Excluded services accounted for about 70 per cent of Medicaid spending, leaving 30 per cent of the budget to be controlled by the priority-setting process (Giacomini 1999, 725–6). 'Because Oregon [in the end] did not ration care based on cost-effectiveness, their basic benefits package fails to maximize health outcomes to Medicaid recipients' (Tengs 1996, 181).

The central idea behind the OHP was that, given fiscal limits, it is better to provide some health insurance for everyone rather than covering only some people for everything. However, the benefits package today is more generous than Oregon's old Medicaid system, and costs for the OHP have grown over the last decade (Oregon Health Services Commission 2001).

Other States. Other U.S. states have tried alternative methods of expanding public coverage of health services to the uninsured. For example, Massachusetts created a basic option for the non-categorical needy called MassHealth. New York's Healthy New York package is for small businesses that do not provide health insurance for their employees and for working, uninsured individuals. Washington's Basic Health Plan gives low-income residents a choice between a managed care–style plan and a less managed plan with higher out-of-pocket costs. Minnesota's MinnesotaCare has a basic benefit that includes single adults without dependent children; initially offering only outpatient services, it recently added inpatient services (Oregon Health Services Commission 2001a).

Despite such efforts, in 2000, 14 per cent of Oregon's, 9 per cent of Massachusetts's, 15 per cent of New York's residents were uninsured, 14 per cent of Washington's and 8 per cent of Minnesota's; the national figure was 14 per cent (Kaiser Family Foundation 2002). As well, there is some evidence that programs to insure low-income adults publicly might not be increasing overall coverage, but rather crowding out private. A study of the expansion of public insurance in four states found that the programs in Oregon and Washington 'resulted in a decline in the number of uninsured and very little crowding out of private insurance,' whereas Tennessee saw 'a decrease in the number of both uninsured persons and privately insured persons,' and Minnesota, 'a decline in the number of privately insured persons and virtually no change in that of uninsured persons' (Kronick and Gilmer 2002, 225).

There seems to be no correlation between how much a state spends on health care and the extent of insurance coverage. State health-care expenditures per capita averaged U.S.$872.64 in 1999: Minnesota ($807.83) and Oregon ($774.18) spent less than the national average, while New York ($1,615.64) and Massachusetts ($1,455.21) were the top two spenders in the country (Kaiser Family Foundation 2002).

Lessons for Canada

Many other industrialized countries have been dealing explicitly with the rationing of health-care services for years. The methods vary from drafting a specific list of services with public involvement (Oregon), through having a national committee make the main decisions, with some public input (United States, United Kingdom, and Australia), through the government's making the decisions, with little public input (Singapore), to the use of guidelines (New Zealand).

All of the above countries have found that it is impossible to set health-care priorities systematically from cost–benefit analysis alone. As well, the delisting of health services is unlikely to produce substantial savings. In both Oregon and New Zealand, explicit priority setting resulted in more services being covered rather than fewer (Coulter and Ham 2000). In the Netherlands, delisting services (long-term in-vitro fertilization, cosmetic surgery, eyeglasses, homeopathic drugs, dental care for those over 18, and several other items) saved the government 4.5 per cent (Williams 1997).

If major savings are a goal of government, delisting is not enough. The prioritizing process, however, is a good way to finance and ensure universal access to interventions that best meet people's needs: 'It is also a matter of equity: in contrast to actuarial private insurance, where every purchaser buys the expected value of the health services needed, public finance is involuntary. It comes from the taxpayers who have a legitimate interest in meeting needs and thereby getting value for their money, but not necessarily in paying for wants' (Musgrove 1996, 56).

The rationale for encouraging democratic deliberation of rationing is that choices in health care involve moral issues, and, more pragmatically, legal challenges to rationing decisions will probably increase, reinforcing the need to make the decision-making process fair and transparent (Coulter and Ham 2000).

Norman Daniels believes that legitimizing limit setting requires what he calls accountability for reasonableness – public access to the rationale for decisions and reasons relevant to meeting the population's health needs with limited resources (Daniels 2000). There are four necessary (but not sufficient) conditions to be met (92):

• *Publicity.* Decisions regarding coverage for new technologies (and other limit-setting decisions) and their rationales must be publicly accessible.

- *Reasonableness*. Rationales for coverage decisions should present a reasonable construal of how the organization should provide 'value for money' in meeting the varied health needs of a defined population under reasonable resource constraints.
- *Appeals*. There must be a mechanism for challenge and dispute resolution regarding limit-setting decisions, including the opportunity to revise decisions in the light of further evidence or arguments.
- *Enforcement*. There must be either voluntary or public regulation of the process to ensure that the first three conditions are met.

Measuring Results: Access, Quality, Cost, and Population Health Status

One of the main purposes of a health-care system is to improve the health of the population, ideally by providing broad access to quality care at a manageable cost. Since Canada's system is mainly publicly funded, it is necessary to discuss what is known about how public financing of services affects their accessibility, quality, and cost. As well, there must be discussion of whether the method of financing health care matters in the pursuit of better population health status.

Deber and colleagues summarized conventional thought in Canada about the financing of health care: 'It is widely recognized that divorcing access to a comprehensive mix of health services from ability to pay inherent in public financing enhances equity. As one moves along the public/private continuum to include more private sector involvement, equity decreases. At the extreme, one has the U.S. system, in which a large proportion of the American public is either uninsured or underinsured for health care' (Deber et al. 1995, part 1).

This argument implies that it is private-sector involvement that decreases equity rather than the fact of individuals' being uninsured, publicly or privately. Being uninsured in the United States does not mean that a person will be denied care when he or she needs it. (By law, neither public nor private hospitals may turn away an indigent patient. For more information, go to www.medlaw.com.) As well, statistics show that many of the uninsured are only temporarily so. For example, the uninsured rate in Minnesota is about 8 per cent, but it declines to 3.1 per cent if one considers people who were uninsured for the entire year of 2001 (Minnesota Department of Health 2002).

However, there are differences in the use of health-care services by the insured and the uninsured and in their health outcomes. For example, uninsured children in the United States were 2.5 times as likely as children with health insurance to be without a recent visit to a physician in 1995–6 (National Center for Health Statistics 1999). As well, from an analysis of 125 peer-reviewed research papers, the Oregon Health Services Commission (2001) concluded that uninsurance is associated with increased mortality (for example, diagnosis of disease at a late and incurable stage); more pain, disability, and suffering (for example, uninsured children are less likely to receive treatment for sore throats, earaches, and asthma); and expensive care (for example, the uninsured are more likely to use the emergency room for care).

Universal insurance, then, is a desirable goal. But there are myriad ways of insuring an entire population, and basic health-status measures, such as life expectancy and infant mortality, do not indicate that one method is particularly better or worse at reducing inequities in health. In Canada, for example, there seems to be queue jumping for non-medical reasons, and evidence suggests that family physicians are not referring the sick and elderly as readily as they should for such treatments as kidney dialysis (Gratzer 1999, 24 and 43). As well, in attempting to balance their fiscal situations, many provincial governments have delisted services, resulting in more people paying for needed services. If having to pay for care is inherently unfair to people with lower incomes, then this 'cost-saving' measure represents increasing inequity in the Canadian system.

Access

In terms of access, there are many studies that seem to indicate that patients wait longer for care in Canada than in countries such as the United States, Sweden, and Germany, but less time than in the United Kingdom and New Zealand.

A study in the 1980s found that Canadians waited longer than Americans for orthopaedic consultation and for surgery (Coyte et al. 1994). Research in the 1990s showed Canadians waiting longer than Americans and Germans for several cardiac procedures (Collins-Nakai, Huysmans, and Skully 1992). According to a 1992 study, Canadians generally waited longer for heart bypasses than Americans or Swedes, but less time than the British (Carroll et al. 1995), and a research project in 1998 indicated that Canadians had shorter waiting times than New Zealanders for bypasses (Jackson, Doogue, and Elliott 1999). Research at Dalhousie University revealed that proper follow-up and diagnosis for patients with gross haematuria (bloody urine) took longer in Canada than in the United States (Moulton 1998).

In the early 1990s the Queen's University Radiation Oncology Research Unit discovered that, for all but emergency care, Canadian patients waited longer for radiation treatment of cancer than did their American counterparts and longer than oncologists considered medically acceptable (Mackillop 1994). A recent report on cancer care by the Cancer Advocacy Coalition (2001) warns that long waiting lists for radiation and the slow approval of new chemotherapy drugs decrease patients' survival and shows that Canadian provinces tend to have higher mortality rates for cancer than American states.

As well, the situation in Canada does not seem to be improving. In an investigation of almost 30,000 breast-surgery patients in Quebec, the median waiting times between diagnosis and surgery rose from 29 days in 1992 to 42 days in 1998 (Mayo et al. 2001). An update for 1998–9 of an audit by the Manitoba Centre for Health Policy and Evaluation of waiting times for eight non-urgent surgical procedures in Winnipeg from 1992 to 1997 detected later increases in the waiting times of six of the eight procedures, including breast-tumour removal and carotid endarterectomies (Currie 2000). While the authors do not draw any conclusions, they note that the trend is of concern.

The Canadian system, which is intended to provide equal access to care, may not be doing so. Low-income people seem less likely to visit medical specialists (Dunlop, Coyte, and McIsaac 2000), and appear to have lower survival rates for cardiac problems (Alter et al. 1999) and cancer (Mackillop et al. 1997).

In 2000, the Canadian Association of Radiologists released a report suggesting that 63 per cent of Canada's X-ray equipment is out of date, as are the majority of diagnostic machines (Canadian Association of Radiologists 2000). Of 25 OECD countries, Canada ranked 19th in terms of magnetic resonance imagers (MRIs) per million people (Esmail 2001). Of 23 OECD members, Canada stood 18th in computed tomography (CT) scans per million people (Esmail 2001). For health-care services (hospital beds, physicians, and other resources), it ranked 5th of eight countries, having more resources available than the United Kingdom, Singapore, and South Africa, for example, but fewer than Germany, Switzerland, the United States, and Australia (Ramsay 2001).

At minimum, such findings challenge the belief that a publicly funded system that prohibits private financing of medically essential services necessarily provides greater and more equal access than one that allows public and private funding. There are problems in Canada and the United Kingdom with waiting lists and survival rates for certain illnesses, for example, but there are Americans who go without health care because of its cost.

A recent survey looked at patients' views on access, quality, and costs of care in Australia, Canada, New Zealand, the United Kingdom, and the United States. The United Kingdom had the largest share of the population waiting four months or more for elective surgery, while Canada had the only statistically significant increase in the number of people waiting four months or more for treatment between 1998 and 2001. However, Canadians and Britons were much less likely to report going without medical care because of costs than were adults in Australia, New Zealand, and the United States (Blendon et al. 2002).

Quality

There are few, if any, indications that can point to whether publicly or privately funded health care is better or worse for a population's health. For example, Toronto's Institute for Clinical Evaluative Sciences in 1999 concluded, after examining some 18 studies of health outcomes in Canada and the United States, that 'none of these studies proved that differences in health outcomes were due solely to differences in the health-care systems of these two countries. As a result, formulation of a distinct hypothesis regarding the relationship(s) between quality of care of each distinct health-care system and outcomes in comparison to each other is unlikely' (Szick et al. 1999, 17).

In the five-country survey mentioned above, respondents in all nations rated physicians' care as excellent or very good. For hospital care, a majority in every country except Britain rated care as excellent or very good. Canadians and Americans with lower incomes were less likely than those with higher incomes to rate their care as excellent or very good; the opposite was true for Britons (Blendon et al. 2002).

In *World Health Report 2000*, the World Health Organization (WHO) (2000) ranked the performance of health-care systems around the world in terms of three goals: good health, responsiveness to people's expectations, and fairness of financial contribution (how much people pay out-of-pocket). In the comparison of overall system performance, Canada ranked better than countries such as the United States and Australia but worse than France, Italy, Singapore, the United Kingdom, Germany, and 20-plus other countries. Being a first attempt at ranking health systems, this document has debatable methodological aspects, and this complex and lengthy report gives no indication that any one country's health-care was unambiguously better than another's. However, the ranking should at least cause people to question whether Canada's system as it stands should be sacrosanct or if Canadians cannot learn from how other countries organize their systems.

Cost

Deber and colleagues state a common view in Canada: 'From both international and Canadian evidence, [is the finding] that exclusive public financing of medically necessary care is also the most economically efficient method. Efficiency is increased through the state's monopsony power over the control of total budgets and over fee and salary negotiations with providers, and through minimizing cost shifting and risk selection. Case studies of Canadian experience reveal that cost escalation is higher in those areas of health care with greater roles for private financing (e.g. drugs, automobile insurance, travel health insurance) than those with public financing and monopsony control (e.g. hospitals). ... The only justification for the mixed financing plans is that they may provide enhanced consumer and provider choice (liberty)' (Deber et al. 1995).

While there is some evidence that governments can increase the efficiency of health-care markets because there are social returns to health, asymmetric information, and other market failures, there is little, if any, evidence that 'exclusive' public financing of medically necessary services is the most economically efficient method. As well, there has been documentation of government failures that are as serious as market failures: poor public accountability, information asymmetry, abuse of monopoly power, and failure to provide public goods (Harding and Preker 2000).

Dr Ake Blomqvist told the Standing Senate Committee on Social Affairs, Science and Technology (2002a, 68): 'If cost containment is a main objective, there would seem to be a prima facie case for extending public sector coverage to encompass a broader range of benefits, for example, by introducing a system of publicly funded Pharmacare, as suggested by the National Forum on Health.' While countries with publicly funded systems *may* be able to control costs by brute force – capping physicians' fees, closing hospitals, and delisting services, for example – better than nations that rely more on private financing, their systems are not necessarily less expensive. Canada spends more on health care than most industrialized countries, all of which allow private-sector financing of medically necessary services.

As well, a recent comparison published in the *British Medical Journal* of Britain's publicly funded National Health Service with California's private, non-profit Kaiser Permanente showed that the per-capita costs of the two systems, adjusted for such aspects as differences in benefits and population characteristics, were similar to within 10 per cent. But Kaiser members experienced more comprehensive and convenient primary-care services and much faster access to specialists' services and hospitals. Kaiser's superior access, quality, and cost performance were attributed to better system integration, more efficient management of hospital use, the benefits of competition, and greater investment in information technology (Feachem, Sekhri, and White 2002).

The struggles faced by Canada's system are numerous: waiting lists, emergency room back-ups, a lack of high-tech medical equipment, limits on newer pharmaceutical treatments, and low provider morale. Many of these issues arise because health care in Canada is organized mainly as a function of government, and therefore increasing costs are problematic. By continuing to demand 'exclusive' public financing of medically necessary services, the federal government is potentially harming Canadians' health and the sector's future prospects (Ramsay and Walker 1996). For such reasons, not only for 'enhanced consumer and provider choice,' mixed financing plans make sense.

Public or Private Financing and Population Health Status

Beyond the Public–Private Debate: An Examination of Quality, Access and Costs in the Health-Care Systems of Eight Countries (Ramsay 2001) reported that, of the many possible determinants, income per capita and literacy have the strongest relationship to health status. Immunization rates are also important. The document concludes that government intervention should focus on (given scarce resources) assuring universal access to and the availability of preventive and basic primary care, even increasing their availability. Beyond this, they should work to ensure that people who cannot afford medical services have access to care when they need it, and they should perhaps require citizens to purchase health insurance for catastrophic events (Ramsay 2001).

World Health Report 2000 states that 'scientific and technical progress ... explained almost half of the reduction in mortality between 1960 and 1990 in a sample of 115 low- and middle-income countries, while income growth explained less than 20 percent and increases in the educational level of adult females less than 40 percent' (WHO 2000, 9). In Europe, the report claims, much of the increase in life expectancy has been the result of modern medical care. But health systems do little to improve health: studies have correlated life expectancy with income per capita but not with numbers of doctors, hospital beds, or health expenditure. And while 'rich' people tend to benefit more from the use of hospital and primary-care services, 'the distribution of primary care is almost always more beneficial to the poor than hospital care.'

None the less, the report advocates for all countries – developed and developing – a universal, publicly financed health system that encompasses everything from road safety through prevention to surgery. 'The ideal is largely to disconnect a household's financial contribution to the health-care system from its health risks and separate it almost entirely from the use of needed services' (36). However, there are extensive studies that show that completely disconnecting use and costs is not necessary to ensuring good health.

One of the most comprehensive studies of health insurance is that of the RAND Corporation (Newhouse 1993). More than 7,000 non-elderly families from six U.S. regions were assigned to different insurance plans and monitored for three to five years. All the plans had a limit on out-of-pocket expenditure and ranged from free care (no coinsurance) to a variety of user-pay plans (with different coinsurance rates for different services). *Total* expenditure for the high-coinsurance group (95 per cent) was well below that of the free-care group (Ramsay 1998). However, the RAND study concluded that the increased use of services by the free-care group had little or no measurable effect on health status and that there was no significant difference between the groups in risk of dying or in measures of pain and worry. In only one instance was the free-care plan better, and that was for low-income people with high blood pressure. However, a 'one-time screening examination achieved most of the gain in blood pressure that free care achieved' (Gratzer 1999, 124–5).

While the RAND report implies that targeted public interventions might be preferable to universal coverage, other analyses, believing the practice ineffective, discount the idea of targeting low-income individuals or even specific diseases (Deaton 2002). Angus Deaton writes, 'It is time that the educational debate was more cognizant of health benefits. As for income, there is a very strong case in poor countries, and among the poor in rich countries, for whom nutrition, nutritional-linked disease and poor housing are important determinants of adult and child health ... [that] a policy of income provision to the poor may well be more effective than spending the same amount of public funds on a weak health-care delivery system' (27–8). Another study discusses the 'fact that many of the conditions driving the need for [acute care] are preventable ought to draw attention to policy opportunities for promoting health' (McGinnis, Williams-Russo, and Knickman 2002, 78).

Results such as these explain why all other industrialized nations have some type of private financing of services considered medically necessary in Canada. Austrian ambulatory patients pay a quarterly fee for physicians' services; inpatients, a fixed fee for all medication. There is a fixed daily fee for Belgian inpatients for all medication received. Germany levies a fixed 'hotel' fee but exempts inpatients from other copayments. Switzerland has an annual deductible for ambulatory care and a fixed daily rate for inpatient stays (National Economic Research Associates 2001).

Most advanced countries attempt to mitigate the potential harmful effects of such cost-sharing measures, which include potential redistribution of income from the poor and sick to the healthy and wealthy and lower use of health services by and worse health status for people with lower incomes. Many studies, going years back, indicate that cost-sharing mechanisms, such as user fees, can harm certain populations (see, for example, Beck 1974; Roemer et al. 1975; Beck and Horne 1980; Evans 1993; and Ramsay 1998).

Because of these types of concerns, an alternative to traditional forms of cost sharing – and one that would maintain the integrity of the Canada Health Act's five principles – has been recommended by some health-care policy analysts and by Alberta's advisory council: medical savings accounts (MSAs). Proponents believe that transferring most of the coverage decisions to individuals and allowing an expanded role for the private sector will make the system more efficient and cost-effective at delivering care, while broadening coverage of services for all citizens. An in-depth discussion of the pros and cons of MSAs is beyond the scope of this paper; however, there are several detailed presentations on how MSAs work in other countries and how they could work in Canada. (See, for example, Standing Senate Committee 2002a; Premier's Advisory Council on Health for Alberta 2001; Gratzer 1999; Litow and Muller 1998; Ramsay 1998; and Massaro and Wong 1996.)

Four Principles for Determining the Extent of Public Financing

Clarify the Purpose of the Health System

'A public health-care system is not there simply to maximize the amount of health in society (however we choose to measure health). It is not there merely to treat disease (however we choose to define disease). It is not there solely to meet health-care needs (however we choose to define health-care needs). And it is not there to ensure equality in health status (however we choose to conceptualize equality). The goal of a public health-care system is a complex composite of a range of goals. It becomes impossible to use a simple maximizing algorithm as a basis for the priority-setting system' (Holm 2000, 31–2).

There are interventions that maintain function at high cost (such as organ transplants), interventions that enhance quality of life (such as Viagra), heroic but marginally effective technologies (such as high-dose chemotherapy), and advances in genetic diagnosis and treatment (Clancy and Danis 2000). As well, observers have associated numerous non-medical factors with health status, such as housing, income, and education. There needs to be agreement on the priorities of the health system.

Decide Which Services to Evaluate

The rationing process produces trade-offs that cut along divisions created by budget structures (fee schedules), institutionalized interests (clinical specialties), ideology (personal versus collective responsibility for illness and care), and information (available evaluation research) (Giacomini 1999). Therefore decision makers should consider the following five questions about each trade-off before proceeding to the evaluation stage (750–1):

- *What is it?* Interventions and technologies with a given label (for

example, heart transplant, prenatal care) may have many manifesta-
tions of practice, function, and effects.

- *What is it for?* At issue may be not the effectiveness of the service, but
  some less tractable question about the medicalization of problems or
  the legitimacy of recipients' needs. Services must be considered in
  terms of public-policy goals and values.
- *How is it situated?* Interventions can be interdependent; restricting
  one may affect another.
- *Whose is it?* Services/technologies have constituencies of innovators,
  marketers, users, and beneficiaries who may influence elements of
  the assessment, such as deciding whether a technology is exempt
  from scrutiny.
- *Who is it for?* The more narrowly defined a technology's boundaries,
  the more burden falls on users to supply the supporting structures
  that make it 'work.' For example, many innovations have not been
  tested on (or adapted to) women.

Evaluate Cost-Effectiveness and Relevance of Programs and Services

Most countries use some form of cost-effectiveness analysis to determine which services to cover publicly. Increasingly, they are also evaluating the relevance of particular services to their system's goals: 'The
most crucial – and controversial – question for evidence-based coverage policy concerns the adequacy of evidence ... One policy is to cover
an intervention unless there is compelling evidence that it is more
harmful than beneficial ... Another standard is the 'best guess': cover if
the preponderance of evidence, whether extensive or meagre, suggests
that the technology is beneficial ... Judging the adequacy of evidence is
often subjective' (Garber 2001, 66–7).

In the United Kingdom, practitioners involved in the priority-setting
process make a judgment about the effectiveness of an intervention if
good-quality evidence is unavailable. In New Zealand, consensus panels of expert professionals and community people are involved in decisions about the effectiveness of some treatments (Edgar 2000). Most
evidence-based coverage processes are flexible, balancing the need for
rigour against limitations in medical knowledge (Garber 2001).

Another concern is that priority-funding lists provide a very diverse
mix of services, and it is often difficult to evaluate the implications in
practice of the trade-offs presented. For example, Oregon covers services relating to treating diabetes, newborn care, and medical therapy

for psoriasis, but not treatment of sexual dysfunction or cancer treatments with little potential to improve chances of survival (Oregon Health Services Commission 2001b).

As well, cost-effectiveness criteria are not generally sufficient to determine whether to insure a health service publicly: 'lifestyle drugs,' such as Viagra, are a case in point. Viagra has been shown to be effective in treating the symptoms of erectile dysfunction in men. However, even if many patients benefited in quality of life, are Canadians willing to close a cardiac surgery unit, for example, in order to fund Viagra publicly (Ferguson 2002b)? In the United Kingdom, Viagra is available from the NHS only for certain clinical conditions. Decision makers there have decided that the NHS is not obliged to subsidize this drug for everyone who might benefit; they have determined that Viagra, in most cases, is not *relevant* to a publicly funded, universal service (New 2000).

Involve the Public

Most Canadians agree strongly with the concept of a mainly publicly funded health-care system and with the principles of the Canada Health Act. However, their support for increased public spending on health care is conditional on the system's being made more efficient, effective, and accountable; they support reducing the scope of coverage if necessary (Vail 2001). As well, 30 to 50 per cent of Canadians are willing to consider options that allow increased private delivery and financing of health care either to preserve the public system or to ensure access to quality care (Vail 2001).

The *Medical Post* reported survey results showing that Canadians are not interested in 'dumping more money in to make the pie bigger,' but 'the idea that governments should fund all health services proven to improve health or quality of life received 90 percent approval' (Milne 2001). As to what these services should be, Canadians favoured diagnostic services, such as MRIs, acute care, long-term care, home and community care, and illness prevention. Lower on the list were health promotion, prescription medications, end-of-life care, and public health.

There are many potential areas for public involvement in the rationing process: for example, in articulating the ethos and values of the system, in deciding which health-care services/treatments should be publicly provided, in determining which groups should receive priority (elderly versus young?), and in figuring out where to locate health-service provision (institution versus community?) (Mullen 2000). One challenge will be to educate citizens on the cost-effectiveness of various programs and services. As the *Medical Post* survey indicated, many Canadians perceive universal access to acute care to be more valuable than access to public health. The importance of perception was evident in Oregon, where the initial deinsurance of organ transplantation was based on the popular belief that transplants are only marginally beneficial. Another common way of cursorily differentiating services is newness versus oldness: transplants and infertility treatments, for example, are included in almost every priority-setting exercise (Giacomini 1999).

Another challenge will be to manage effectively the various lobby groups in Canada. Practitioners – chiropractors and massage therapists, in British Columbia's most recent delisting exercise, for instance – have protested decreased public funding of the services that they provide. Hospital employees have raised concerns over initiatives to provide auxiliary services privately. Physicians and hospitals have resisted attempts to cap their budgets. Local residents have complained loudly when a hospital is closed in their area. These are but a few of the many groups that place demands on limited public funds.

The reasonableness and transparency of the approach to rationing are most important. The public can participate in varying degrees, but, at the least, the information and criteria informing priority-setting decisions must be readily available. Once funding decisions have been made – which procedures to cover, or which practice guidelines to implement – individuals (patients, providers, and those directly affected by the policy/choice) must have the right to challenge the decisions.

REFERENCES

Alberta Health and Wellness. 2002. *Alberta Health Care Insurance Plan/Benefits.* 31 May. www.health.gov.ab.ca/ahcip/benefits.htm, 12 June 2002.
Alter, David A., et al. 1999. 'Effects of Socioeconomic Status on Access to Invasive Cardiac Procedures and on Mortality after Acute Myocardial Infarction.' *New England Journal of Medicine* 341: 1359–67.
Angus Reid Group. 1997. *Canadians' Perceptions of the Health Allowance System: Key Findings.* Oct. www.nextcity.com/cpi/empowerment/Arkeyfindings. html, 28 Dec. 2001.

Arnold, Tom. 2001. 'Majority Open to Mix of Public, Private Health,' *National Post Online*, 13 July. www.nationalpost.com/, 24 July 2001.

Australian Department of Health and Aged Care. 2000. *Portfolio Budget Statements, 2001–2*, 9 May. www.health.gov.au, 29 January 2002.

– 2002. *Medicare Benefits Branch Home Page*, 18 Jan. www.health.gov.au/haf/branch/mbb/index.htm, 28 January 2002.

Baxter, David. 2002. 'Population Matters: Demographics and Health Care in Canada.' In David Gratzer, ed., *Better Medicine: Reforming Canadian Health Care*. Toronto: ECW Press, 135–72.

Baxter, David, and Andrew Ramlo. 1998. *Healthy Choices: Demographics and Health Spending in Canada, 1980 to 2035*. Vancouver: Urban Futures Institute.

Beck, R.G. 1974. 'The Effects of Co-payment on the Poor.' *Journal of Human Resources* 9: 129–42.

Beck, R.G., and J.M. Horne. 1980. 'Utilization of Publicly Insured Health Services in Saskatchewan, during and after Copayment.' *Medical Care* 18, No. 8: 787–806.

Blendon, Robert J., et al. 2002. 'Inequities in Health Care: A Five-Country Survey.' *Health Affairs* 21, no. 3: 182–91.

Brimacombe, Glenn G., Pedro Antunes, and Jane McIntyre. 2001. *The Future Cost of Health Care in Canada, 2000 to 2020: Balancing Affordability and Sustainability*. Ottawa: Conference Board of Canada.

British Columbia Ministry of Health and Ministry Responsible for Seniors. 2002. *Medical and Health Care Benefits*, 6 May. www.healthservices.gov.bc.ca/msp/infoben/benefits.html, 12 June 2002.

British Medical Association (BMA). 1999. *Healthcare Funding Review*. Dec. web.bma.org.uk/public/polsreps.nsf/htmlpagesvw/hcfund, 28 January 2002.

Bureau of TennCare. 2002. *Tennessee Enrolment in TennCare*. 5 May. www.state.tn.us/tenncare/ enrol-co.htm, 9 June 2002.

Canadian Association of Radiologists. 2000. *Outdated Radiology Equipment: A Diagnostic Crisis*. Special Ministerial Briefing. Saint Laurent, Que.: Canadian Association of Radiologists.

Canadian Institute of Actuaries. 1995. *Troubled Tomorrows: The Report of the Canadian Institute of Actuaries' Task Force on Retirement Savings*. Toronto: Canadian Institute of Actuaries.

– 2001. *Health Care in Canada: The Impact of Population Aging*. Submission to the Standing Committee on Social Affairs, Science and Technology, 21 March. Toronto: Canadian Institute of Actuaries.

Canadian Institute for Health Information (CIHI). 2001. *Total Health Care Spend-*

ing Surpasses $100 Billion, Reports CIHI. 18 Dec. www.cihi.ca/medrls/ 18dec2001.shtml, 29 Jan. 2002.

Cancer Advocacy Coalition. 2001. *Report Card 2001 on Cancer Care in Canada.* 13 Dec. www.canceradvocacycoalition.com, 9 June 2002.

– 2002. *Mortality/Incidence Rates, 1993–1997.* www.canceradvocacycoalition. com, 9 June 2002.

Carroll, R.J., et al. 1995. 'International Comparison of Waiting Times for Selected Cardiovascular Procedures.' *Journal of the American College of Cardiology* 25: 557–63.

Clancy, Carolyn M. and Marion Danis. 2000. 'Setting Priorities "American Style."' In Angela Coulter and Chris Ham, eds., *The Global Challenge of Health Care Rationing.* Buckingham: Open University Press, 52–9.

Collins-Nakai, R.L., H.A. Huysmans, and H.E. Skully. 1992. 'Task Force 5: Access to Cardiovascular Care: An International Comparison.' *Journal of the American College of Cardiology* 19: 1477–85.

Conference Board of Canada. 2001. 'Finding a Future for Canada's Health Care System.' *Performance and Potential, 2001–2002.* Ottawa: Conference Board of Canada.

Coulter, Angela, and Chris Ham. 2000. 'Introduction: International Experience of Rationing (or Priority Setting) and Where Are We Now?' In Angela Coulter and Chris Ham, eds., *The Global Challenge of Health Care Rationing.* Buckingham: Open University Press, 1–12, 233–50.

Coyte, Peter, et al. 1994. 'Waiting Times for Knee Replacement Surgery in the United States and Ontario.' *New England Journal of Medicine,* 20 Oct.

Currie, R.J. 2000. *Manitoba Centre for Health Policy Report: Waiting Times for Surgery: A Second Look.* Nov. www.umanitoba.ca/centres/mchp/reports_ 97–00/waits2.htm, 9 June 2002.

Cutler, David M., and Mark McClellan. 2001. 'Is Technological Change in Medicine Worth It?' *Health Affairs* 20, no. 5: 11–29.

Daniels, Norman. 2000. 'Accountability for Reasonableness in Private and Public Health Insurance.' In Angela Coulter and Chris Ham, eds., *The Global Challenge of Health Care Rationing.* Buckingham: Open University Press, 87–106.

Deaton, Angus. 2002. 'Policy Implications of the Gradient of Health and Wealth.' *Health Affairs* 20, no. 2: 13–30.

Deber, R., et al. 1995. *The Public/Private Mix in Health Care,* Parts 1 and 2. Ottawa: National Forum on Health. wwwnfh.hc-sc.gc.ca/publicat/ issuesm/deber1.htm/ and wwwnfh.hc-sc.gc.ca/publicat/issuesm/ deber2.htm/, 20 Jan. 2002.

Doan, Ngan. 2001. *Minnesota Care Disenrollee Survey.* Presentation. St Paul's: Minnesota Department of Health.

Dunlop, Sheryl, Peter C. Coyte, and Warren McIsaac. 2000. 'Socio-economic Status and Utilisation of Physicians' Services: Results from the Canadian National Population Health Survey.' *Social Science and Medicine* 51, no. 1: 123–33.

Edgar, Wendy. 2000. 'Rationing Health Care in New Zealand – How the Public Has a Say.' In Angela Coulter and Chris Ham, eds., *The Global Challenge of Health Care Rationing*. Buckingham: Open University Press, 175–91.

El Feki, Shereen. 1998. 'Profile – Canadian Healthcare Struggles with Its Five Pillars of Faith.' In *Healthcare International, 1st Quarter 1998*. London: Economist Intelligence Unit, 34–66.

Emmerson, Carl, Christine Frayne, and Alissa Goodman. 2000. *Pressures in U.K. Healthcare: Challenges for the NHS*. London: Institute for Fiscal Studies.

Esmail, Nadeem. 2001. 'Canada's Abysmal Health Technology Record.' *Fraser Forum*, Nov. 24–6.

Evans, Bob. 1993. 'User Fees for Health Care: Why a Bad Idea Keeps Coming Back.' Health Policy Research Unit 93: 9D. Vancouver: Health Policy Research Unit, University of British Columbia.

Feachem, Richard G.A., Neelam K. Sekhri, and Karen L. White. 2002. 'Getting More for Their Dollar: A Comparison of the NHS with California's Kaiser Permanente.' *British Medical Journal* 324: 135–41.

Ferguson, Brian. 2002a. E-mail. Associate professor, Department of Economics, University of Guelph. 7 Jan.

– 2002b. E-mail. 13 Jan.

Frew, Stephen A. 2001. *Consolidated Omnibus Budget Reconciliation Act (COBRA)/Emergency Medical Treatment and Active Labor Act (EMTALA) Resources Executive Summary* 2.9. April. www.medlaw.com/handout.htm, 31 Jan. 2002.

Fries, James F., et al. 1993. 'Reducing Health Care Costs by Reducing the Need and Demand for Medical Services.' *New England Journal of Medicine* 329: 321–5.

Fuchs, Victor R., and Harold C. Sox, Jr. 2001. 'Physicians' Views of the Relative Importance of Thirty Medical Innovations.' *Health Affairs* 20, no. 5: 30–42.

Garber, Alan M. 2001. 'Evidence-Based Coverage Policy.' *Health Affairs* 20, no. 5: 62–82.

Giacomini, Mita K. 1999. 'The *Which*-Hunt: Assembling Health Technologies for Assessment and Rationing.' *Journal of Health Politics, Policy and Law* 24, no. 4: 715–58.

Goodman, John C. 2001. 'Characteristics of an Ideal Health Care System.' *Policy Report* 242. Dallas: National Center for Policy Analysis, April. www.ncpa.org/pub/st/st242/, 8 June 2002.

Government of New Brunswick. 2002. *Public Health and Medical Services: Intro-duction*. www.gnb.ca/0394/coverage-e.asp, 12 June 2002.

Government of Quebec. 2001. *Health*. 2 Nov. www.gouv.qc.ca/Vision/Sante/Sante_en.html, 20 Nov. 2001.

Gratzer, David, ed. 1999. *Code Blue: Reviving Canada's Health-Care System*. Toronto: ECW Press.

– 2002. *Better Medicine: Reforming Canadian Health Care*. Toronto: ECW Press.

Griffiths, Sian, John Reynolds, and Tony Hope. 2000. 'Priority Setting in Prac-tice.' In Angela Coulter and Chris Ham, eds., *The Global Challenge of Health Care Rationing*. Buckingham: Open University Press, 203–13.

Ham, Chris. 1996. 'Learning from the Tigers: Stakeholder Health Care.' *Lancet* 347: 951–3.

Harding, April, and Alexander S. Preker. 2000. *The Economics of Public and Private Roles in Health Care: Insights from Institutional Economics and Organiza-tional Theory*. Washington, DC: World Bank.

Health Care Financing Administration (HCFA). 2001a. *Medicaid*. www.hcfa.gov.medicaid/ medicaid.htm, 28 Jan. 2002.

– 2001b. *Medicaid Services*. www.hcfa.gov/medicaid/mservice.htm, 28 Jan. 2002.

– 2001c. *Medicare*. www.hcfa.gov.medicare/medicare.htm, 28 Jan. 2002.

– 2001d. *Medicare Coverage Policy – Coverage Process*. www.hcfa.gov/coverage/ 8a2.htm, 28 Jan. 2002.

– 2001e. *Medicare Coverage Policy – Home Page*. www.hcfa.gov/coverage/, 28 Jan. 2002.

– 2001f. *Your Medicare Benefits: Your Health Care Coverage in the Original Medi-care Plan for ... Part A (Hospital Insurance), Part B (Medical Insurance) Including Preventive Services*. Baltimore: United States Department of Health and Human Services.

Health Insurance Commission. 2001. *About Medicare*. 13 Dec. www.hic.gov.au/ yourhealth/our_services/am.htm, 29 Jan. 2002.

Herrick, Devon. 2001. 'Uninsured by Choice.' *Briefing Analysis* 379. 15 Nov. Dallas: National Center for Policy Analysis.

Holm, Søren. 2000. 'Developments in the Nordic Countries – Goodbye to the Simple Solutions.' In Angela Coulter and Chris Ham, eds., *The Global Challenge of Health Care Rationing*. Buckingham: Open University Press, 29–37.

Hsiao, William C. 1995. 'Medical Savings Accounts: Lessons from Singapore.' *Health Affairs* (Summer), 260–6.

Hunter, Justine. 2001. '36% Back Two-Tier Health: Poll.' 7 July. *National Post Online*. www.nationalpost.com/, 24 July 2001.

Jackson, N.W., M.P. Doogue, and J.M. Elliott. 1999. 'Priority Points and Cardiac Events While Waiting for Coronary Artery Bypass Surgery.' *Heart* 81: 367–73.

Kaiser Family Foundation. 2002. *State Health Facts Online.* www.statehealth-facts.kff.org/, 9 June 2002.

Klein, Rudolph, and Alan Williams. 2000. 'Setting Priorities: What Is Holding Us Back – Inadequate Information or Inadequate Institutions?' In Angela Coulter and Chris Ham, eds., *The Global Challenge of Health Care Rationing.* Buckingham: Open University Press, 15–26.

Kronick, Richard, and Todd Gilmer. 2002. 'Insuring Low-Income Adults: Does Public Coverage Crowd Out Private?' *Health Affairs* 21, no. 1: 225–38.

Lichtenberg, Frank R. 2001. 'Are the Benefits of Newer Drugs Worth Their Cost? Evidence from the 1996 MEPS.' *Health Affairs* 20, no. 5: 241–51.

Litow, Mark E., and Stacey V. Muller. 1998. *Feasibility of Health Care Allowances in Canada.* Toronto: Consumer Policy Institute.

Lyons, William, and William F. Fox. 2001. *The Impact of TennCare: A Survey of Recipients.* Knoxville: Tenncare.

Mackillop, W.J. 1994. 'Waiting for Radiotherapy in Canada and the U.S.' Presented at the 36th Annual American Society for Therapeutic Radiology in San Francisco, 3 Oct.

Mackillop, W.J., et al. 1997. 'Socioeconomic Status and Cancer Survival in Ontario.' *Journal of Clinical Oncology* 15: 1680–9.

Manitoba Health. 2002. *Manitoba Health Services Insurance Plan.* www.gov.mb.ca/health/ mhsip/index.html, 16 Nov. 2001.

Marmot, Michael. 2002. 'The Influence of Income on Health: Views of an Epidemiologist.' *Health Affairs* 20, no. 2: 31–46.

Martin, Douglas K., and Peter A. Singer. 2000. 'Priority Setting and Health Technology Assessment: Beyond Evidence-Based Medicine and Cost-Effectiveness Analysis.' In Angela Coulter and Chris Ham, eds., *The Global Challenge of Health Care Rationing,* Buckingham: Open University Press, 135–45.

Massaro, Thomas, and Yu-Ning Wong. 1996. 'Medical Savings Accounts: The Singapore Experience.' Policy Report 203. Dallas: National Center for Policy Analysis.

Mayo, Nancy E., et al. 2001. 'Waiting Time for Breast Cancer Surgery in Quebec.' *CMAS* 164: 1133–38.

McGinnis, Michael J., Pamela Williams-Russo, and James R. Knickman. 2002. 'The Case for More Active Policy Attention to Health Promotion.' *Health Affairs* 20, no. 2, 78–93.

McMahon, Fred, and Martin Zelder. 2002. 'Making Health Spending Work.' Public Policy Sources 54. Vancouver: Fraser Institute.

Miller, Tom. 1996. 'MSAs: Panacea or Placebo?' *Competitive Enterprise Institute Update Article*. 7 Jan. www.cei.org/UpdateReader.asp?ID=261, 26 April 2001.

Milne, Celia. 2001. 'More Questions Than Answers in Health Funding.' *Medical Post Online* 37, no. 37: www.medicalpost.com/, 28 Dec. 2001.

Minnesota Department of Health and the School of Public Health, University of Minnesota. 2002. *Minnesota's Uninsured: Findings from the 2001 Health Access Survey.* April. St Paul's: Minnesota Department of Health.

Moulton, Donalee. 1998. 'Bladder Cancer Survival Affected by Long Canadian Waiting Lists.' *Medical Post*, 12 July, 5.

Mullen, Penelope M. 2000. 'Public Involvement in Health Care Priority Setting: Are the Methods Appropriate and Valid?' In Angela Coulter and Chris Ham, eds., *The Global Challenge of Health Care Rationing*. Buckingham: Open University Press, 163–74.

Musgrove, Philip. 1996. *Public and Private Roles in Health: Theory and Financing Patterns*. Washington, DC: World Bank.

National Center for Health Statistics. 1999. *Health, United States, 1999, with Health and Aging Chartbook*. Hyattsville, MD: National Center for Health Statistics.

National Economic Research Associates. 1997. *The Health Care System in Singapore*. London, UK: National Economic Research Associates.

– 2001. 'Funding U.K. Health Care.' *Breaking News*, 8 June. www.nera.com/_template.cfm?c=6168&o=3583, 28 Jan. 2002.

National Forum on Health. 1995. *The Public and Private Financing of Canada's Health System*. Ottawa: Health Canada. wwwnfh.hc-sc.gc.ca/publicat/public/, 10 Jan. 2002.

New, Bill. 2000. *What Business Is the NHS In? Establishing the Boundary of a Health Care System's Responsibility*. London: Institute for Public Policy Research.

Newfoundland Department of Health and Community Services. 1999. *Medical Care Plan and Newfoundland Hospital Insurance Plan*. www.gov.nf.ca/mcp/html/, 12 June 2002.

Newhouse, J.P. 1993. *Free for All? Lessons from the RAND Health Insurance Experiment*. Cambridge, Mass.: Harvard University Press.

New Zealand Ministry of Health. 2001a. *Guide to Eligibility for Publicly Funded Personal Health and Disability Services in New Zealand*. www.moh.govt.nz/moh.nsf/wpgIndex/About-FAQs+Contents, 29 Jan. 2002.

– 2001b. *An Overview of the Health and Disability Sector in New Zealand*. Wellington: Ministry of Health.

Nova Scotia Department of Health. 2001. *Insured Health Services in Nova Scotia*. Halifax: Department of Health.

Oberlander, Jonathan, Theodore Marmor, and Lawrence Jacobs. 2001. 'Rationing Medical Care: Rhetoric and Reality in the Oregon Health Plan.' *Canadian Medical Association Journal* 164, no. 11: 1583–7.

Office of Medical Assistance Programs, Oregon Department of Human Services. 2001. *The Oregon Health Plan: It May be for You.* 2 April. www.omap.hr.state.or.us/ohp/3256_0401.html, 28 Jan. 2002.

Ontario Ministry of Health and Long-Term Care. 2000. *OHIP Facts.* 1 Sept. www.gov.on.ca/MOH/english/pub/ohip/services.htm, 20 Nov. 2001.

Oregon Health Services Commission. 2001a. *Oregon Health Services Commission Report: Prioritized List of Packages for OHP Standard.* Salem: Office of Oregon Health Policy and Research.

– 2001b. *Prioritized List of Health Services.* 1 Oct. www.ohppr.state.or.us/hsc/index_hsc.htm, 28 Jan. 2002.

Premier's Advisory Council on Health for Alberta. 2001. *A Framework for Reform.* Dec. www2.gov.ab.ca/home/health_first/documents/, 10 Jan. 2002.

Prince Edward Island Department of Health and Social Services. 2001. *Hospital and Medical Services Insurance.* Charlottetown: Department of Health and Social Services.

Ramsay, Cynthia. 2001. *Beyond the Public–Private Debate: An Examination of Quality, Access and Costs in the Health-Care Systems of Eight Countries.* Vancouver: Western Sky Communications Ltd.

– 1998. *Medical Savings Accounts: Universal, Accessible, Portable, Comprehensive Health Care for Canadians.* Vancouver: Fraser Institute.

Ramsay, Cynthia, and Michael Walker. 1996. 'A Thriving Health Care Sector Could Contribute to a Healthy Economy.' *Fraser Forum,* Oct. Vancouver: Fraser Institute, 17–21.

Roemer, M., et al. 1975. 'Copayments for Ambulatory Care: Penny-Wise and Pound-Foolish.' *Medical Care* 13, no. 6: 457–66.

Saskatchewan Health. 2000. *Coverage.* www.health.gov.sk.ca/ps_coverage_full.html, 16 Nov. 2001.

– 2001. *The Action Plan for Saskatchewan Health Care.* Regina: Saskatchewan Health.

Sawyer, Douglas M., and John R. Williams. 1995. 'Core and Comprehensive Health Care Services: 3. Ethical Issues.' *CMAJ* 152. www.cma.ca/cmaj/vol-152/issue-9/1409.htm, 20 Jan. 2002.

Scandlen, Greg. 2001. 'Propping Up SCHIP: Will This Program Ever Work?' *Briefing Analysis* 371. 7 Sept. Dallas: National Center for Policy Analysis.

Singapore Ministry of Health, Strategic Planning Branch, Policy and Development Division. 2001. *About the Ministry of Health in Singapore.* Feb. www.gov.sg/moh/mohinfo_a.html, 14 Nov. 2001.

Standing Senate Committee on Social Affairs, Science and Technology. 2002a. *Volume Five: Principles and Recommendations for Reform – Part 1. The Health of Canadians – The Federal Role.* Ottawa: The Senate, April.

– 2002b. *Volume Three: Health Care Systems in Other Countries. The Health of Canadians – The Federal Role.* Ottawa: The Senate, Jan.

– 2002c. *Volume Two: Current Trends and Future Challenges. The Health of Canadians – The Federal Role.* Ottawa: The Senate, Jan.

Strategic Policy Directorate, Population and Public Health Branch. 2001. *The Population Health Template: Key Elements and Actions that Define a Population Health Approach.* July draft. Ottawa: Health Canada.

Syme, S. Leonard, Bonnie Lefkowitz, and Barbara Kivimae Krimgold. 2002. 'Incorporating Socioeconomic Factors into U.S. Health Policy: Addressing the Barriers.' *Health Affairs* 20, no. 2, 113–18.

Szick, Sharon, et al. 1999. 'Health Care Delivery in Canada and the United States: Are There Relevant Differences in Health Outcomes?' Toronto: Institute for Clinical Evaluative Sciences.

Tengs, Tammy O. 1996. 'An Evaluation of Oregon's Medicaid Rationing Algorithms.' *Health Economics* 5: 171–81.

Tuohy, Carolyn Hughes. 2002. 'The Costs of Constraint and Prospects for Health Care Reform in Canada.' *Health Affairs* 21, no. 3: 32–46.

United Kingdom Department of Health. 2001. *The NHS Plan: A Plan for Investment, A Plan for Reform.* 27 July. doh.gov.uk/nhsplan/, 28 Jan. 2002.

Vail, Stephen. 2001. *Canadians' Values and Attitudes on Canada's Health Care System: A Synthesis of Survey Results.* Ottawa: Conference Board of Canada.

Walker, Michael, and Greg Wilson. 2001. *Waiting Your Turn: Hospital Waiting Lists in Canada.* Vancouver: Fraser Institute.

Walters, David J., and Donald A. Morgan. 1995. 'Core and Comprehensive Health Care Services: 2. Quality of Care Issues.' *CMAJ* 152. www.cma.ca/cmaj/vol-152/issue-8/1199.htm, 20 Jan. 2002.

Washington State Health Care Authority. 2002a. *2002 Basic Health Member Handbook.* Olympia: Washington State Health Care Authority.

– 2002b. *How Much Will Basic Health Coverage Cost?* www.wa.gov/hca/basichealth.htm, 9 June 2002.

Williams, John R. 1997. 'CMA's Core-Services Framework Featured at International Conference.' *Canadian Medical Association Journal* 156. www.cma.ca/cmaj/vol-156/issue-8/1192.htm, 20 Jan. 2002.

Williams, John R., and Michael Yeo. 2000. 'The Ethics of Decentralizing Health Care Priority Setting in Canada.' In Angela Coulter and Chris Ham, eds., *The Global Challenge of Health Care Rationing,* Buckingham: Open University Press, 123–32.

Wilson, Ruth, Margo S. Rowan, and Jennifer Henderson. 1995. 'Core and Comprehensive Health Care Services: 1. Introduction to the Canadian Medical Association's Decision-Making Framework.' *Canadian Medical Association Journal* 152. www.cma.ca/cmaj/vol-152/issue-7/1063.htm, 20 Jan. 2002.

Witt, Julia. 2002. E-mail. PhD candidate, Department of Economics, University of Guelph. 14 Jan.

World Health Organization. 2000. *The World Health Report 2000: Health Systems: Improving Performance*. Geneva: WHO.

7 Delivering Health Care: Public, Not-for-Profit, or Private?

RAISA B. DEBER

Defining Terms

The appropriate mix between public and private health care has become a topic of considerable heat; the intention of this paper is to clarify the discussion. On the one hand, many recent provincial reports examining health care have suggested more 'privatization.' Perhaps the strongest recent such statement has come from the Premier's Advisory Council on Health for Alberta, which argued that the current system 'operates as an unregulated monopoly where the province acts as insurer, provider and evaluator of health services.' None the less, that report echoes similar language from other organizations (Preker and Harding 2000; Preker, Harding, and Travis 2000; Crowley, Zitner, and Faraday-Smith 2002; Zitner and Crowley 2002). It recommends that 'we can't regulate to perfection. It's time to open up the system, take the shackles off, allow health authorities to try new ideas, encourage competition and choice, and see what works and what doesn't' (Premier's Advisory Council 2001, 4–5).

This debate is not confined to Canada. Internationally, however, it has generated considerably more heat than light. Countries use a wide variety of delivery mechanisms and models; because particular features are embedded within wider systems, one cannot directly extrapolate performance across systems (Organisation for Economic Co-operation and Development 1987; 1994; Marmor 2001). Nevertheless, the advocates of more private-sector involvement argue that this is essential to preserving a universal and sustainable health-care system and that private delivery within 'public–private partnerships' is likely to be more efficient and can help obtain better value for money (Kelly and Robinson 2000; Arnold 2001; Commission on Public Private Partnerships 2001). Yet opponents of for-profit delivery point to a host of potential difficulties with greater use of the private sector for delivery, including worries about the compatibility of the values inherent in health care with those underlying markets (Relman 1992; Woolhandler and Himmelstein 1997; Fuller 1998a, b; Himmelstein et al. 1999; Kushner 1999; Arvay Finlay 2000; Evans et al. 2000; Taft and Steward 2000; Heyman 2001; Rachlis et al. 2001). Policy initiatives such as Alberta's Bill 11 have become emblematic of the disputes on the appropriate role of for-profit delivery within a publicly funded system (Fuller 1998a; Alberta Health 2000; Arvay Finlay 2000; CCPA 2000, Armstrong 2000; Choudhry 2000; Plain 2000; Rachlis 2000b).

The two sides have been talking past one another, using similar terms to mean very different things. Because individuals are rarely assigned randomly to public, not-for-profit (NFP), private-for-profit small business (FP/s), or private-for-profit corporate (FP/c) providers, the evidence is often contentious, with advocates of the various positions often resorting to claims that various organizations are or are not comparable. There is remarkably little disinterested information, and a plethora of papers state positions without benefit of supporting evidence. Before evaluating the evidence about public and private delivery, then, we should define our terms, while recognizing fully that this paper on occasion superimposes a conceptual framework other than that used by the authors being cited.

Elements of Health-Care Systems: Financing, Delivery, and Allocation

Health-care systems are commonly divided into several components. Although various writers may use slightly different nomenclatures and break down these functions in slightly different ways, they all distinguish between how services are paid for – which I term *financing* – and how they are organized, managed, and provided – which I call *delivery* (OECD 1987; Donahue 1989; Deber et al. 1998). Systems may also explicitly incorporate other elements – such as planning, monitoring, and evaluating – or leave these to the workings of market forces. 'Privatizing' health care may accordingly involve changes in financing (for example, budget reductions and user fees – activities that Bendick terms 'load shedding') and/or in delivery (for example, vouchers, contracting out, grants and subsidies, and public–private partnerships) (Bendick 1989; Kamerman and Kahn 1989).

The missing link connecting financing and delivery – sometimes termed *allocation* – refers to the incentive structures set up to manage flow of funds from those who pay for care to those who deliver it. Saltman et al. place allocation approaches on a continuum (Saltman and von Otter 1992; 1995; Deber et al. 1998; Saltman, Figueras, and Sakellarides 1998). At one end, 'patients follow money,' as funders allocate global budgets to providers. At the other end, 'money follows patients,' as providers depend on attracting clients. Unfortunately for those hoping for clear prescriptions for reform, no one allocation model can ensure cost control, client responsiveness, and delivery of high-quality, appropriate care; instead, one often faces policy trade-offs (McFetridge 1997). None the less, there is clearly room for improvement.

This paper concentrates on delivery rather than on financing or allocation – that is, on the best way to *deliver* health care, regardless of how it is paid for. However, whereas approximately 70 per cent of Canadian health expenditures comes from public sources, it focuses on particular sectors. Comprehensive services under the Canada Health Act receive almost all their money from the public sector, with the Canadian Institute for Health Information (CIHI) estimating the public share at 99 per cent of expenditures for physicians' services, 90 per cent for hospital care, and variable but considerable portions of such other services as pharmaceuticals, home care, and rehabilitation (CIHI 2000a; Deber 2000). Public policy clearly has more interest in how best to deliver services paid for with public money, if only to ensure accountability for the use of public funds. I therefore concentrate on assisting in answering the question of what difference it makes how we choose to deliver publicly financed services. However, as we see below, certain forms of delivery may prove more compatible with certain approaches to financing; financing and delivery turn out to be separate, but linked matters. Neither will this paper deal with the underlying values involved, even though these clearly shape policy. I take on a more limited role. Deng Xiaoping observed that it does not matter whether a cat is black or white as long as it catches mice; I examine the evidence for predicting the relative performance of various delivery options.

Table 7.1
Categories of health-care systems

	Public (collective payment)	Private (individual payment)
Public-sector delivery	National Health Service (e.g., United Kingdom)	User fees for public services
Private-sector delivery	Public insurance	Private insurance

Levels and Characteristics of Public and Private

Although we tend to speak loosely of 'public' and 'private,' each term contains multiple meanings and multiple levels (Starr 1989; Ovretveit 1996; Canadian Healthcare Association 2001). As Starr notes (1989), the terms are usually paired to denote such oppositions as open versus closed, government versus markets, or the whole versus the part. Starr cautions that because the terms do not have consistent meanings in different institutional settings, it is risky to generalize about the merits of privatization as public policy beyond a particular institutional or national context. The boundaries between public and private are not always clear; a number of organizations, often highly regulated and/or dependent on public funds, profess public-service objectives and can be classified as either public or private, depending on definitions. Examples include workers' compensation, sickness funds that finance health insurance in certain European countries, and even regional health authorities (RHAs) in many Canadian provinces. One has to look not only at the ownership structure but also at the broad framework of incentives that determine how these institutions behave.

One can combine the public–private and the financing–delivery dimensions to create a 2×2 table (Table 7.1) (Deber et al. 1998; Donahue 1989). In Canada, the public financing–public delivery cell (like Britain's National Health Service) includes most public health departments (whose employees usually work for some level of government), as well as provincial psychiatric hospitals and, in some provinces, home care. Private financing–public delivery captures both publicly delivered services that rely heavily on user fees (for example, public transit, non-privatized post offices), as well as such health-care examples as pay beds in National Health Service hospitals in Britain (Higgins 1988; Ovretveit 1996). Most physician and hospital care in Canada is in the public financing–private delivery cell, while the 30 per cent of privately financed care (for example, much of pharmaceuticals, rehabilitation, dental care, and complementary and alternative medicines) is largely in the private financing–private delivery quadrant.

The distinction between public and private, however, blurs important distinctions *within* each category. The next section categorizes various forms of public and private delivery and summarizes arguments from the relevant literature, in full recognition that such organizations tend to be heterogeneous.

Public Delivery
It is well recognized that public encompasses at least four distinct levels:

- federal (national government)
- sub-national (state/provincial governments)
- regional governments/authorities
- local governments

Many of the fiercest battles are taking place within the public sector, as various levels of government dispute roles, responsibilities, and who should pay for what.

In terms of service delivery, public organizations seem to have the following characteristics:

- Their employees are members of the civil service of that jurisdiction.
- They are more likely to have unionized workforces.
- They may have a monopoly on certain types of service provision.
- If the government unit is small, they may find it more difficult to justify (or attract) the critical mass of expertise needed for certain activities.
- They are bound by civil-service rules and procedures about a host of issues, including formal procurement and bidding procedures.
- Their operations are subject to transparency and disclosure provisions.
- They cannot raise capital by issuing equity (although they may be able to float bonds). Instead, they must satisfy voters that their claim to tax revenues is warranted.
- They have a number of goals that must be balanced, of which the

financial bottom line/efficiency is only one. (These goals may include provision of 'good jobs' in areas of high unemployment. Other authors suggest that public delivery tends to emphasize universal coverage, uniform services and quality, and uniform prices, which may in turn lessen bottom-line efficiency while serving other goals.)

- Depending on the accounting procedures in place, they may have difficulties in spreading capital expenditures over many years or otherwise depreciating capital assets (for example, some jurisdictions require the full cost of capital programs to be brought into a single year's budget).
- They are not likely to attract charitable donations or volunteer labour.

Accordingly, although the evidence is mixed, they are often viewed as being bound into 'silo thinking' (that is, unable to co-operate across organizational barriers), more rigid/less flexible/less nimble, less effective, and more complacent (because of the absence of competition). Certainly, they have more difficulty in using part-time or temporary help to manage peak service periods or in spreading equipment/capital costs over many jobs. The requirements for accountability may inhibit the ability to take risks, and hence to innovate. Technology may be more antiquated. In recent years, the search for efficiency has led to proposals that government separate policy from delivery, concentrate only on core functions, and put its efforts into 'steering' (managing policy development and providing leadership) rather than 'rowing' (directly delivering services) (Osborne and Gaebler 1992; Skelly 1996; Ford and Zussman 1997; Preker and Harding 2000). Developed and developing nations have privatized many formerly public organizations (Hatry 1983; DeHoog 1984; Carroll, Conant, and Easton 1987; Donahue 1989; Kamerman and Kahn 1989; Clutterbuck, Kernaghan, and Snow 1991; Kemp 1991; McFetridge 1997; Yergin and Stanislaw 1998)

In some countries, including Britain and Sweden, health care has traditionally been delivered by the public sector. The National Health Service (NHS) in Britain owns and operates hospitals, and its personnel work for the national government. Swedish hospitals are run by their county councils. In contrast, in Canada, very little delivery of health care occurs within the public sector. As we saw above, there are exceptions, including services to the military and northern or Aboriginal communities (federal employees), provincial psychiatric hospitals, and public health. None the less, any analysis of delivery in Canada must begin with the recognition that most of it is already private.

Private Delivery
It is less commonly recognized that *private* also encompasses many levels. In this paper, we concentrate on four major levels of the private sector – private not-for-profit, for-profit small business, private for-private corporate, and private delivery by families and individuals. We now look at the characteristics of each in turn.

Private Not-for-Profit (NFP) Delivery. This heterogeneous category of organizations has a variety of names, including non-profit, not-for-profit, voluntary, community, and the 'third sector.' These bodies may receive their revenues from a combination of charitable contributions, government contracts, and/or fees for services that they provide. They may employ skilled workers or rely on volunteers. They may work closely with government or at arm's length. Indeed, they may carry out publicly determined purposes. At one extreme, they become quasi-public. For example, in British Columbia, home support workers may be employed by Community Health Councils, which some observers classify as public (Pollak 2000). These councils are a component of the province's RHAs; in turn, they are among the nearly 700 'public agencies' to whose boards the provincial government makes at least one appointment (Government of British Columbia Board Resourcing and Development Office 2002). None the less, many of these 'public' agencies are not subject to the financial or administrative requirements of the provincial government and in our terms are private NFPs.

NFP organizations have the following characteristics.

- They are not part of government and so not bound by most of their 'red tape' (although the recent trend towards 'accountability' may increase such formal requirements and move them closer to the public end of the continuum).
- Although they can run a 'surplus' of revenue over expenditures, they cannot distribute this surplus to individuals in the form of profits. They can spend it in other ways, including higher wages or 'perks' to employees and managers, training/education, research, community service, or subsidizing less profitable services. Some, but not all, of these activities might be judged as 'public goods,' which benefit the community.

- They receive special tax exemptions from government.
- They can draw on volunteers and receive charitable contributions, as well as grants and contributions from governments.
- They are motivated by multiple objectives, rather than by just the financial bottom line.
- They can go bankrupt.

NFP firms have played a critical role in education, health, and social services in most countries; in Canada, they are the dominant form of organization within these sectors. Most proposals for 'privatization' represent a shift within private delivery from NFP to for-profit (FP) organizations. This category reveals the importance of distinguishing between financing and delivery. Canada's 'public' hospitals are often erroneously classified as part of the public sector, instead of being recognized as NFPs, with independent, community-based boards of directors and a long tradition of service to their communities. Some authors confound financing and delivery and argue that hospitals are public because they receive about 90 per cent of their budgets from public-sector sources. The CIHI reports that 99 per cent of expenditures for physicians' services come from public sources, but the distinction between physicians who work for government (for example, in provincial psychiatric hospitals) and those in private practice is still clear. Further confusion may arise in provinces such as Ontario, which classifies 'public hospitals' within the MUSH (municipalities, universities, schools, and hospitals) sector, because they receive provincial transfers, thus blurring municipalities and public schools, which are indeed public, with universities and hospitals, which are not. Hospital (and university) management has considerable autonomy to determine its mix of staff and services, whereas public school principals do not.

The distinction between public and NFP is crucial, largely because many of the arguments made against public delivery do not fully apply to NFPs. However, the distinction is becoming less clear in some provinces, particularly as they start to demand greater accountability for public funds. Regionalization in all provinces other than Ontario has replaced many formerly independent hospital boards with RHAs. This move towards regionalization has further blurred this distinction. Although in theory RHAs remain private organizations, whose employees do not work for government, some provinces have sought to exert more and more control over their day-to-day operations. Recognizing that the line can be blurry, however, does not eradicate it, although it may suggest more careful balancing of new accountability requirements against flexibility and responsiveness.

Private For-Profit Small Business (FP/s) Delivery. This category of organizations includes small business/entrepreneurs that are privately owned (often by the health professionals delivering the service) but need not answer to shareholders. In Canada, this group includes virtually all physicians' services other than those delivered by salaried hospital employees, as well as many other providers (for example, physiotherapy clinics). It also encompasses many clinics and small hospitals, such as Ontario's Shouldice Hospital (Shouldice Hospital 2002) and CROS private cancer clinic (Office of the Provincial Auditor General of Ontario 2001). The United States also has a sizeable number of FP/s hospitals (Cutler 2000). Until recently, most private hospitals in Britain also fell into this category (Higgins 1988). So do most private hospitals in other European countries, such as France (Poullier and Sandier 2000).

Characteristics of these FP/s businesses include the following:

- They pay taxes.
- They can go bankrupt.
- They are not bound by the 'red tape' of government and can be more flexible and nimble.
- They are often not bound by the 'red tape' and accountability requirements of NFP status.
- They usually cannot receive charitable donations or the services of volunteers.
- They are not required to provide a return on investment to shareholders.

The evidence reviewed suggests that many of the often-expressed concerns about the implications of FP delivery may not apply fully to the FP/s category. In some cases, they differ from NFPs only in whether they deem a surplus 'profit.'

Private For-Profit Corporate (FP/c) Delivery. The FP/c category of investor-owned delivery is what is often referred to by critics of 'privatization.' The prime duty of management is to maximize the return on investment and ensure profits for individuals holding shares. Thus providing high-quality care becomes a means to an end (running a successful business), rather than an end in itself. FP/c organizations have the following characteristics:

• They are expected to provide a return on investment to their share-holders.
• They have access to capital through issuing equity.
• They cannot attract charitable donations or volunteer labour.
• They pay taxes.

Basic economics tells us that the incentives for such organizations are thus to maximize revenues and minimize costs; this is what is *meant* by efficiency. As Evans reminds us, 'From the outset, however, it is important to emphasize that profit per se is associated with neither moral turpitude nor additional costs' (Evans 1984, 211). Responding to their incentives implies that FP/c organizations should skimp on care, albeit only to the extent that this would not harm their business (Cutler 2000). A major policy dilemma is that it is not always easy to distinguish between efficiency and skimping. The literature discusses mechanisms to ensure that profit maximization does not harm quality, including transparency (provision of information to consumers) and regulatory controls, in the expectation that such mechanisms raise the cost of poor practice, either indirectly (a poor reputation may harm 'sales') or directly (through lawsuits or regulatory penalties). These in turn imply considerable administrative costs to regulators and assume that quality is easily measured.

Traditionally, FP/cs have not played a major role in any developed country in such health-care sectors as hospitals and physicians' services, although they dominate such sectors as pharmaceuticals and are very active in laboratory testing. More recently, in the United States such organizations have also assumed dominant positions in certain markets for hospitals, health maintenance organizations (HMOs), and insurance (although most U.S. hospitals are still NFP). In Canada, the potential entry of FP/cs has evoked considerable concern, particularly as various international trade agreements may make such experiments irreversible (Manga 1988; Martin 1993; CCPA 2000; Sanger 2000; Marmor 2001).

Delivery by Individuals and Families. Finally, although this paper deals only with formal organizations, as any parent or caregiver can testify, individuals and their families provide a considerable amount of care. When individuals are very ill, this desire to help can place considerable burdens on caregivers (Armstrong, et al. 1994; Armstrong and Armstrong 1996; Hayes et al. 1997; Hollander 1997; CCPA 2000; Coyte 2000; Pollak 2000; Armstrong, Armstrong, and Coburn 2001). Most discussions about private delivery are not referring to individuals, families, and friends or, for the most part, to the NFP sector. The debate about 'public versus private' is often mislabelled – the most passionate arguments are really about 'not for profit' versus 'for profit.'

Health Sectors and Direct versus Indirect Funding

Health care is not homogeneous. In one analysis, Deber and colleagues divided Canadian health care into 16 different sectors, only some of which are covered under provincial health insurance plans: acute hospital care; chronic hospital care; ambulatory/outpatient care (including physician's services); laboratories and radiology; capital costs; ancillary benefits (dental, vision, physiotherapy, chiropractic and podiatry); ambulance and transportation; nursing homes/homes for the aged; home care; rehabilitation care; drugs; assistive devices; mental health; public health/health promotion; education/training of health professionals; and planning, research and management (Deber, Adams, and Curry 1994). The CIHI database has information on up to 38 'uses of funds,' although it reports its data only for hospitals, other institutions, drugs (prescription and non-prescription), physicians, other professionals (dental, vision, and other), other institutions, capital, public health and administration, and other health spending (prepayment health administration, research, and other) (CIHI 2000b).

However defined, these sectors vary in the way they deliver care, the roles of various types of delivery organizations, and the potential implications of different models. Like all organizations, service providers constantly face 'make or buy' decisions – deciding which goods employees will make and which the organization will buy (Shelanski and Klein 1995; Preker, Harding, and Travis 2000). Thus even public organizations will still obtain many goods and services from private-sector companies; for example, even the largest local government still purchases telephone services or paperclips from outside providers. Public funds can accordingly flow to different organizations either *directly* (for example, by provision of funds to provide a particular service) or *indirectly* (for example, by purchase of goods and services). Accordingly, one cannot provide simple answers about the 'best' form of delivery model. The answer inevitably will be, 'It depends.'

Appendix A reviews the literature for a number of sectors to provide some guidance about relevant factors and the circumstances under which one might prefer various modes of delivery. The framework presented above, however, shows that it is important to distinguish two separate questions about delivery. First, why (or why not) use public as opposed to private delivery? Second, if one is using private delivery, why (or why not) select an FP as opposed to an NFP?

Evaluating Success

Evaluation of success depends heavily on the criteria being used and on whose viewpoint matters. For example, for recipients of services, the key questions are:

- What services are being delivered (including such considerations as quality and timeliness)?
- To whom are they being delivered?
- What is the effect of those services?

Although payers and providers also are interested in outcomes, they face different questions:

- Which resources are being used to provide those services, in terms of:
  - mix of resources?
  - volume of each resource?
  - cost of each resource?
- What is the fiscal bottom line (profit/loss)?

Accordingly, there are in-built conflicts between payers and providers. Payers wish to minimize their costs, while individual providers wish to ensure 'good jobs at good pay.'

Of course, life is not that simple. One obvious example is that minimizing short-run costs may not be sustainable over the long term. If those employing providers squeeze down wage and benefit levels, they may create a labour shortage; basic labour economics would predict that they would then have to increase wages (and/or improve working conditions) in order to attract workers. Evaluating efficiency thus requires paying some attention to how savings are being obtained. There are a series of 'win-win' possibilities. These include increasing appropriateness, improving inflexible bureaucratic rules, and improving quality. Most parties agree that providing services to people who do not need them (or are unlikely to benefit from them) is pure waste. Similarly, poor quality is rarely cost-effective – having to repeat an X-ray because the first one has been lost benefits no one except the seller of X-ray films. However, other purported efficiencies may instead result from incomplete accounting (particularly if organizations being compared do not provide the same services or serve the same client groups) or from changes to the costs of resources.

One study considering public versus private provision of services suggested eight evaluation criteria (Hatry 1983):

- What is the cost of the government service? (Full costing would need to include the administrative costs associated with monitoring contracts.)
- What is the financial cost to citizens, particularly if the delivery mechanism is a private monopoly?
- What range of choices is available to service clients?
- What is the quality/effectiveness of service, including considerations of possible fraud or corruption?
- What are the potential distributional effects? Who gains? Who loses?
- What is the staying power of the provider and the potential for service disruption (strikes? bankruptcies?)?
- Is the approach reversible if it doesn't work well?
- What is the feasibility/ease of implementation – including legal constraints – and what are interest-group reactions?

For health care, one might want to add definitions of services being purchased (for example, does laboratory testing extend only to the test, or does it also include interpreting and communicating the results, and assisting in ensuring that test ordering is appropriate?). In addition, the homogeneity/heterogeneity of services to be provided and the population to be served needs assessment.

Interpreting Our Results

Competition, Contestability, Complexity, and Measurability

Most scholars who have attempted to compare public and private delivery of services have concluded that any differences in efficiency relate less to differences between public and private ownership than to the extent of competition (Osborne and Gaebler 1992). The debate thus shifts somewhat from the merits of privatization to the merits of competition (Saltman 1995). Competition is the lifeblood of economics – it refers to the interactions between two or more sellers or buyers in a single market, each attempting to get or pay the most favorable price. Under circumstances of perfect competition, no single buyer or seller can dominate the prices to be paid. Economists assume that, given perfect information, Adam Smith's famous invisible hand ensures optimal distribution of resources and an efficient price, as purchasers shop around for the best price, while sellers seek out buyers who place the highest value on their services. Under such circumstances, government regulation would not be necessary. Competition is not equivalent to private ownership; monopolies can exist with private ownership, while competition can exist within a system of public ownership and administration.

In practice, however, not all markets can function in this textbook manner. One key issue relates to the production characteristics needed to generate particular goods and services. Two World Bank economists have developed a theory in terms of two such characteristics, which they term *contestability* and *measurability* (Preker and Harding 2000); it is similar to the framework suggested by Vining and Globerman (1999): 'Contestable goods are characterized by low barriers to entry and exit from the market, whereas non-contestable goods have high barriers such as sunk cost, monopoly market power, geographic advantages, and "asset specificity" (Preker and Harding 2000, 10).

Asset specificity refers to the relative lack of transferability to other uses of assets intended for use in a given transaction. Highly specific assets represent sunk costs that have relatively little value beyond their use in a specific transaction. For example, the equipment and skills involved in open heart surgery would have few alternative uses. The concept of contestability builds on earlier work by Baumol and Willig; economists adopting this view argue that it is not necessary for government to regulate even natural monopolies, as long as barriers to entry are low enough that higher prices can attract new competitors (Preker and Harding 2000). In short, a contestable market is easy to enter and to exit.

It is easier to sustain a competitive market when contestability is high. For example, it would appear relatively simple for firms offering home-making services to enter and exit a market. A firm losing a contract would go out of business; those gaining contracts could hire the now available workers. In contrast, one is unlikely to want to encourage excess capacity for open heart surgery in order to allow for such competition, if only because of the need to maintain sufficient volumes to ensure quality outcomes.

Measurability relates to 'the precision with which inputs, processes, outputs, and outcomes of a good or service can be measured' (Preker and Harding 2000). Monitoring performance is easiest when measurability is high. For example, it is relatively simple to specify the performance desired for conducting a laboratory test or collecting garbage. In contrast, it would be more difficult to specify the activities to be expected of a general practitioner and hence more difficult to monitor his or her performance and to ensure quality.

This observation is consistent with the findings of Bendick, who examined the efficacy of the privatization of publicly delivered social services within a framework of public financing (Bendick 1989). He concluded that privatization to FPs tended to be efficient for services where goals were measurable, easily monitored, and easily evaluated (for example, garbage collection). He noted that evidence also indicated that NFP deliverers had a better record in providing services in the interest of clients beyond what was precisely specified in contracts. Accordingly, where problems are complex, such as health and social welfare programs, and where the processes to be employed are not well understood, he recommended privatizing programs to NFPs rather than to FPs – an approach that he refers to as the empowerment of mediating institutions.

One can argue about the degree of contestability and measurability of particular health-care items. The theory becomes less comfortable, however, when one begins to consider what makes a market more or less contestable. It is well recognized that high capital investment can present a major barrier to entry; one does not casually set up an automated laboratory, for example. Similarly, professionalism can also represent barriers to entry – one cannot practise as a health professional without considerable training, and registration/licensure in that jurisdiction. Competition thus presupposes excess capacity or, at the very least, the ability of new capacity to appear and disappear depending on the results of the competition. This runs contrary to the emphasis that most countries have placed on controlling costs through controlling supply and leads to some suspicion that competition may not be particularly effective in reducing costs under many circumstances.

Some observers have linked increased capacity to growth of waste and duplication (Higgins 1988).

More alarming, however, is the implication of reducing barriers to exit. The theory notes that contestability is hampered by the existence of organizations (or individuals) that consumers wish to retain as care providers, even though they might be able to purchase services elsewhere for less money. Preker and Harding state explicitly that a number of factors that we might consider inherently desirable – such as expertise and a good reputation – can also reduce contestability. 'Once incumbents have invested in activities that result in expertise or generate trust, they enjoy a significant barrier to entry for other potential suppliers, thereby lowering the degree of contestability' (Preker and Harding 2000). It is unclear whether policy makers wish to encourage disposable providers, rather than retention and encouragement of excellence.

Another important production factor is *complexity* – that is, whether the goods and services stand alone or require co-ordination with other providers. Even laboratory tests that are highly measurable gain much of their value by being embedded within a system of care, in which providers order tests appropriately and are aided in interpreting and acting on their results. Similarly, even the most routinized tasks within a hospital have requirements not common in normal business environments – for example, food service within a hospital must take account of dietary restrictions, and cleaning staff must take account of hazardous materials. Union concerns that contracting out support services might endanger patients' care may be self-serving, but also contain a large grain of truth (Hospital Employees' Union 2001).

Why (or Why Not) Public Delivery?

As for employing public or private delivery, a number of powerful international agencies have suggested that public delivery is inherently less efficient than private. This is the language of 'public sector monopoly' (Preker and Harding 2000; Preker, Harding, and Travis 2000). 'Public monopolies exhibit the usual negative features. First, monopoly suppliers often reduce output and quality, while raising prices. The excess in prices over and above what the market would normally bear – *rents* – leads to allocative inefficiency or a net deadweight welfare loss to consumers who have to forgo the consumption of other goods ... Second, monopoly suppliers have strong incentives to lower expenditures through decreased output when staff members benefit from the financial residuals' (Preker and Harding 2000, 19).

This issue of 'rents' is a critical one and would seem to be associated with monopoly in general, whether public or private. Advocates of one style of delivery tend to point to abusive examples under the other – often those activities that can be subsumed under the label 'corruption.' Hence Preker and Harding suggest that 'a manifestation of such rents is the informal user charges that are commonly levied on patients and their families in public health facilities,' describing these in terms of 'accepting bribes or peddling influence' (Preker and Harding 2000). Yet trade unions like to speak of the fraud that has been found in some examples (largely U.S.) of FP delivery (Sutherland 2001). Advocates on both sides tend to stretch the definition of fraud and corruption by mentioning in the same paragraphs activities that do not seem as inherently objectionable. Thus Preker et al. mention in the same passage 'public sector workers requiring bribes in order to do their job' and 'workers negotiating through collective bargaining better wages and working conditions than other employers might pay' (Preker and Harding 2000).

Because incentive structures have consequences, these issues would appear to relate more strongly to the nature and effectiveness of monitoring activities than to the delivery mode per se. Certainly, there are honest and dishonest individuals in all walks of life. What incentive structures have been set up, and how is compliance measured and monitored? In general, it does not seem advisable to create incentive structures that penalize best practices and assume that providers will be so altruistic that they will work against their own economic best interests.

Where Can FP Firms Make Their Profits?

Health care is not exactly like other goods and services. Apart from the emotional/moral implications of dealing with potentially life-threatening conditions, and the reluctance of many people to assume that their life and well-being are just another commodity (Marmor, Schlesinger, and Smithey 1987), economists stress 'asymmetry of information'; unlike in most commercial relationships, the patient usually must rely on the provider to tell him or her which services to purchase (Evans 1984; Rice 1998; Deber 2000). Professional ethics thus emphasize providers' role as agents for their patients. In contrast, FP firms are expected to provide a return on investment to shareholders. Payers for health care wish to purchase needed care at 'best quality, best price.' For these goals to be compatible, FPs have to offer care at rates and quality compatible with those that public or NFP providers could offer. The literature suggests possible ways in which FPs could make their profits, some (but not all) of which would also be acceptable for society (Deber 1998). These include the following eight methods.

Strong Economies of Scale
This particularly applies to services subject to 'make or buy' considerations, where individual organizations can benefit from amortizing costs over a larger population base than would typically be found in a single organization. Public organizations, by definition, are confined to a particular jurisdiction; smaller communities thus stand to gain considerable potential efficiencies of scale. These economies can apply to capital expenditures or to specialized expertise. These factors appear particularly likely in highly measurable services with many potential customers to absorb fixed costs. Although NFPs could accomplish similar goals, history suggests that they are more likely to have difficulties obtaining capital and evoking co-operation from other providers.

Better Management
A related set of factors involves FPs' ability to provide expertise otherwise not affordable. This issue is particularly relevant for small communities/organizations dealing with larger corporations (see Appendix). However, monitoring activities is key to ensuring that benefits do not accrue solely to the FP.

Freedom from Labour Agreements
To the extent that public or not-for-profit organizations offer better wages or working conditions than the minimum necessary to attract 'good enough' workers, there is an obvious profit potential in driving down labour costs, including deskilling. This is one reason for strong union opposition to the shift to the private sector (Heyman 2001). Competition can force NFPs to 'race to the bottom' and impose similar measures.

Overly aggressive control over wages and working conditions can be counterproductive. To the extent that unattractive conditions encourage workers to leave and discourage new entrants (for example, to nursing), such measures can lead to labour shortages and ultimately increase costs. None the less, breaking union agreements and hiring workers at lower rates are a major theme among proponents of FP delivery. Whether this constitutes efficiency I leave to the reader.

Evasion of Cost Controls

Even though government can still borrow money at a lower cost than the private sector, all parties may find it expedient to replace capital costs by operating costs. In public–private partnerships for capital development (see Appendix) the full costs will not appear on a government balance sheet. To the extent that government is short-sighted, blocks access to capital, or refuses to fund technological improvements, it creates incentives to step around it and move to private partners, even if long-term costs rise considerably. Justifications for public–private partnerships often claim that new facilities would not otherwise have been built, rather than citing actual savings.

Similarly, some procedures, though highly beneficial, have high marginal costs. Hip and knee implants are a notable example. To the extent that funding cutbacks lead to arbitrary limitations on how many such procedures take place, demand will be felt in a private tier. The case can (and, in this author's view, should) be made for modifying allocation formulas to ensure that the publicly funded system is continuing to meet genuine needs in a timely manner, but this may be easier said than done. Paradoxically, the success of cost containment may have led to pressures to provide wanted services, higher remuneration for providers, and more 'creature comforts' outside the formal system of expenditure control. Under such circumstances, private delivery is sought out precisely because it will increase expenditures over what government is willing to allocate explicitly.

Sacrifice of Difficult-to-Measure Intangibles

In the absence of clearly defined outcomes, FPs will probably devote less money to activities that, though important, are not required of them. Obvious examples include teaching (and training the next generation of providers), research, quality assurance, and ties to the community. The Appendix notes such examples as laboratory services in Walkerton (in which FP/c firms did less reporting), CROS (which does not do teaching or research), and the different activities of NFP versus FP women's health centres.

Risk Selection / Cream Skimming

Any organization has an incentive to avoid 'unprofitable' patients. However, if it is also expected to offer a return on investment to its shareholders, that incentive is magnified. FPs tend to be more responsive to such incentives. In general, most U.S. studies tend to equate 'unprofitable' with being unable to pay for care – usually, being low income and/or uninsured/underinsured (Marmor, Schlesinger, and Smithey 1987). The evidence cited confirms that FPs are less likely to offer services on which they will not make a profit (Marmor, Schlesinger, and Smithey 1987). In Canada, the existence of a single payer means that determining which services are most lucrative depends on what government is willing to pay, rather than on which patients could afford to pay.

The term *cream skimming* describes a number of situations. The private dialysis clinic is happy to perform uncomplicated dialysis, while transferring the brittle diabetic to an NFP hospital. This division of labour may be appropriate, particularly if the uncomplicated cases do not require the hospital's expensive infrastructure. FPs tend to locate where profits seem most likely; for example, private ambulance companies do not appear anxious to serve remote northern communities. Here, other sectors (either public or NFP) must take over the less attractive business niches. Finally, the private FP tier, performing uninsured services, may none the less not assume the full costs of its care if it sends all complications back to the publicly funded system. In vitro fertilization to assist infertile couples to have children may be a 'private' service offered only to those able to pay, but the resulting babies are delivered at public expense, including the high costs of those requiring neonatal intensive care.

Risk selection/cream skimming is accordingly not inappropriate, as long as several key conditions are met. First, costing should recognize the differences in populations being served, rather than assuming that average costs apply across the board. It is misleading, and unfair, to conclude that 'private is best' if private treats only good risks or routine cases. Second, there must be enough patients and providers to maintain the infrastructure to provide the services and serve the clients that the FP sector is reluctant to address. Under some circumstances (for example, in large cities), there would be enough volume to support both. In others, the FP may succeed at the expense of high-needs groups in the community. Here again, one size will not fit all.

Dubious Practices
Another issue in U.S. studies is conflict of interest by providers (Donaldson and Currie 2000). Despite professional codes of ethics, there is a conflict between incentive structures that reward providers for increasing services, cost controls that attempt to minimize such services, and quality assurance mechanisms that seek to ensure that services maximize health outcomes. To the extent that incentive structures are too powerful, governments have had to introduce regulatory frameworks, which in turn increase red tape (and costs) and may hamper clinical autonomy. Although its extent is unclear, fraud, particularly among some of the more aggressive U.S. FPs, would also come under this heading.

Low Bids to Drive Out Competitors, Then Higher Charges?
Where quasi-monopolies exist, and barriers to entry are high, there have been reports of FPs giving low bids to drive out competitors and then charging higher, monopoly prices. Evaluation clearly must consider both short- and long-run costs and consequences.

Revenue Generation outside the Publicly Funded System
A critical insight arises from Donaldson and Currie's (2000) thorough review of the literature on public purchase of private surgical services from FP and NFP providers. Private facilities did not depend on publicly financed business; most of their revenues came through private purchase of care through private insurance. Thus, contrary to the rhetoric implying that the only issue was whether 'public' or 'private' delivery could offer better and more efficient care, the business plans of most such organizations depended on the existence of a parallel private system for payment. Sometimes this parallel system offered enhanced services (including shorter waits), and sometimes, other services not insured by the public plan. But the examples reviewed by Donaldson and Currie suggest that 75 to 85 per cent of patients of private clinics in England, Wales, Sweden, Australia, and New Zealand paid privately. A thorough analysis of private medicine in Britain reached a similar conclusion (Higgins 1988). This finding leads to the issues – beyond the scope of this paper – of impact on costs, access, and waiting lists for those individuals remaining within the publicly financed system. Similarly, Wendy Armstrong of the Consumer Association of Canada, Alberta branch, observes: 'The real problem we

have found in Alberta with our over 50 private investor owned day surgery clinics is that private delivery and private payment ultimately walk hand in hand – because they really aren't more efficient or cheaper unless they provide less or charge more on top of the public reimbursement. It also has become pretty apparent that privatization walks hand in hand with commercialization. It appears that you can't give the responsibility to deliver medical care to commercial interests and not expect them to adopt all the commercial trappings including aggressive marketing, focus on increased sales, and pursuit of returns (profit). In such an environment, even the community controlled facilities start taking on these values.'

On reflection, we can see that it is difficult to envision private provision from public funds within a competitive model; the financial risk to providers would appear excessive. The proposal that FP services be allowed to compete in the market as long as all funds come from public sources is particularly unrealistic. Similarly, proposals that FPs be allowed to relieve the pressure on inadequate 'public' resources carry with them the assumption that NFP delivery will remain inadequate in perpetuity. Should NFP hospitals improve their productivity and eliminate waiting lists, the market for the private services would vanish, regardless of how well they had performed. Investors would accordingly appear to require greater guarantees of revenues, given good performance, in order to justify making any capital commitments. Indeed, the public–private partnership (P3) arrangements described in the Appendix are characterized by such provisions. In turn, such guarantees would appear to remove any incentive (or even any ability) of the public or NFP sectors to improve their services. It would also imply that competitive markets, if set up, would be unlikely to persist, since such guarantees would leave little room for new competitors to enter the market unless barriers to entry were low. In short, FP firms would appear to require either a guaranteed stream of public revenue and/or the ability to generate additional revenues from private sources. Funding and delivery are linked.

Lessons Learned

Comparisons Are Difficult

Most attempts to compare costs and outcomes in various organizational styles are bedevilled by problems in making comparisons across organizational forms:

Heterogeneity of Organizations
The categories FP, NFP, and public are remarkably heterogeneous, and good and poor performance can be found within each (Gray 1999).

Differences in Services Offered. For the most part, FPs do not offer the same service as do their public or NFP counterparts. FPs tend to occupy niche markets, providing only high-volume (or profitable) services. Efforts to 'control' for those differences often overadjust; real differences end up looking statistically insignificant. For example, teaching hospitals are unlikely to be FPs. FP laboratories specialized in high-volume procedures, leaving specialized testing to NFP hospital-based labs. As we saw above, there is no inherent problem with this specialization, particularly when the population base is large enough to sustain it, but cost comparisons must (and often do not) take these differences into account.

Differences in Clientele. Similarly, FPs wish to serve clients who are willing and able to afford their services and who are most profitable. FP dialysis clinics may not take diabetics with major co-morbidities. This market segmentation can be termed 'cream skimming,' but it is problematic only if pricing is unfair or the 'buttermilk' cannot be served. This might occur, for example, if the clinic serving the high-volume care left the organizations serving the more complex cases without the critical mass or resources to deliver those services (Griffin, Cockerill, and Deber 2001).

Differences in Cost Structure. FPs pay taxes, and NFPs do not. There may also be differences in access to (and cost of) capital. The calculations about the merits of the private finance initiative (PFI) described in the Appendix depend heavily on the choice of 'discount rate' – that is, how much we adjust future costs (and benefits) of resources invested to reflect the fact that future benefits are worth less than those that can be consumed immediately.

   A complex issue is how to report costs. Conventionally, many studies look at average costs. However, this may be inappropriate, particularly when there are high fixed costs (for example, for equipment and staff). In such situations, simply reporting average costs does not capture economies (and diseconomies) of scale. When a facility cannot be closed (for example, an emergency room serving a remote community or a unit offering highly specialized expertise), moving cases to 'lower-cost' alternatives requires those fixed costs to be spread across a smaller number of patients. This may explode average costs at the original facility and lead to a *less* efficient system.

Differences in Regulatory and Market Environments. The regulatory and market environments within which these organizations function vary considerably. Affluent neighbourhoods attract different clients, with different needs, regardless of organizational form. Since FPs are un-likely to locate where clients could not pay for their services, considerable confounding of organization type and other characteristics is likely. Similarly, firms behave very differently in highly competitive markets than when they have a quasi-monopoly on service provision.

Comparisons Are Not Impossible

There are none the less systematic differences in the incentives and values inherent in organizational forms. Marmor (Marmor, Schlesinger, and Smithey 1987) argues that the success of organized corporate institutions represents 'the incremental decline of a service ethos – more naked in one sector, more camouflaged in the other,' and he sees the challenge as being 'to discover rules of the medical game that constrain the vices of both rampant commercialism and complacent professionalism.' Thus public or NFP firms may have little incentive to improve efficiency or client service. In contrast, FPs are in business to make a profit and are thus more likely to respond to financial incentives. In theory, firms can maximize profits in a number of ways, depending on whether they are competing on quality or price. Economic theory would predict that FPs would be more responsive than NFP or public organizations to incentives to target the most profitable services and client groups, to minimize costs, and to maximize revenue.

The empirical results reported in the Appendix are all in the predicted direction; FPs are indeed more responsive to these market signals. Similarly, the empirical results support the theoretical prediction that maintenance of quality varies with the extent to which potential customers can observe it; invisible factors are more likely to be ignored. Thus firms marketing to providers (for example, physicians) have different incentives to maintain quality than those marketing directly to patients or third-party payers; in consequence, quality differences are greater in the nursing-home sector than among hospitals. FPs seek to maximize revenue by increasing charges when the reimbursement plan so allows or by decreasing costs where that is feasible. (Often their NFP competitors in that market soon follow suit.) Cost comparisons accordingly depend on the regulatory and reimbursement environment.

The incentives inherent in a corporate structure, all other things being equal, appear inimical to many desired outcomes. FPs have an incentive to maximize the amount that they bill payers (thus increasing total health-care spending) and to minimize quality of care (unless this will harm their business), labour costs, and spending on non-profitable activities (including particular services, client groups, and such activities as teaching, research, and community service). These tendencies can be controlled, but only through fairly elaborate and costly measurement and monitoring of performance. 'The interests of government and of its contractors simply diverge on some fundamental points. The government would like to pay as little as possible ... while suppliers would like to earn as much as possible. Each party prefers stability and would rather shift risk to the other. Each wants the other to fulfill commitments precisely, while retaining flexibility for itself. The craft of contracting is to devise covenants that bring divergent purposes into something approaching alignment' (Donahue 1989, 115).

Competition and Co-operation Must Be Balanced

Competition runs somewhat counter to another highly advocated trend – that of greater co-operation among providers. Considerable emphasis has been placed on the need to integrate and co-ordinate services. Competition, in contrast, sets up providers as rivals. Best practices can become trade secrets, and information is less likely to be shared. How to reconcile these conflicting imperatives (co-operate or compete) has received little consideration.

Measuring and Monitoring of Performance Are Essential

An overwhelming theme of the material reviewed is the importance of being able to measure and monitor performance. Many studies end at this point. However, further examination reveals that such measurement and monitoring are neither simple nor inexpensive.

Measuring and Monitoring of Performance Can Be Costly and Difficult

Whereas certain services, such as refuse collection, are relatively 'straightforward, immediate, measurable, monitorable, and technical' (Bendick 1989), others are not. As the World Bank has noted, it is difficult to measure performance for many – indeed most – health care services (Preker and Harding 2000; Preker, Harding, and Travis 2000). The literature reviewed in the Appendix suggests that NFP providers are most likely to provide high-quality services under such circumstances, whereas FP/c firms have a strong incentive not to go beyond the levels specified in their contracts. Furthermore, many economists concur that it is difficult for consumers to assess the quality of the care that they receive (Evans 1984; Rice 1998; Sloan 2000).

Donaldson's review of over 2,000 references concluded that *no* study reviewed had a system in place to monitor costs, quality of care, or outcomes in private providers (Donaldson and Currie 2000). Performance monitoring in theory was often called for; in practice it rarely occurred.

Regulatory policy always gives rise to tension between the need to protect and the desire to increase flexibility and reduce the costs and burden of 'administrivia.' For example, how specific should regulations be concerning the number and skills of staff members, their training, their relationships with referring professionals, their handling of pharmaceuticals, their physical plans, the food that they serve, and so on? How capable are regulators of observing and enforcing these rules? Where does cost exceed benefit?

Certainly, there are perennial complaints about insufficient data for monitoring, particularly after a service moves outside direct government control. This is not a public–private issue per se, but one of ensuring accountability within alternative delivery experiments. For example, the Auditor General of Ontario has found that the data being collected were inadequate to evaluate the performance of NFP Community Care Access Centres (Office of the Provincial Auditor General of Ontario 1998b).

Donahue's excellent assessment of the privatization debate clarifies how very difficult it is to write good contracts, particularly when the desired outputs are difficult to specify precisely (Donahue 1989). One chapter reviews the history of weapons procurement by the Pentagon and notes: 'There are several impediments to straight-forward contracting that bedevil the acquisition of all but the most standardized military goods. First, when there is uncertainty over the mission a weapon is to fulfill, or over the technology involved, the government enters into contracts that are incompletely specified and subject to revision. Second, because contracts are incomplete and changeable, competitive bids are, at best, tentative and, at worst, meaningless. Third, once the government has selected a supplier, it has only the feeblest sanctions to deter poor performance, since there are usually formidable barriers against replacing contractors' (114). Donahue goes on: 'There are almost no weapons acquisition problems that cannot be overcome by better procedures, closer oversight, and more complete evaluation. But the indignant calls for procedural reform that follow every scandal miss the point that contracting *itself* is costly. The more completely rules, obligations, and procedures are defined in order to enforce accountability, the higher the price in time, money, and flexibility. Herein lies one of the Pentagon's most important, and most poignant, lessons for advocates of expanding the private sector's role in the public's business' (108).

The seemingly endless cycles of reform thus range between the much-ridiculed sixteen-page specifications for a metal whistle and efforts to relax regulations that end up in new procurement fiascos. The higher the stakes, the more ferocious the competition. Because 'only a few firms have the expertise, equipment, and capital to even contemplate bidding,' competition may be 'cataclysmic' – 'winners will flourish; losers may perish' (Donahue 1989). Uncertainties about the value of what is being purchased increase incentives and opportunities for interested parties 'to manipulate perceptions of common need' and to politicize spending decisions (Donahue 1989).

In a privatized delivery system, much control over staffing and purchasing escapes from government control. It may no longer be clear who establishes the mandate, defines the nature of the service, or calculates costs to the consumer of service, or what experimentation with delivery methods is allowed (Ford and Zussman 1997). As Langford notes, 'Whatever contracts may say, in reality, contractors often end up defining the clients to be served and the quality and quantity of the service being provided' (Ford and Zussman 1997). He adds: 'How much tolerance will there be among private sector partners in particular, who are putting up their own money, information and equipment for the program design "add-ons" that are peculiar to government (e.g., external reporting, media management, freedom of information regulations, labour relations requirements, official language regulations, equity considerations)?' (Ford and Zussman 1997). Firms operating in multiple jurisdictions also resist having to work with different regulatory regimes and often seek exemption from government mandates within individual states (Kleinke 2001).

Complying with accountability regulations may be too costly for many smaller providers. As Wendy Armstrong observes: 'The problem with RFPs is that the inclusion of requirements like incredibly expensive ISO or CSA standards – or providing a full range of products – drive out small competitors and local competitors (including community run agencies) in every industry – not just home care or health care' (personal communication, 12 Nov 2001).

Changing Delivery Structures Alters Power Relationships

Any system of resource allocation creates winners and losers. Advocates of private delivery often assume that this move will weaken the bargaining position of unionized labour; to the extent that there are labour shortages, this view may be naïve. It is less often recognized that private delivery can in fact strengthen the constituency for particular programs and make it more difficult to reduce their budgets. Several studies of privatization have concluded that suppliers can forge effective political coalitions to protect and to increase program funding (Bendick 1989; Donahue 1989). The precise impact varies from case to case; but power relationships are likely to be affected and, with them, the nature and level of resource allocation.

Experiments Should Not Be Irreversible

One ongoing issue relates to the effect, if any, of international trade agreements on public–private partnerships. For example, lawyer Steven Shrybman has noted the expansive reading that some court decisions have given to 'expropriation,' which might allow investors to seek damages under NAFTA or WTO procedures for such eventualities as contract cancellation for non-performance and introduction of public-health or regulatory measures (Shrybman 2001a). These disputes would be settled by international tribunals, under their rules; local or provincial governments would not have standing. Advocates of such partnerships disagree (Fasken Martineau DuMoulin LLP 2001).

None the less, considerable uncertainty exists. What is more disquieting is the possibility that experimentation with for-profit private delivery might be a one-way valve – that is, there would be no way to reverse the experiment even if the results proved disappointing.

Health Human-Resource Issues Must Be Dealt With

Although the focus of this paper is not on change management, or labour shortages, many advocates of privatization base their arguments on the belief that existing labour agreements are too inflexible and/or too expensive. The language of 'public-sector monopoly' refers less to the form of management (which, as we saw above, is neither public sector nor a monopoly) than to centralized bargaining for a unionized workforce. To many of these writers, the primary advantage of privatization appears to be breaking the power of the trade unions. Plans that seek to mitigate inefficiencies in work rules and allow flexibility and empowerment may be highly worthwhile. Plans that expect primarily to transfer public resources from workers to investors are unlikely to win long-term support or to be particularly wise public policy.

For-Profit Delivery Requires Predictable Revenue Streams

As I noted above, FP delivery seeks predictable revenue streams. An examination of partnerships for transportation observed that when private-sector partners invest money in new facilities, they want government 'to commit to a policy framework for the duration of the partnership that will not endanger the financial viability of the new facility' (Ford and Zussman 1997). One possibility is guaranteed funding (for example, the P3 initiatives); more common is a parallel private revenue stream. At present, the scope for parallel private financing of medically necessary physician and hospital services is small, because of the provisions of the Canada Health Act and the strong views of the Canadian public. However, extra charges to insured persons for insured services are prohibited only for care deemed medically required, and the dividing line between what is necessary and what is not is not always clear. Thus a clinic may provide a mixture of insured and uninsured services. To the extent that prices paid by the publicly funded system are well controlled, there are clear incentives to expand the uninsured services available and even to push for private financing to top up public money (Donaldson and Currie 2000).

Barriers to Meeting Patients' Demands Can, and Must, Be Addressed

One key justification frequently put forward for private FP facilities has been NFPs' inability to meet patients' needs. The CROS clinic described in the Appendix was necessary only because existing facilities were unable to mobilize the personnel needed to operate an additional shift within their clinics. The private market in Britain capitalized on the difficulty that NHS hospitals had in giving patients their choice of hospital dates (Higgins 1988). At present, considerable administrative waste motion exists, frustrating providers, patients, and funders. Hospitals and agencies often do not receive final information about the money that they will receive from the province until well into the fiscal year – a sure prescription for inefficiency. Other barriers may arise from inflexible labour or budgetary arrangements. Constant crisis has burned out workers and managers, while efficiency drives have eroded the flexibility needed for innovation. Morale is low. Regardless of what decisions are made about delivery – and the material reviewed does not leave this author sanguine about the benefits of FP/c delivery except under highly defined circumstances – the client focus of the existing system must be addressed with some urgency. In theory, there is no reason why existing NFPs cannot be as nimble, innovative, and flexible as their FP counterparts. Discovering why they are not, and making the appropriate changes, would appear to be both essential and desirable.

Appendix: What the Literature Shows: Case Studies in Delivery

This Appendix summarizes some of the voluminous literature on the implications of various delivery modes. Authors who have tried to synthesize even tightly defined sectors have confronted several thousand references. This review is not comprehensive, although I have sought to locate and analyse the key references and review articles, with an emphasis on Canada, the United Kingdom, and the United States.

A Note on Statistical Analysis

Many of the studies reviewed rely on statistical analysis of varying degrees of sophistication. In all such studies, the analyst uses statistics to understand variations in a *dependent variable* (or criterion variable) as a function of variations in one or more *independent variables* (or predictor variables). The analysis may or may not *control* for other variables, which, though unrelated to the hypothesis being tested, are also likely to affect the dependent variable.

For example, assume that one is measuring how effective a new drug is at controlling blood pressure. In this case, the dependent variable is blood pressure, and the independent variable is whether the patient is taking the new drug or something else (possibly including a placebo). Clearly, there will be considerable variation in the dependent variable; not all patients have the same blood pressure. The *science* of statistical analysis seeks to clarify whether the differences *between* groups are greater than the differences *within* them.

The *art* of statistical analysis, however, lies in the choice of variables. In the blood pressure example, what, if anything, should the analyst control for? Age? Sex? How high the initial blood pressure was? Presence of other co-morbid conditions, such as diabetes or renal failure? The relationship will get larger, or smaller, depending on which controls are used. This issue is particularly problematic in   non-experimental designs, where cases are not assigned randomly. Consider attempting to evaluate the impact of education on future income. Clearly, education is intertwined with other factors, including parental income, residence, work habits, and future occupation. Equally clearly, these factors are not identical – one can find people with very high incomes and very little education (for example, certain athletes) and others with a great deal of education and very little income (for example, graduate students). Should one control for occupation in trying to assess the relationship? If one does so, to the extent that education strongly affects which occupation an individual will be able to have, this 'overcontrols' and removes much of the relationship that one wishes to investigate. As we see below, selecting which variables to control for strongly influences many of the studies reported below, particularly those attempting to compare public, NFP, and FP hospitals.

Privatization of Local Government Activities

Local governments are responsible for providing or ensuring the provision of a host of services, ranging from collecting garbage to maintaining police and fire protection. Service delivery absorbs a high proportion of local-government expenditures. Under fiscal pressure, governments throughout the world have shown increased interest in an array of 'alternative service delivery' (ASD) models. Public organizations are expected to follow democratic principles and adhere to broader policy objectives, but also to be efficient and customer-focused. The extensive literature on new approaches to local service delivery considers a variety of mechanisms, including changes in financing (for example, user fees, franchises), management (for example, improving productivity), and delivery (Hatry 1983; DeHoog 1984; Kemp 1991; Skelly 1996; Ford and Zussman 1997). These mechanisms include shifts from public to private delivery of publicly funded services – 'contracting out.' An overview of such models found them to be largely responding to the perceived rigidities of government: 'In essence, has it become easier to solve the internal problems of government by moving innovative organizations/programs outside of the formal system?' (Ford and Zussman 1997).

Evaluation of these programs is relatively sparse. Hatry's comments still apply: 'Unfortunately, little systematic, objective evaluation of most of these alternatives is available. Most available information is descriptive, anecdotal, and advocacy or public-relations oriented. Information on the consequences of the use of these approaches, when mentioned at all, is usually provided by the government that undertook the action, and such information is usually limited to assessments in the first year of the activity – before longer-term consequences have been identified' (Hatry 1983, 9).

The success stories reported often resulted from improving the management of revenues rather than controlling costs – for example, adjusting accounting and billing systems to maximize reimbursements from the state and federal governments. These gains tended to be higher in smaller organizations that could not otherwise afford highly specialized expertise. Other advantages of contracting out were avoiding large initial costs, allowing benchmarking to compare multiple competing suppliers, and avoiding bureaucratic problems within government.

However, Donahue's review of evaluations of local service contracting in the United States, including a 1984 study for the federal Department of Housing and Urban Development's Office of Policy Development and Research, found that much of the savings came from lowering wage costs. In only one example – the capital-intensive task of laying asphalt – did the private sector pay higher wages; for the other services, between 18 per cent and 75 per cent of the additional costs in the public sector came from wage differentials. In addition, monthly benefit costs for municipal employees averaged $553 a month, as compared to $368 for contractors. Donahue concluded: 'Delegating certain functions to private firms usually saves tax dollars, and much of these savings comes at the expense of public employees. What remains to be done is to weigh the joint implications of these two facts' (1989, 145).

Hatry concluded that there were indeed success stories but that the results were ambiguous: 'A shift in either direction, either from municipal to private or from private to municipal, would likely lead to reduced costs. The rationale is that when a local government is willing to make such a substantial shift, its previous condition is likely to be so inefficient that any change would lead to an improvement' (1983, 25).

Provincial auditors general in Canada have examined a number of such experiments. Although a lesson consistently drawn in the literature was the importance of carefully monitoring contractors' performance (Hatry 1983), paradoxically, when governments are too weak to manage programs internally, they are often too weak to manage external contracts. In a number of cases, governments have failed to specify expectations clearly and have ended up paying considerably more than expected and/or getting far less. In New Brunswick, a leasing arrangement for the Evergreen School was estimated to have cost the province $774,576 more than it would have had it done the work itself, with no savings in operating costs realized (Office of the Auditor General of New Brunswick 1998). In Ontario, a contract between the provincial Ministry of Community and Social Services and Anderson Consulting to support transformation of the former Family Benefit and General Welfare Assistance programs also led to huge cost overruns and estimated expenses far higher than would have been the case had government workers delivered the services (Whorley 2001). The provincial legislature's Standing Committee on Public Accounts and the auditor general have issued scathing reports (Office of the Provincial Auditor General of Ontario 1998a; 2000).

In contrast, when outcomes could be clearly defined, contracting out has realized efficiencies. However, a review of solid-waste contracting among 327 Canadian municipalities revealed substantial public–private differences only in communities with a population of under 10,000, which were able to take advantage of economies of scale and management efficiencies by contracting out services. The author concluded that the main gains came from competition, rather than from public or private delivery per se (McDavid 2001).

A number of these experiments resemble the military-procurement examples cited by Donahue (1989), in that the sunk costs become so high that government becomes reluctant to abandon the existing vendor, even as expectations are not met. Donahue noted other lessons learned from the military in his conclusions.

The studies also stressed the need for government to monitor the activities and performance of the private-sector companies, while expressing concern about its capacity to do so. Whorley (2001, 340) concluded that 'the success of collaborative arrangements is threatened when public actors enter as the subordinate player' and expressed 'concern about power imbalance, divergent interests, [and] the appropriate allocation of benefits and accountability.'

Public–Private Partnerships (the Private Finance Initiative)

Governments in many countries have been experimenting with public – private partnerships (P3) arrangements. They have justified these efforts usually as a way of enhancing access to capital in an era when government has been unwilling to provide such resources directly. Students of P3 have categorized such arrangements, depending on the nature of risk transferred between public and private sectors. At one extreme is outsourcing or contracting out. At the other, government sells public assets outright to the private organization ('privatization'). Between lie an array of such options, including BOO (build, own, operate), BOT (build, operate, transfer), BOOT (build, own, operate, transfer), and DBFO (design, build, finance, operate) (Bennett Jones 2001).

One of the more enthusiastic experiments with, in effect, contracting out the construction of hospitals has been occurring in the United Kingdom. Unlike Canada's arrangements, the National Health Service (NHS) was founded on public delivery; the NHS absorbed most existing hospitals into the public sector, subject to management directives from the government, and its employees became part of the national civil service (Higgins 1988). British experiments thus began with asking, 'Why/why not public delivery?' before considering the role of FP versus NFP organizations. The Conservatives introduced the Private Finance Initiative (PFI) in 1992 as a way both to secure more capital than would otherwise be available and to bring private-sector efficiencies to the procurement process. As many observers have noted (Gaffney, et al. 1999a, b, c; Pollock, et al. 1999; Boyle and Harrison 2000b; Harrison 2001), the first rationale appears largely spurious. Although Third World governments have problems in obtaining capital, Britain (and indeed Canada's provincial governments) have no such situation. For the most part, they can borrow at lower rates of interest than private partners.

Several British observers have scrutinized the ability of these arrangements to obtain better 'value for money (VFM), affordability, efficient allocation of risks, and the ability to retain a strategic overview of health service provision within a framework accountable to the public at large' (Boyle and Harrison 2000b, 6). Since the PFI, though introduced in 1992, had not yet delivered a new hospital as of 2000, it was difficult to evaluate its success. Some authors are highly negative (Gaffney et al. 1999a, b, c; Pollock et al. 1999); Boyle and Harrison (2000a) term the benefits 'unproven': 'Evaluation of some aspects of its impact is therefore inevitably a speculative matter. Judgments can turn on fine points of disagreement around issues where there is a high level of uncertainty. This created scope for political reasoning rather than economic evaluation to be the effective determinant of the balance of public and private finance.' Boyle and Harrison (2000b) note that in the one case examined by the National Audit Office, it was unable to determine whether there were any savings at all: 'Moreover, even if the basic VFM (value for money) conclusions were accepted, cost savings between the PFI option and the PSC (Public Sector Comparator) almost entirely depend on the kind of things that are included in the transfer of risk to the private sector, and how these have been costed. Finally, claims that the PFI would introduce substantial innovation in the design and running of health care buildings seem largely illusory' (Boyle and Harrison 2000b, 14).

This analysis brings us back to the difference between encouraging a private role and encouraging competition. In four of the first fifteen PFI contracts, there proved to be only one final bidder. Not surprisingly, the costs of successful bids under such circumstances increased substantially from initial estimates (Boyle and Harrison 2000b). The authors also point to the high transaction costs inherent in managing the competitive bid process, including payments to consultants, which would raise the final price. They explain that there are two types of risks in such arrangements, only one of which advocates of PFIs have emphasized: 'On the supply side there are the risks of building procurement which are common to most large development projects: that the structure is not available on time and within costs, and that what is delivered diverges from the intended design specification. There is also the maintenance of the building and associated services – to a specified quality – over the lifetime of its use by the NHS client. The risk transfer element of the PFI process has focused on these supply-side risks: on construction delay and cost overrun, unavailability of parts of the hospital, and the failure of facilities management to meet contract standards.' But there is more to the story. 'Meanwhile the public sector retains the uncertainty of the demand side risk. Moreover, by taking on a 30-year contract for services, there is an additional risk for the public sector. If the demand for hospital services were to decline dramatically, then the NHS trust is tied into an agreement for maintenance and facilities management services over and above any cost of producing the building itself. If this were a public sector procurement, then in the worst case scenario, the facility could be allowed to run down at no expense to the trust other than – in PFI terms – the availability fee.' Assessments have ignored these factors. 'This is a potential risk that has not been factored into the equation when comparing the two options. There are examples – Dartford & Gravesham is one – where the contract allows for the charge to be reduced in the event of lower utilisation, but only if the consortium is able to avoid costs' (Boyle and Harrison 2000b).

In Canada, cost containment by governments has generated a large, pent-up demand for capital and made hospitals and other public agencies increasingly desperate. In addition, accounting rules in provinces such as Ontario have required hospitals to expense all capital contributions in the year of funding; neither has that province funded depreciation. In consequence, capital costs have not been amortized or reflected in operating costs (CIHI 2001). Not surprisingly, hospitals have looked elsewhere for capital investment, even if the long-term cost might be higher.

Accordingly, some hospitals have been considering P3 arrangements. British Columbia has proposed building a private institution in Abbotsford, to the dismay of unions (Hospital Employees' Union

2001). A recent report for the Ontario Hospital Association's Committee on Hospital Capital Development incorporates enthusiastic reports on British, Australian (Victoria), and U.S. (Veterans' Administration hospitals) examples (Bennett Jones 2001) but concentrates on the risks of construction-cost overruns, ignoring the demand-side risks identified in the British evaluations. (The PFI would lock participating hospitals into specified costs over the lifetime of the contract; even in an economic downturn, the partners would have first call on hospital resources, regardless of other priorities.) In British Columbia, the government has decided to finance long-term-care institutions through what it calls P3 initiatives, which have evoked concern from some analysts (Vogel 2000, Rachlis 2000a).

Strictly speaking, the descriptions being used by Canadian advocates of P3 arrangements do not apply to the Canadian health-care system. Bennett Jones's report begins with the debatable assumption that the systems in Britain and Australia are 'highly analogous to the Ontario system,' thus equating NFP and public entities and bypassing any complexities of the three-way relationships among government and its NFP and FP/c partners.

Assessment of such arrangements is complicated. For example, private companies in general cannot borrow money as cheaply as government can, although this factor is less important, given current low interest rates. Yet they may be able to build more efficiently. The extent to which private efficiency can offset higher interest rates will clearly vary across situations. The University Health Network, in Toronto, financed recent facility renovations through a bond issue, priced at a slightly higher interest rate than comparable Ontario bonds (Bennett Jones 2001). Other PFI examples cost more than they would have under traditional procurement approaches; however, the existence of the PFI allowed the hospitals to be built now, rather than waiting for government money to become available (Bennett Jones 2001). In effect, the PFI arrangements shift building costs from capital to operating budgets and take them 'off the books' for government. There is reason to believe that total costs will be higher, but the total is easier to shield from public accountability. Thus judgments about the merits of such arrangements are based on policy rather than accounting considerations.

Some authors observe that private-sector operators are somewhat risk averse and reluctant to build a hospital without a guarantee that their lease payments would continue, regardless of changes of government or in patterns of service use (Bennett Jones 2001). The communities that most need hospital care may not be those in a position to pay market prices. Australia's first large P3 project – the La Trobe hospital – was a failed experiment; the private-sector company operating the facility lost money and eventually returned it to the government (Bennett Jones 2001). The report describing this example indicated a major lesson learned: 'Ensure that a good location is picked. La Trobe which was in an isolated area suffering from a crash in the town's industry, was a poor choice for sustaining a vibrant hospital' (Bennett Jones 2001). Its residents may not have agreed.

Recently, the auditors general in a number of Canadian provinces have expressed some concern about P3 arrangements (Office of the Auditor General of New Brunswick 1998; Office of the Auditor General of Nova Scotia 1997; 1998; 1999; Office of the Provincial Auditor General of Ontario 1998a; 2000; 2001). Considerable concern has also arisen as to whether P3 arrangements will have implications under international trade obligations, which may make experiments irreversible (Fasken Martineau DuMoulin LLP 2001; Shrybman 2001a; b).

Acute General Hospitals

In Canada, almost all (98 per cent) hospitals are NFPs, with a residual sector of small FP facilities that ante-dated medicare and were allowed to continue. One prominent experiment with FP management of an NFP hospital occurred in 1984 in Hawkesbury, Ontario (population about 10,000), following merger of three local hospitals into two. Ontario requires that hospitals and their communities provide a portion of capital expenditures, and the hospital was unable to raise its share. The province accordingly sponsored a competition, using a request for proposals (RFP) to find an operator that would cover the community's share of capital, in exchange for a ten-year management contract for all non-clinical services. The only qualified bidder was a U.S. company, American Medical International (AMI), then a chain of 130 hospitals operating in 13 countries. Although it was able to achieve some economies of scale in operating costs (for example, IT systems), the management contract was not renewed, and Hawkesbury General Hospital returned to NFP management (Bennett Jones 2001).

In contrast, U.S. hospitals have many types, usually grouped into three categories: public (primarily Veterans' Administration hospitals, and municipal hospitals in poor, inner-city neighbourhoods), NFP (often run by religious or charitable organizations), and FP (often run by large, publicly traded chains, which are expected to give a return on investment to their shareholders). As of 1994, 60 per cent of 'nonfederal short-term general hospitals' were NFP, 28 per cent public, and 12 per cent FP, mostly owned by large, publicly traded corporations (Sloan 2000). A number of articles have reviewed the literature. Comparisons of performance are extremely complex, since the three types of hospitals prove not to be interchangeable. They often serve different patient populations and provide different services. Analyses hence differ in factors controlled for, while critiques generally suggest yet other controls that might have been useful.

Accordingly, some comparative analyses conclude that FPs perform better, while others take similar data to conclude that they are worse, and still others find no significant differences. Woolhandler and Himmelstein found that FPs had the highest charges, with NFPs in the middle, and public the lowest (Woolhandler and Himmelstein 1997; 1999; Himmelstein, Woolhandler, and Hellander 2001). They suggest that the higher administrative charges from the FPs account for much of the cost difference (Rachlis 2000a). Silverman found that spending on the U.S. Medicare program was highest in communities where all hospital beds were in FPs (Silverman, Skinner, and Fisher 1999). In contrast, Zelder concluded that 'of the 15 studies reviewed, 8 showed that private hospitals performed better, 3 found that public hospitals performed better, and 4 revealed no difference in performance.' Some of his analyses combined FPs and NFPs, while others separated these out. Zelder attributed the superior showing of private hospitals to their ability to avoid paying high wages to unionized employees, particularly those doing such non-professional tasks as cleaning and meal preparation (Zelder 2001).

As I noted above in the section on statistics, the question of which factors should be controlled for can critically affect conclusions. For example, teaching hospitals are known to have higher costs and better outcomes. Yet because there were no FP teaching hospitals in the U.S. database used by these studies, controlling for teaching status selectively removed the most complex cases from the analysis. Similarly, FPs maximize profits by adjusting their case mix and labour costs; they also tend to be smaller. Yet one important study by Robinson and Luft first 'controlled for a wide range of differences among hospitals, including number of competitors, case-mix, size, occupancy, and labour costs' (i.e., most dimensions on which FPs would differ from NFPs) before concluding that 'for-profits had significantly lower cost per admission and per day than non-profits' (Zelder 2001). Another of the studies cited by Zelder (by Ferrier and Valdmanis) as showing the greater efficiency of FPs controlled for such factors as 'quality (defined as a hospital's excess mortality), hospital size and occupancy rate, and the proportion of services provided to outpatients and in intensive care.' A national study of 981 U.S. hospitals in the early 1980s by Shortell and Hughes found 'no difference in quality measured in terms of mortality by ownership;' but Hartz et al., 'using fewer covariates,' Hartz et al. found higher mortality in FP than in NFP hospitals (Sloan 2000). All teaching hospitals in Sloan's sample were either public or NFP; controlling for this factor thus excluded many of the most complex cases from the FP sample (Sloan et al. 1998).

Clearly, analysts can differ as to which factors to control for and which might seem sufficiently associated with ownership type to remain in the comparison. The point is not that one analysis is right and the other wrong, but that such comparisons are rarely value neutral.

Donaldson and Curie conclude that, 'faced with the same financial pressures, for-profit facilities respond differently compared with not-for-profits, to the detriment of patient care' (2000). For example, private hospitals in Los Angeles performed more Caesarean deliveries for Medicaid patients (Gregory et al. 1999). One paper widely cited in support of the conclusion that there are systematic differences between FP and NFP providers is an examination of U.S. patients with end-stage renal disease. Early praise for FP clinics (Lowrie and Hampers 1981) had led to a proliferation of such organizations; subsequent evaluation found that those treated in FPs had a higher crude mortality rate and a lower likelihood of being placed on the waiting list for a renal transplant (which, if successful, would remove them from the need for dialysis), as compared with NFPs (Garg et al. 1999). However, a number of letters to the editor of the *New England Journal of Medicine* argued variously that the researchers had too small a sample, did not properly adjust for case mix, did not consider distance to a transplantation centre, used old data that did not account for changes in delivery of dialysis, did not control for affiliation with academic programs, or did not properly control for co-morbidity. Another letter reported that a separate, independent analysis had come to similar conclusions, though with smaller differences (a 5–7 per cent higher mortality rate, rather than the 20 per cent reported by Garg et al.). Clearly, there is always one more control that might be performed.

Both supporters and opponents of FP delivery note that these organizations tend to reduce labour costs and are much less likely to employ unionized workers (Zelder 2001). Whether this is good or bad, of course, depends substantially on the commentator's views.

These conflicting interpretations reinforce the difficulty of defining 'better' performance. For example, one study analysed by Zelder focused only on profits from treating elderly patients and assumed that, since all hospitals were dealing with the same reimbursement formula, the higher profits among FPs must have represented lower costs. In the absence of outcome data, it then equated lower costs with better performance (Zelder 2001). One review of FPs versus NFPs noted that study results were inconsistent and differences small; FPs tended to have a higher cost per day, but shorter stays, meaning that the difference in cost per admission fluctuated around zero (Marmor, Schlesinger, and Smithey 1987). Furthermore, when physicians control the delivery of care, there was no measurable difference in quality of care between FPs and NFPs (Marmor, Schlesinger, and Smithey 1987). The analyses performed under the auspices of the (U.S.) National Bureau of Economic Research (NBER) (Cutler 2000) found FPs more financially successful than NFPs, but much of the difference resulted from skill at increasing public-sector reimbursement. They also found that NFP hospitals in the same market followed closely behind and adopted similar approaches.

Some studies have examined the performance of NFPs that have 'converted' to FPs. Once so converted, a hospital can pay out future surpluses in the form of profits to shareholders (although past surpluses must be transferred to other charitable uses). FPs can then raise working capital through equity instruments not available to NFP or public institutions. Government may also benefit in terms of increased revenues, because FPs lose their former tax exemptions, although there are potentially offsetting losses from changes in the 'public goods' (such as care to the indigent) that they may have provided.

Sloan's case study of hospital conversions in North Carolina, South Carolina, and Tennessee was affected by small sample sizes (which made it difficult to reach statistical significance) but also discovered changes in the predicted direction. Moving from NFP to FP status decreased the probability that a hospital would run certain potentially unprofitable programs, such as AIDS, community health, rehabilitation, open heart surgery, or skilled nursing units. It increased the probability of having home health (at the time quite lucrative), sports medicine, or magnetic resonance imaging (MRI), and increased emergency-room visits (Cutler 2000). However, the conversion also brought in capital resources and allowed service improvements. Interpretation of the results is complicated, because hospitals that converted were by no means a random sample. In general, the research shows that those NFPs converting had poorer financial performance, a high debt load, and an organizational culture oriented more to business (Cutler and Horwitz 1998; Cutler 2000). Indeed, six of the ten cases studied by Sloan were relatively small hospitals in small communities that were otherwise at risk of closing; merely changing ownership did not make them particularly profitable (Cutler 2000).

An extensive analysis of private health care in the United Kingdom finds similar differences between FP and public facilities. Higgins (1988) traces the evolution from a 'cottage industry' of small, non-corporate FPs providing relatively simple care (FP/s organizations) to profit-seeking business enterprises. The difficulties of comparing across jurisdictions were also evident; for example, in Britain the key advantage to patients in 'going private' was not earlier admission (queue jumping), but the ability to plan admission dates (which many Canadian patients already can do). There was no evidence that the private alternative reduced waiting lists, and some anecdotal evidence to the contrary. Higgins concludes: 'On balance, the evidence suggests that public systems of care (such as the NHS) may be relatively cost-effective and moderately successful in controlling costs but at the price of under-investment in important facilities and services. Private systems, on the other hand, are often characterised by waste, for which patients (or their insurers) have to pay in the form of higher prices, over-provision of services and under-occupancy of beds.'

Similarly equivocal results emerge from a major study of the U.S. literature comparing public, NFP, and FP hospitals, psychiatric hospitals, nursing homes, and managed-care companies conducted by the Institute of Medicine in 1986 and updated in 1999 (Gray 1999). The initial review had concluded that 'studies generally showed that expenses were similar at nonprofit and for-profit hospitals. However, depending upon method of payment (cost-based or charge-based reimbursement), the costs to purchasers were from 8–24 percent higher in for-profit hospitals than in nonprofit hospitals' (Gray 1999). This is consistent with the finding that FPs were better at maximizing reimbursement, although NFPs soon discovered and exploited the same loopholes (Cutler and Horwitz 1998; Cutler 2000; Sloan 2000). Recognizing that comparisons were complicated because no teaching hospitals were FP (although several have since converted), Gray (1999) concluded:

- 'Nonprofits care for more uninsured patients than for-profits, though not as much as public hospitals.' However, the extent of such care varied considerably.
- 'Nonprofit hospitals provide a wider array of services than do for-profit hospitals, including services focused on vulnerable populations (e.g., HIV/AIDS) or services that lose money.'
- Quality differences were small but tended to favour NFPs. Cost differences were smaller once the incentive system was changed (i.e., the US Medicare system phased out its cost-based reimbursement formula), but markups and costs to purchasers remained higher in FPs.
- NFP psychiatric hospitals 'had fewer quality violations and complaints and higher staff/patient ratios' than did FPs, while expenses of FPs 'were either similar to or higher than those of nonprofits.' 'Performance differences between for-profit and nonprofit psychiatric hospitals regarding community benefit activities (e.g., uncompensated care) depended upon the extent of pressure and influence by communities, regulators, and professionals.'

The summary results suggest that FPs are slightly more expensive than public or NFP hospitals and more likely to serve a niche market that investors believe can be profitable. However, to the extent that health professionals (particularly physicians) control care, there are unlikely to be major differences in quality. Competition tends to lower the differences, largely by forcing private NFPs 'to be increasingly similar to their for-profit counterparts' (Sloan 2000).

Although in this paper I have not systematically reviewed other OECD systems, many of their hospitals are public or NFP, and most of their FPs fall into the FP/s category. For example, more than two-thirds of hospital care in France is provided by public hospitals (which are part of the civil service), most of the 'private' hospitals are NFPs, FPs tend to be small and occupy niche markets, and both public and NFP hospitals have been operating under budget caps for 15 years (Poullier and Sandier 2000). Although several FP/c hospitals have been established in recent years, they do not appear to constitute a major portion of the market. For example, the fourth largest private hospital company in France owned only eight facilities, with net annual revenues of U.S.$75 million (Universal Health Services 2001).

Nursing Homes

A number of studies of nursing homes express concerns about the quality implications of FP delivery (Tarman 1990; Spector, Selden, and Cohen 1998). Marmor, Schlesinger, and Smithey (1987) summarized over a dozen such studies of U.S. nursing homes in their 1987 study; they used different databases and different measures of costs, none the less reaching the same conclusion: 'Controlling for characteristics of patients, range of services provided, and other attributes of the facility, for-profit homes have average costs 5 to 15 percent lower than their nonprofit counterparts.' These lower costs appeared to translate directly into lower quality – 'for-profit facilities are disproportionately represented among institutions offering the very lowest quality care' (Marmor, Schlesinger, and Smithey 1987, 230).

Gray's review concluded similarly: 'Expenses per patient day were higher in nonprofit than in for-profit nursing homes, but charges were similar and for-profits were more profitable. The distribution of costs differed by type, with nonprofits spending more on patient care and for-profits having higher "ownership costs" (interest, depreciation, rent). Most studies of nursing home quality favored nonprofits, using such measures as care planning, quarterly review of patients, room conditions, and quality of living environment' (Gray 1999). These findings appear to persist in current work; a recent study concluded that 'investor-owned nursing homes provide worse care and less nursing care than do not-for-profit or public homes' (Harrigan, et al. 2001).

Why are the differences in quality between FP and NFP so much more striking in the nursing-home sector than among hospitals? A number of economists have suggested 'asymmetric information' – that is, the difficulty that most consumers of such services have in distinguishing between high- and low-quality care. Some writers have hypothesized that NFP can accordingly stand as a proxy for better quality. Others propose that transparency and scrutiny are essential. In the hospital sector, clinicians may enforce adequate standards of care. In contrast, nursing homes may be under less scrutiny. Chou compared the care for nursing-home residents who were visited by a spouse or child within one month of admission with those who were not. Two of his four quality indicators showed larger differences between for-profit and NFP homes for those residents without familial eyes on the staff. He concludes: 'The NFP nondistribution constraint will soften the incentive to exploit those aspects of quality of service which are hard to monitor. On the contrary, for-profit homes are more likely to take advantage of their patients to make a profit' (Chou 2002).

Consistent with this view, other authors have observed that the availability of cost-cutting mechanisms often depends on regulatory factors – that is, the extent to which 'outside bodies' are willing to set constraints on the workings of market forces. For example, in B.C., 'the unionization of B.C. staff in both for-profit and NFP facilities has limited the ability of private employers to pay substandard wages' (Vogel 2000, 39). However, the province did not control staffing levels, and 'several [for-profit] facilities were ordered to close in B.C. in the late 1990s due to poor staffing levels and inadequate care, including lack of nutritional supports and incontinence supplies' (Vogel, 2000, 39).

Managed-Care Companies

Managed-care organizations combine the insurance and delivery function; although details vary, customers agree to seek care only from associated providers. In return, the organization can use the buying power associated with its client base to negotiate better rates from providers. The best-known type is the (U.S.) health maintenance organization (HMO). Initially, HMOs were NFPs that employed salaried physicians and emphasized (at least in theory) preventive medicine. As costs increased, the United States placed increasing emphasis on managed care; it has largely replaced the older style of insurance (which merely paid bills) in much of the country.

Although attacking HMOs is a popular sport in the United States, the HMO industry includes both NFP and FP companies. Kleinke (2001), who helped build one of the companies and describes himself as a former 'true believer in the managed care revolution,' summarized some of his objections to the industry. One indicator of 'customer dissatisfaction' is leaving one's HMO. Disenrolment rates are much lower in 'fiercely not-for-profit MCOs like Kaiser and Group Health,' which he links to corporate responses to incentives to maximize return to shareholders. The industry refers to the proportion of revenues spent for medical services as the 'medical loss ratio' – all resources spent for care are seen as coming directly out of shareholders' pockets. In his view, the for-profits use 'aggressive adverse-risk avoidance, highly differential premium rating, and constant enrollment turnover' (Kleinke 2001, 70–1). Quoting Kuttner (1998a; b), Kleinke notes that the average medical loss ratio for NFP HMOS was 90 per cent; for most FP plans, it was 80 per cent; and for 'some of the most ferociously managed MCOs,' as low as 60 per cent. Organizations 'that spend as little as it was 80, 70, or only 60 percent of the premium dollar on medicine are not managing care. Instead, they are managing money, and doing it quite well' (Kleinke 2001, 71).

Gray's review of the literature showed that 'nonprofits in 1996 spent more of the premium dollar on medical expenses, had higher member satisfaction, provided more appropriate services to patients with six conditions, and performed better on measures of prevention' (Gray 1999). Himmelstein and colleagues found lower performance by FPs than by NFPs on all fourteen of the quality indicators being used by the National Committee for Quality Assurance (Himmelstein et al. 1999).

Managed care suggests another lesson from the literature reviewed. Competition can lead to a 'race to the bottom' and cause NFPs to behave in ways similar to their FP rivals (Gray 1997). Kleinke argues that Kaiser and Group Health were dragged 'into a bidding war that resulted in significant losses for everybody, the for-profits included, in the late 1990s' (Kleinke 2001, 72). As a result, 'socially oriented HMOs [had to] embrace practices they once abhorred just to stay in business.' (Kuttner 1998a).

Social Services / Residential Care

Although some authors have suggested that business discipline could improve the delivery of social services (Carroll, Conant, and Easton 1987), such services also tend to have 'low measurability,' which the literature suggests could make them vulnerable to stinting on the more difficult to measure outcomes. In the 1980s, Knapp compared the relative efficiency of public, private NFP, and private FP providers of publicly funded residential child care in the United Kingdom (Knapp 1986). Controlling for technologies of care and characteristics of clients revealed that private (both FP and NFP) bodies appeared more cost effective than the public sector, largely part because they paid lower wages and could tap charitable donations. However, the study did not look at outcomes, particularly the long-term effects of care on children and their families. Judge, who compared private-sector provision of residential care for the frail elderly in England and Wales to public provision, initially saw private provision as good value for money (Judge 1986). Subsequent work found private FP provision less expensive than public (NHS) or NFP (consortia among the NHS and voluntary providers) in providing mental-health services (Knapp et al. 1998; Knapp et al. 1999), but it also performed least well on quality of care (Knapp et al. 1999). Different sectors supported different clienteles, complicating comparisons (Knapp et al. 1998). In Canada, an increasing proportion of residential care falls outside the public sector (Chambers et al. 1992), including a growing market for unregulated retirement homes.

Ambulatory Clinics

Alberta's Bill 11, like Ontario's Independent Health Facilities Act (Lavis et al. 1998), allows public financiers to purchase clinical services from FP providers. Accordingly, private clinics (usually private FP clinics) are hotly contested. Two Canadian studies reported that allowing private surgery increased waiting lists within the public (NFP) sector (DeCoster et al. 1999; W. Armstrong 2000); although other explanations might apply, studies in other systems have reached similar conclusions (Donaldson and Currie 2000). Indeed, Alberta's auditor-general and its medical regulator both recently called for more stringent controls on the contracting out of certain clinical services (Weber 2001).

Many commentators see Toronto's Shouldice Hospital as emblematic of the value that FP clinics could offer. Established by Dr Shouldice in 1945, this 89-bed private hospital employs 12 surgeons and repairs 7,000 abdominal-wall hernias per year. It has an excellent reputation, attracting clients from around the world. It does not appear to be owned by shareholders; we would label it FP/s. It is licensed and inspected by Ontario's Ministry of Health and Long Term Care and provides its services without additional charge to Ontario residents (except for the premium for semi-private rooms, which NFPs also charge). The hospital is proud of its activities in training and research (Shouldice Hospital 2002). It is thus noteworthy for not appearing to respond to the fiscal incentives of maximizing profits; it instead exemplifies a 'focused factory' offering high-quality care within a niche market. There are clearly limits to how many such facilities can be established, which will depend on the catchment area and the need for the procedure. However, it does not appear to exemplify FP corporate medicine; the clinic appears proud of activities (such as rehabilitation, follow-up, training, and research) that are rare at companies attempting to maximize their bottom line.

Similarly, in 2001, the NFP Cancer Care Ontario (CCO) contracted with Canadian Radiation Oncology Services (CROS), an FP/s under the direction of Dr Tom McGowan (formerly a top clinician/manager with CCO), initially to treat breast cancer patients who would otherwise have been referred, at far higher cost, to the United States (CROS 2001). This FP clinic was needed because of complex failures (at the provincial, CCO, and clinic levels) in dealing with the numbers of patients requiring treatment. At the time, there was spare capacity of the necessary equipment for radiation treatment and diagnosis, but a shortage of personnel willing to work for CCO wages. The private clinic accordingly used the facilities of a large NFP teaching hospital (Toronto's Sunnybrook Regional Cancer Centre), operating a second shift weekdays between 6:30 p.m. and 10:30 p.m. Most of their 80 employees worked in the NFP cancer clinics during the day. The FP clinic was able to pay $50 per hour for overtime work; evidently, the NFP clinic was unable to find the flexibility in its wage structure to do the same.

Cost comparisons between CROS and CCO are complex. CROS treated only patients with breast and prostate cancer within a narrow range of treatment protocols, leaving the more complex cases to the NFPs. It did not do teaching or research, which are a major part of CCO's mandate. It relied on the services of the teaching hospital for all unexpected events, such as managing cardiac arrests, and purchased other key resources (such as machine maintenance and treatment planning) on an incremental-cost (per patient) basis. Auditors have battled over the appropriate cost comparisons. The FP is far cheaper than sending overflow patients to the United States ($3,500, versus $18,000). Whether it is cheaper than care in NFPs is unclear. The conflicting reports raise such issues as the appropriateness of comparisons based on average costs, given that much of the cost structure is based on the fixed costs of having the facility, equipment, and trained staff. (Changes in volume treated thus affect average costs far more than they do the marginal costs of treating one more, or one less, patient.) The reports also raise such issues as the appropriate balance of clinical versus academic responsibilities, differences in case mix, and differences in costs to patients (Office of the Provincial Auditor General of Ontario 2001; Bryant and Pepler 2002; Elitzur 2002).

The overall merits of such FP models are thus highly debatable. Analysis must separate out the short-run implications this clinic (which appears to have been run by sincere individuals meeting a genuine need) and the longer-run consequences for the cancer-care system. Organizationally, it falls within the FP/s category run by health professionals; the evidence reviewed suggests that such models, unlike FPcs, do not appear particularly susceptible to incentives to skimp on care or quality. On the basis of the material reviewed, the clinic appears to have delivered high-quality care to patients who need it and have introduced more innovative uses of non-physician health professionals than the NFPs. Two key policy questions involve why the NFPs were unable to find the flexibility to handle these patients without contracting with CROS and how (and whether?) to remove similar barriers to innovation within the NFP sector. The implications of the FP model for the rest of the system are also unclear; would staff at the CCO clinics agree to work overtime when they could receive higher remuneration at CROS? Finally, once the principle of FP operation is accepted, how to ensure that corporate FP clinics whose activities appear less benign cannot move into the newly created markets?

The literature reviewed suggests that ambulatory clinics are subject to the same pressures as hospitals to avoid unprofitable services and clients. Khoury, Weisman, and Jarjoura (2001) examined 296 NFP and 108 FP women's health centres in the United States. Using data from the 1994 National Survey of Women's Health, they found that the NFPs outperformed the FPs on several outcome measures: serving underserved women, delivering comprehensive primary-care services, providing training for health professionals and education services for clients and the community, and involving the community in governance. Similarly, FP dialysis clinics are said to treat only routine cases, leaving the complex ones to hospitals. This specialization is not in itself objectionable but can complicate cost comparisons, particularly if average costs are used to compute reimbursement.

Finally, under some circumstances, FP delivery can operate by the same 'buyer beware' rules as the free market, sacrificing such professional niceties as ensuring that care is given on the basis of need, rather than just of willingness to pay. Laser eye surgery has been a classic example. Although the laser equipment is costly, the same equipment and staff can serve individuals with cataracts (a medically necessary, if elective, procedure insured by the health-care system) and the large market of near-sighted individuals who would like to eliminate the need to wear glasses or contact lenses (a procedure not deemed medically necessary). In a critical examination, Guyatt noted that the dominant form of laser surgery – laser-assisted in situ keratomileusis (LASIK) – took about 10 minutes per eye. Most clinics were performing about 20 procedures per day and charging $2,000 per eye (Guyatt 2001). The high profit potential attracted not only physician-run clinics, but also several large corporations, which then employed opthalmologists to do the surgery. The increased capacity then led to price wars and behaviour more common in the marketplace than in traditional health-care organizations. Some of these firms ran hard-sell advertisements, including 'buy one, get one free' offers. Guyatt argues that they underplayed the risks of surgery, overstated benefits, and aggressively recruited customers from optometrists (including offering them financial incentives for each referral). Ultimately, the leading firms overexpanded, merged, and declared bankruptcy. The final nail came when their major surgeon, unpaid, resigned.

The negative impact spread beyond customers of these firms. Although data were only anecdotal, Guyatt suggests that the boom in laser eye surgery increased waiting times for patients with higher medical needs (Guyatt 2001). This is not unexpected; if there is not a surplus of health personnel, the staff (and time) devoted to privately funded care can often be at the expense of the 'medically necessary' care being delivered by the publicly funded system. Thus private clinics, if not well managed, can also drain off resources. In addition, there are suggestions that many patients were harmed by the procedure rather than benefiting from it. And the publicly funded system absorbed many of the 'repair' costs.

Laboratory Services

Laboratory services are relatively well suited to private provision. The tests are well defined. Quality-assurance procedures can be established, and performance measured and monitored. Many tests can take place in large, automated facilities, which need substantial capital investment but promise considerable economies of scale for common, routinized tests. In Canada, they can be offered in organizations that are public (for example, public health laboratories), NFP (for example, hospital labs), FP small business (for example, physicians' offices), or corporate FP (for example, commercial labs). Barriers to entry are considerable; at present, three private companies have nearly 90 per cent of the business (Browne 2000). Since hospital laboratories are part of hospital global budgets, there are strong incentives to out-source testing and gain the resulting budgetary flexibility.

Obtaining cost data is difficult because corporate balance sheets are not subject to the same disclosure requirements as public or NFP organizations. Conversations with individuals involved in laboratory services suggested that FPs are able to extract a premium for their services. For example, on 1 July 1995, Alberta was able to combine its funding for hospital lab services (about $150 million per year) with private fee-for-service billing for such services (about $90 million per year) and negotiate a 30 per cent reduction in costs. This was held out as a success story; however, even at this reduced level (which is below that being paid in such provinces as Ontario) per-capita costs are still considerably higher than those in Atlantic Canada, which had no private FP labs at all.

The example of laboratory services clarifies the importance of defining properly what services are being purchased. Clearly, costs are less for routine tests than for the more complex procedures often carried out in hospitals. Provided that costing is done accurately and that results are reported quickly and accurately, there would be no apparent reason not to capture economies of scale (although these might also be attainable within an NFP organization). However, a 'test' is only one component of a larger service – such tests must also be interpreted, and their results communicated. According to the *Report of the Walkerton Inquiry* (O'Connor 2002), one major cause of the public-health catastrophe, in which contaminated drinking water killed seven people and sickened more than 2,300, was a failure of regulation. The local officials responsible for testing and maintaining the water system were both incompetent and dishonest. Provincial government reductions eliminated public testing of drinking water. The FP firm that had assumed responsibility for testing Walkerton's water was staffed by individuals who could perform the tests but were not trained microbiologists. And they did not forward test results to regulatory bodies. In consequence, the severity of the outbreak was underestimated, with devastating consequences to the health of the community (O'Connor 2002). The report insists on proper regulatory mechanisms: 'When government laboratories conducted all of the routine drinking water tests for municipal water systems throughout the province, it was acceptable to keep the notification protocol in the form of a guideline under the ODWO [Ontario Drinking Water Objectives] rather than in a legally enforceable form – that is, a law or regulation.' But 'the entry of private laboratories into this sensitive public health area in 1993, and the wholesale exit of all government laboratories from routine testing of municipal water samples in 1996, made it unacceptable to let the notification protocol remain in the form of a legally unenforceable guideline. This was particularly so since, at the time, private environmental laboratories were not regulated by the government. No criteria had been established to govern the quality of testing, no requirements existed regarding the qualifications or experience of laboratory personnel, and no provisions were made for licensing, inspection, or auditing by the government' (O'Connor 2002).

One of many lessons of Walkerton is that the FP provider gained 'efficiencies' by focusing narrowly on the actual testing; it was not required to provide such (in retrospect, essential) intangibles as interpreting results or notifying affected parties.

Home Care

Home care is another sector in which all three modes of delivery can coexist (Ontario Home Health Care Providers' Association 2001). For example, publicly financed home care in British Columbia can be delivered by RHAs (which some of the analyses term 'public'), charitable organizations, or FP businesses (Pollak 2000). There are relatively low barriers to entry or exit. Workers delivering homemaking services tend to earn little and to leave for better-paying jobs. Even professionals, such as nurses, PTs, or OTs, can in theory move relatively easily between companies. Accordingly, home care is a sector that has seemed relatively well suited for experiments with competition.

Ontario has sought to test the managed-competition model for the purchase of home-care services (Baranek, Deber, and Williams 1999; Williams et al. 1999). In the former non-system, care was provided by a mixture of NFP (for example, the Victorian Order of Nurses, Saint Elizabeth) and FP providers. In 1996, the province began to set up 43 Community Care Access Centres (CCACs) and gave them fixed budgets, with a mandate to ensure that care was purchased on a 'best quality, best price' basis. In turn, the CCACs issued requests for proposals (RFPs). The consequences on the sector have been severe (Browne 2000; Sutherland 2001; Williams et al. 2001). Some of the complaints that have arisen could apply to any sort of delivery model, regardless of ownership; labour objects to what it sees as duplication and unproductive procedures and to the disparity in compensation levels (found in Ontario, although not in some other provinces) between the hospital and home-care sectors. Other complaints refer to any competitive model, again regardless of ownership: time spent monitoring the system, communication/co-ordination difficulties, impaired teamwork, lack of 'critical mass,' chilling effect on ability to criticize care, downward pressure on wages and working conditions (leading to increased turnover and diminished continuity of care), and the undermining of trust between agencies (Browne 2000). However, a number do relate specifically to private delivery, including difficulty in obtaining accurate data when FPs keep much of their information secret and the possibility of fraud, heightened because one of the FP agencies (Olsten) had recently paid $61 million to the U.S. Department of Justice for criminal violations in its U.S. home-care billings (Sutherland 2001).

The balance between competition and co-operation is crystal clear in home care. Shapiro (2002) recently synthesized all the 'innovative' home-care studies in Canada funded by the Health Transition Fund. She observed that a recurring problem involved trying to provide services via external organizations, whether they be FPs or NFPs. In effect, the formalization of relationships was seen to impinge on flexibility in a number of ways. It was difficult to provide continuity of care, to set up more flexible time arrangements (for example, by using full-time workers to serve a number of clients in a senior citizens' apartment building), or to have closer, more informal contact with providers in other organizations to exchange information on clients.

Thus, even in this market with low barriers to entry and exit, competition was proving to have adverse effects on the sector. These experiments with competition (regardless of ownership type) have made clear the importance of properly defining expected outcomes. For example, a destabilized workforce may lead to high turnover (with ominous implications for both training costs and continuity of care) and to difficulty in attracting enough competent workers. Shapiro (1997) examined the shift of home-care services in Manitoba after the province contracted out to a U.S. FP (Olsten) a portion of these services previously provided through public-sector workers. This move drew widespread opposition from health-care workers and the public. After a one-year trial period, the project was abandoned on the grounds that the FP delivery was more expensive than publicly delivered care (Shapiro 1997; Vogel

2000; Rachlis, 2000a; and Pollak 2000). Quality was also endangered; Shapiro found that the turnover rate increased from 15–25 per cent for workers in the public sector to 50 per cent in the FP company.

In summary, the literature reviewed stresses the complexity of comparing public, NFP, and FP delivery and the importance of making clear which elements of the delivery system are being referred to.

NOTE

The literature is voluminous, and this paper has merely scratched the surface. Enormous thanks are due to the many colleagues who assisted me by suggesting material, including Owen Adams, Wendy L. Armstrong, Lillian Bayne, Andrea Baumann, Glenn Brimacombe, Adalsteinn D. Brown, Marcy Cohen, Brian Lee Crowley, P.J. Devereaux, Colleen Flood, Colleen Fuller, Carole Kushner, Jonathan Lomas, Ted Marmor, Tom McCowan, Michael Mendelson, Larry Nestman, Michael Rachlis, Thomas Rathwell, Paddy Rodney, Leslie Roos, Noralou Roos, Evelyn Shapiro, William Tholl, and A. Paul Williams, plus several who asked not to be formally recognized. They are not responsible for the interpretations made. I would also like to thank CIHR for funding assistance.

REFERENCES

Alberta Health. 2000. *Bill 11, Alberta's Health Care Protection Act: A Stronger Health System for the Future*. Tabled in the Alberta Legislature, 2 March.

Armstrong, Pat, and Hugh Armstrong. 1996. *Wasting Away: The Undermining of Canadian Health Care*. Toronto: Oxford University Press.

Armstrong, Pat, Hugh Armstrong, and David Coburn. 2001. *Unhealthy Times: Political Economy Perspectives on Health and Care in Canada*. Don Mills, Ont.: Oxford University Press.

Armstrong, Pat, et al. 1994. *Take Care: Warning Signals for Canada's Health System*. Toronto: Garamond Press.

Armstrong, Wendy. 2000. *The Consumer Experience with Cataract Surgery and Private Clinics in Alberta: Canada's Canary in the Mine Shaft*. Report published by the Consumers' Association of Canada (Alberta), Jan.

Arnold, Tom. 2001. 'Majority Open to Mix of Public/Private Health: Poll Reveals "Dichotomy."' *National Post*, 13 July. www.nationalpost.com

Arvay Finlay. 2000. *Canada Health Act and Alberta Bill 11*. Prepared for the Canadian Union of Public Employees, 8 March.

Baranek, Pat, Raisa B. Deber, and A. Paul Williams. 1999. 'Policy Trade-offs in "Home Care": The Ontario Example.' *Canadian Public Administration* 42, no. 1, 69–92.

Bendick, Marc, Jr. 1989. 'Privatizing the Delivery of Social Welfare Services: An Ideal to Be Taken Seriously.' In Sheila B. Kamerman and Alfred J. Kahn, eds., *Privatization and the Welfare State*. Princeton, NJ: Princeton University Press, 97–120.

Bennett Jones. 2001. *Public–Private Partnerships for Ontario Hospital Capital Projects*. Background report prepared by Bennett Jones LLP for the Ontario Hospital Association's Committee on Hospital Capital Development, Aug.

Boyle, Sean, and Anthony Harrison. 2000a. *Investing in Health Buildings: Public–Private Partnerships*. King's Fund, Private Finance Initiative in the NHS, May. www.kingsfund.org.uk

– 2000b. *PFI in Health: The Story So Far*. King's Fund, Private Finance Initiative in the NHS. www.kingsfund.org.uk

Browne, Paul L. 2000. *Unsafe Practices: Restructuring and Privatization in Ontario Health Care*. Ottawa: Canadian Centre for Policy Alternatives.

Bryant, Murray J. and Eileen Pepler. 2002. *Report to the Members of the Public Accounts Committee, Ontario Legislative Assembly*. Jan.

Canadian Healthcare Association. 2001. *The Private–Public Mix in the Funding and Delivery of Health Services in Canada: Challenges and Opportunities*. Ottawa: CHA Press.

Canadian Institute for Health Information (CIHI). 2000a. *National Health Expenditure Trends, 1975–2000*. National Health Expenditure Database. Ottawa: CIHI.

2000b. *NHEX Definition*. Composition of Total Health Expenditures by Source of Finance. www.cihi.ca/facts/nhex/defin.htm

– 2001. *Canada's Health Care Providers*. Toronto: CIHI and Institute for Work and Health.

Canadian Radiation Oncology Services (CROS). 2001. *Bringing Radiation Oncology Closer to Home: Report of Canadian Radiation Oncology Services First Six Months of Operation, February–August 2001*. Nov.

Carroll, Barry J. Ralph W. Conant, and Thomas A. Easton. 1987. *Private Means, Public Ends: Private Business in Social Service Delivery*. New York: Praeger.

CCPA (Canadian Council for Policy Alternatives). 2000. *Health Care, Limited: The Privatization of Medicare*. A synthesis report prepared by the CCPA for the Council of Canadians, in collaboration with the Canadian Health Coalition.

Chambers, Larry W., et al. 1992. *The Organization and Financing of Public and Private Sector Long Term Care Facilities for the Elderly in Canada. Report on Part*

1: Survey of the Provinces. Centre for Health Economics and Policy Analysis Working Paper Series 92-13, McMaster University, Hamilton. April.

Chou, Shin-Yi. 2002. 'Asymmetric Information, Ownership and Quality of Care: An Empirical Analysis of Nursing Homes.' *Journal of Health Economics* 21: 293–311.

Choudhry, Sujit. 2000. 'Bill 11, the Canada Health Act and the Social Union: The Need for Institutions.' *Osgoode Hall Law Journal* 38 (31 July): 39–99.

Clutterbuck, David, Susan Kernaghan, and Deborah Snow. 1991. *Going Private: Privatisations around the World*. London: Mercury Books.

Commission on Public Private Partnerships. 2001. *Building Better Partnerships: The Final Report of the Commission on Public Private Partnerships*. London: Institute for Public Policy Research.

Coyte, Peter. 2000. *Home Care in Canada: Passing the Buck*. Dialogue on Health Reform. www.hcerc.utoronto.ca

Crowley, Brian L., David Zitner, and Nancy Faraday-Smith. 2002. *Operating in the Dark: The Gathering Crisis in Canada's Health Care System*. Halifax: Atlantic Institute for Market Studies (AIMS).

Cutler, David M. 2000. *The Changing Hospital Industry: Comparing Not-for-Profit and For-Profit Institutions*. Chicago: University of Chicago Press.

Cutler, David M., and Jill R. Horwitz. 1998. *Converting Hospitals from Not-for-Profit to For-Profit Status: Why and What Effects?* Working Paper 6672, National Bureau of Economic Research. www.nber.org

Deber, Raisa B. 1998. 'Public and Private Places in Canadian Healthcare.' *Hospital Quarterly* 1, no. 2: 28–9, 31.

– 2000. 'Getting What We Pay For: Myths and Realities about Financing Canada's Health Care System.' *Health Law in Canada* 21, no. 2: 9–56.

Deber, Raisa B., Orvill Adams, and Lynn Curry. 1994. 'International Healthcare Systems: Models of Financing and Reimbursement.' In Jack A. Boan, ed., *Proceedings of the Fifth Canadian Conference on Health Economics*. Regina: Canadian Plains Research Center, 76–91.

Deber, Raisa B., et al. 1998. 'The Public–Private Mix in Health Care.' In National Forum on Health, ed., *Striking a Balance: Health Care Systems in Canada and Elsewhere*. Sainte-Foy, Que.: Éditions MultiMondes, 423–545.

DeCoster, Carolyn, et al. 1999. 'Waiting Times for Surgical Procedures.' *Medical Care* 37, no. 6 Suppl, JS187–JS205.

DeHoog, Ruth H. 1984. *Contracting Out for Human Services: Economic, Political, and Organizational Perspectives*. Albany: State University of New York Press.

Donahue, John D. 1989. *The Privatization Decision: Public Ends, Private Means*. New York: Basic Books.

Donaldson, Cam, and Gillian Currie. 2000. *The Public Purchase of Private Surgical Services: A Systematic Review of the Evidence on Efficiency and Equity.* Institute of Health Economics Working Paper 00-9. Edmonton.

Elitzur, Ramy. 2002. *Review of the Report by the Provincial Auditor on the Canadian Radiation Oncology Services.* 22 Jan.

Evans, Robert G., 1984. *Strained Mercy: The Economics of Canadian Health Care.* Toronto: Butterworths.

Evans, Robert G., et al. 2000. *Private Highway, One-Way Street: The DeKlein and Fall of Canadian Medicare?* Centre for Health Services and Policy Research, University of British Columbia, HPRU 2000:3D. Vancouver. March.

Fasken Martineau DuMoulin LLP. 2001. *Comments of Fasken Martineau DuMoulin LLP on the Shrybman Opinion: Submission to the Walkerton Inquiry, Part 2.* Prepared for the Canadian Council for Public–Private Partnerships.

Ford, Robin, and David Zussman. 1997. *Alternative Service Delivery: Sharing Governance in Canada.* Toronto: KPMG and IPAC.

Fuller, C. 1998a. *Canada's Health Care Crisis: More and More Health Care Services Being Privatized.* Canadian Centre for Policy Alternatives Monitor, March.

– 1998b. *Caring for Profit: How Corporations Are Taking over Canada's Health Care System.* Vancouver: New Star Books.

Gaffney, Declan, et al. 1999a. 'NHS Capital Expenditure and the Private Finance Initiative: Expansion or Contraction?' *BMJ* 319: 48–51.

– 1999b. 'PFI in the NHS: Is There an Economic Case?' *BMJ* 319: 116–19.

– 1999c. 'The Politics of the Private Finance Initiative and the New NHS.' *BMJ* 319, no. 7204: 249–53.

Garg, Pushkal P., et al. 1999. 'Effect of the Ownership of Dialysis Facilities on Patients' Survival and Referral for Transplantation.' *New England Journal of Medicine* 341, no. 22: 1653–60.

Government of British Columbia Board Resourcing and Development Office. 2002. *Board Resourcing and Development Office – Home Page.* www.fin.gov.bc.can/abc/index.htm, 1 March 2002.

Gray, Bradford H. 1997. 'Conversion of HMOs and Hospitals: What's at Stake?' *Health Affairs* 16, no. 2: 29–47.

– 1999. *The Empirical Literature Comparing For-profit and Nonprofit Hospitals, Managed Care Organisations and Nursing Homes: Updating the Institute of Medicine Study.* Washington, DC: Coalition for Nonprofit Healthcare. www.cnhc.org/Report3.pdf

Gregory, Kimberly D., et al. 1999. 'Cesarean Deliveries for Medicaid Patients: A Comparison in Public and Private Hospitals in Los Angeles County.' *American Journal of Obstetrics and Gynecology* 180, no. 5: 1177–84.

Griffin, Pat, Rhonda Cockerill, and Raisa B. Deber. 2001. 'Potential Impact of Population-Based Funding on Delivery of Pediatric Services.' *Annals of the Royal College of Physicians and Surgeons of Canada* 34, no. 5: 272–9.

Guyatt, Gordon H. 2001. 'Laser Eye Surgery: A Disturbing Model for Private Health-Care Delivery.' *Annals of the Royal College of Physicians and Surgeons of Canada* 34, no. 3: 157–9.

Harrigan, Charlene, et al. 2001. 'Does Investor Ownership of Nursing Homes Compromise the Quality of Care? *American Journal of Public Health* 91, no. 9: 1–5.

Harrison, Anthony. 2001. 'Public–Private Partnerships within Health Care since the NHS Plan.' In John Appleby and Anthony Harrison, eds., *Health Care UK 2001 – Autumn – The King's Fund Review of Health Policy.* London: King's Fund Publishing, 63–81.

Hatry, Harry P. 1983. *A Review of Private Approaches for Delivery of Public Services.* Washington, DC: Urban Institute Press.

Hayes, Virginia E., et al. 1997. *Services for Children with Special Needs in Canada.* Report prepared for the Canadian Association for Community Care and Health Canada, Oct. Victoria: Health Network, Canadian Policy Research Networks.

Heyman, George. 2001. *A Presentation to the Select Standing Committee on Health.* President, B.C. Government and Service Employees' Union, 7 Nov.

Higgins, Joan. 1988. *The Business of Medicine: Private Health Care in Britain.* London: Macmillan Education.

Himmelstein, David, Steffie Woolhandler, and Ida Hellander. 2001. *Bleeding the Patient: The Consequences of Corporate Health Care.* Monroe, Maine: Common Courage Press.

Himmelstein, David U., et al. 1999. 'Quality of Care in Investor-Owned vs. Not-for-Profit HMOs.' *JAMA* 282: 159–63.

Hollander, Marcus J. 1997. *Assessing the Impacts of Health Reforms on Seniors: Part 1. A Synthesis Report of Health Reforms and Seniors' Perceptions of the Health System.* Report prepared for the National Advisory Council on Aging, Ottawa, Dec.

Hospital Employees' Union. 2001. *Build Hospitals for People, Not for Profits.* Presentation to the B.C. Select Standing Committee on Health, 8 Nov.

Judge, K. 1986. 'Value for Money in the British Residential Care Industry.' In Anthony J. Culyer and B. Jonsson, eds., *Public and Private Health Services: Complementarities and Conflict.* Oxford: Basil Blackwell, 200–18.

Kamerman, Sheila B., and Alfred J. Kahn. 1989. *Privatization and the Welfare State.* Princeton, NJ: Princeton University Press.

Kelly, Gavin, and Peter Robinson. 2000. *A Healthy Partnership: The Future of Public Private Partnerships in the Health Service*. London: Institute for Public Policy Research.

Kemp, Roger L. 1991. *Privatization: The Provision of Public Services by the Private Sector*. Jefferson, NC: McFarland and Company.

Khoury, Amal J., Carol S. Weisman, and Chad M. Jarjoura. 2001. 'Ownership Type and Community Benefits of Women's Health Centres.' *Medical Care Research and Review* 58, no. 1: 76–100.

Kleinke, J.D. 2001. *Oxymorons: The Myth of a U.S. Health Care System*. San Francisco: Jossey-Bass.

Knapp, M. 1986. 'The Relative Cost-effectiveness of Public, Voluntary and Private Providers of Residential Child Care.' In Anthony J. Culyer and B. Jonsson, eds., *Public and Private Health Services: Complementarities and Conflict*. Oxford: Basil Blackwell, 171–99.

Knapp, Martin, et al. 1998. 'Public and Private Residential Care: Is There a Cost Difference?' *Journal of Health Services Research and Policy* 3, no. 3: 141–8.

– 1999. 'Private, Voluntary or Public? Comparative Cost-effectiveness in Community Mental Health Care.' *Policy and Politics* 27 no. 1: 25–41.

Kushner, Carol. 1999. *In Search of the Greenest Grass: A Comparative Analysis of Recent Funding Announcements and Recommendations for Home Care Services in the New City of Toronto*. Report prepared by the Toronto-area CCACs.

Kuttner, Robert. 1998a. 'Must Good HMOs Go Bad? First of Two Parts: The Commercialization of Prepaid Group Health Care.' *New England Journal of Medicine* 338, no. 21: 1558–63.

– 1998b. 'Must Good HMOs Go Bad? Second of Two Parts: The Search for Checks and Balances.' *New England Journal of Medicine* 338, no. 22: 1635–9.

Langlois, Kathy. 1997. 'A Saskatchewan Vision for Health: Who Really Makes the Decisions?' In Robin Ford and David Zussman, eds., *Alternative Service Delivery: Sharing Governance in Canada*. Toronto: KPMG and IPAC, 173–84.

Lavis, J.N., et al. 1998. 'Free-standing Health Care Facilities: Financial Arrangements, Quality Assurance, and a Pilot Study.' *CMAJ* 158, no. 3: 359–63.

Lowrie, Edmund G., and C.L. Hampers. 1981. 'The Success of Medicare's End-Stage Renal-Disease Program: The Case for Profits and the Private Marketplace.' *New England Journal of Medicine* 305, no. 8: 434–8.

Manga, Pran. 1988. *The Canada–U.S. Free Trade Agreement: Possible Implications on Canada's Health Care Systems*. Discussion Paper No. 348 prepared for the Economic Council of Canada, Ottawa, May.

Marmor, Theodore R. 2001. 'Comparing Global Health Systems: Lessons and Caveats. In Walter W. Wieners, ed., *Global Health Care Markets: A Comprehen-*

sive Guide to Regions, Trends, and Opportunities Shaping the International Health Arena. San Francisco: Jossey-Bass, 7–23.

Marmor, Theodore R., Mark Schlesinger, and Richard W. Smithey. 1987. 'Nonprofit Organizations and Health Care.' In Walter W. Powell, ed., *The Nonprofit Sector: A Research Handbook.* New Haven, Conn.: Yale University Press, 1–35.

Martin, Brendan. 1993. *In the Public Interest? Privatization and Public Sector Reform.* Atlantic Highlands, NJ: Zed Books.

McDavid, James C. 2001. 'Solid-Waste Contracting-out, Competition, and Bidding Practices among Canadian Local Governments. *Canadian Public Administration* 44, no. 1: 1–25.

McFetridge, D.G. 1997. *The Economics of Privatization.* C.D. Howe Institute Benefactors Lecture, Toronto, 22 Oct.

O'Connor, Dennis R. 2002. *Report of the Walkerton Inquiry: The Events of May 2000 and Related Issues. Part One: A Summary.* Toronto: Ontario Ministry of the Attorney General.

Office of the Auditor General of New Brunswick. 1998. 'Special Report for the Public Accounts Committee, Evergreen and Wackenhut Leases.' *1998 Auditor General's Report, Chapter 14.* www.gnb.ca

Office of the Auditor General of Nova Scotia. 1997. 'Education and Culture: Public–Private Partnerships for School Construction.' *1997 Auditor General's Report*, Chapter 8. www.gov.ns.ca/audg/1997ag.htm

– 1998. 'Education and Culture: Public–Private Partnerships for School Construction Follow-up Review.' *1998 Auditor General's Report*, Chapter 7. www.gov.ns.ca/audg/1998ag.htm

– 1999. 'Education: Public–Private Partnerships (P3s) for School Construction – Follow-up Review.' *1999 Auditor General's Report*, Chapter 5. www.gov.ns.ca

Office of the Provincial Auditor General of Ontario. 1998a. 'Ministry of Community and Social Services, Business Transformation Project/Common Purpose Procurement.' *1998 Annual Report*, Chapter 3.01. www.gov.on.ca/opa/english/r98t.htm

– 1998b. 'Long Term Care Community-Based Services Activity.' *1998 Annual Report*, Chapter 3.05. www.gov.on.ca/opa/english/r98t.htm

– 2000. 'Follow-up of Recommendations in the 1998 Annual Report.' *Special Report on Accountability and Value for Money.* www.gov.on.ca

– 2001. *Special Audit for the Standing Committee on Public Accounts: Cancer Care Ontario.* 13 Dec.

Ontario Home Health Care Providers' Association. 2001. *Private Sector Delivery of Home Health Care in Ontario.* June. www.ohhcap.on.ca/docs

Organisation for Economic Co-operation and Development (OECD). 1987. *Financing and Delivering Health Care: A Comparative Analysis of OECD Countries.* Paris: OECD.

– 1994. *The Reform of Health Care Systems: A Review of Seventeen OECD Countries.* Paris: OECD.

Osborne, David E., and Ted Gaebler. 1992. *Reinventing Government: How the Entrepreneurial Spirit Is Transforming the Public Sector.* Reading, Mass.: Addison-Wesley.

Ovretveit, John. 1996. 'Beyond the Public–Private Debate: The Mixed Economy of Health.' *Health Policy* 35: 75–93.

Plain, Richard. 2000. *The Privatization and Commercialization of Public Hospital Based Medical Services within the Province of Alberta: An Economic Overview from a Public Interest Perspective.* Department of Economics, University of Alberta, Medicare Economics Group, March.

Pollak, Nancy. 2000. 'Cutting Home Support: From 'Closer to Home' to 'All Alone.' Without Foundation, Part 3. In Marcy Cohen and Nancy Pollak, eds., *Without Foundation: How Medicare Is Undermined by Gaps and Privatization in Community and Continuing Care,* Victoria: Canadian Centre for Policy Alternatives.

Pollock, Allyson M., et al. 1999. 'Planning the "New" NHS: Downsizing for the 21st century.' *BMJ.* 319: 179–84.

Poullier, Jean-Pierre, and Simone Sandier. 2000. 'France.' *Journal of Health Politics, Policy and Law* 25, no. 5: 899–905.

Preker, Alexander S., and April Harding. 2000. *The Economics of Public and Private Roles in Health Care: Insights from Institutional Economics and Organizational Theory.* World Bank Group Documents and Reports, Working Paper No. 21875.

Preker, Alexander S., April Harding, and Phyllida Travis. 2000. '"Make or Buy" Decisions in the Production of Health Care Goods and Services: New Insights from institutional Economics and Organizational Theory.' *Bulletin of the World Health Organization* 78, no. 6: 779–89.

Premier's Advisory Council on Health for Alberta. 2001. *A Framework for Reform.* Report of the Premier's Advisory Council on Health, Edmonton, Dec.

Rachlis, Michael M. 2000a. 'The Hidden Costs of Privatization: An International Comparison of Community Care.' In Mary Cohen and Nancy Pollak, eds., *Without Foundation: How Medicare Is Undermined by Gaps and Privatization in Community and Continuing Care.* Victoria: Canadian Centre for Policy Alternatives.

– 2000b. *A Review of the Alberta Private Hospital Proposal.* Ottawa: Caledon Institute of Social Policy, March.

Rachlis, Michael, et al. 2001. *Revitalizing Medicare: Shared Problems, Public Solutions*. Study prepared for the Tommy Douglas Research Institute, Jan.

Relman, Arnold S. 1992. 'What Market Values Are Doing to Medicine.' *Atlantic Monthly*, March, 99–106.

Rice, Thomas. 1998. *The Economics of Health Reconsidered*. Chicago: Health Administration Press.

Saltman, Richard B. 1995. *The Public–Private Mix in Financing and Producing Health Services*. Mimeo report prepared for the World Bank, Washington, DC, Feb.

Saltman, Richard B., Josep Figueras, and Constantino Sakellarides. 1998. *Critical Challenges for Health Care Reform in Europe*. Philadelphia: Open University Press.

Saltman, Richard B., and Casten von Otter. 1992. *Planned Markets and Public Competition: Strategic Reform in Northern European Health Systems*. Philadelphia: Open University Press.

– 1995. *Implementing Planned Markets in Health Care: Balancing Social and Economic Responsibility*. Buckingham: Open University Press.

Sanger, Matt. 2000. *Reckless Abandon: Canada, the GATS and the Future of Health Care: Executive Summary*. Ottawa: Canadian Centre for Policy Alternatives.

Shapiro, E. 1997. *The Cost of Privatization: A Case Study of Home Care in Manitoba*. Ottawa: Canadian Centre for Policy Alternatives.

– 2002. *Sharing the Learning: The Health Transition Fund Synthesis Series: Home Care*. Ottawa: Health Canada, 2002.

Shelanski, H.A., and P.G. Klein. 1995. 'Empirical Research in Transaction Cost Economics – A Review and Assessment.' *Journal of Law, Economics and Organization* 11, no. 2: 335–61.

Shouldice Hospital. 2002. *Shouldice Hernia Centre Home Page*. www.shouldice.com, 1 March 2002.

Shrybman, Steven. 2001a. *Canada's International Trade Obligations and Municipal Government Authority: Response to the Canadian Council for Public–Private Partnerships*. Prepared for the Canadian Union of Public Employees.

– 2001b. *A Legal Opinion Concerning the Potential Impact of International Trade Disciplines on the Proposed Public–Private Partnership Concerning the Halifax Harbour Solutions Project*. Prepared for the Canadian Union of Public Employees, Ottawa, 17 Sept.

Silverman, E.M., J.S. Skinner, and E.S. Fisher. 1999. 'The Association between For-profit Hospital Ownership and Increased Medicare Spending.' *New England Journal of Medicine* 341, no. 6: 444–6.

Skelly, Michael J. 1996. *Alternative Service Delivery in Canadian Municipalities*. Toronto: ICURR Publications.

Sloan, Frank A. 2000. Not-for-profit Ownership and Hospital Behavior. In Anthony J. Culyer and Joseph P. Newhouse, eds., *Handbook of Health Economics*. Amsterdam: Elsevier Science, 1141–74.

Sloan, Frank A., et al. 1998. *Hospital Ownership and Cost and Quality of Care: Is There a Dime's Worth of Difference?* Working Paper 6706, National Bureau of Economic Research. Cambridge, Mass. www.nber.org

Spector, William D., Thomas M. Selden, and Joel W. Cohen. 1998. 'The Impact of Ownership Type on Nursing Home Outcomes.' *Health Economics* 7: 639–53.

Starr, Paul. 1989. 'The Meaning of Privatization.' In Sheila B. Kamerman and Alfred J. Kahn, eds., *Privatization and the Welfare State*. Princeton, NJ: Princeton University Press, 15–48.

Sutherland, Ross. 2001. *The Costs of Contracting Out Home Care: A Behind the Scenes Look at Home Care in Ontario*. CUPE Research, Feb. www.cupe.ca/www/305/the cost of home care.

Taft, Kevin, and Gillian Steward. 2000. *Clear Answers: The Economics and Politics of For-Profit Medicine*. Edmonton: Duval House Publishing.

Tarman, Vera Ingrid. 1990. *Privatization and Health Care: The Case of Ontario Nursing Homes*. Toronto: Garamond Press.

Universal Health Services. 2001. *Universal Health Services, Inc., Acquires Fourth Largest Private Hospital Company in France*. Press release. www.uhsinc.com/releases/release63.htm

Vining, Aidan R., and Steven Globerman. 1999. Contracting-out Health Care Services: A Conceptual Framework. *Health Policy* 46: 77–96.

Vogel, Donna, 2000. 'Unfulfilled Promise: How Health Care Reforms of the 1990s Are Failing Community and Continuing Care in BC.' In Marcy Cohen and Nancy Pollak, eds., *Without Foundation: How Medicare Is Undermined by Gaps and Privatization in Community and Continuing Care*. Victoria: Canadian Centre for Policy Alternatives.

Weber, Bob. 2001. 'Privatization Worries Alberta Auditor-General.' *Globe and Mail*, 10 Oct., A16.

Whorley, David. 2001. 'The Andersen–Comsoc Affair: Partnerships and the Public Interest.' *Canadian Public Administration* 44, no. 3: 320–45.

Williams, A. Paul, et al. 1999. 'Long Term Care Goes to Market: Managed Competition and Ontario's Reform of Community-Based Services.' *Canadian Journal on Aging* 18, no. 2: 125–51.

– 2001. 'From Medicare to Home Care: Globalization, State Retrenchment and the Profitization of Canada's Health Care System.' In Pat Armstrong, Hugh Armstrong, and David Coburn, eds., *Unhealthy Times: Political Economy Perspectives on Health and Care in Canada*. Don Mills, Ont.: Oxford University Press, 7–30.

Woolhandler, Steffie, and David U. Himmelstein. 1997. 'Costs of Care and Administration at For-Profit and Other Hospitals in the United States.' *New England Journal of Medicine* 336: 769–74.

– 1999. 'When Money Is the Mission: The High Costs of Investor-Owned Care' (editorial). *New England Journal of Medicine* 341, no. 6: 444–6.

Yergin, Daniel, and Joseph Stanislaw. 1998. *The Commanding Heights: The Battle between Government and the Marketplace That Is Remaking the Modern World.* New York: Simon and Schuster.

Zelder, Martin. 2001. *How Private Hospital Competition Can Improve Canadian Health Care.* Public Policy Sources No. 35. Vancouver: The Fraser Institute. www.fraserinstitute.ca

Zitner, David, and Brian L. Crowley. 2002. *Public Health, State Secret.* Research Report. Halifax: Atlantic Institute for Market Studies (AIMS), Jan.

PART THREE

FEDERAL–PROVINCIAL FISCAL DYNAMICS

8 Increasing Provincial Revenues for Health Care

MELISSA RODE AND MICHAEL RUSHTON

The *Interim Report* of the Commission on the Future of Health Care in Canada (Romanow Commission) outlines four options (2002, 26–7) for keeping Canada's health-care system fiscally sustainable:

- providing more revenue to allow a basically sound system that has recently been somewhat underfunded to 'catch up'
- searching for new revenue sources to deal with rapidly increasing costs, owing to an aging population and the supply and demand of new health technologies
- looking for ways to use the private provision of insurance and services to supplement the system
- improving service delivery within the system

This paper focuses on the first and second options, comparing the enhanced use of existing revenue sources with finding new ones. We do not mean in any way to rule out the other two options as possibilities, perhaps superior ones. But we leave to other investigators the questions of whether the system is underfunded and whether more efficient use of private or public health-care resources is possible.

After outlining key concepts in the analysis of health-care funding – efficiency and equity – we construct an argument in four parts. First, we reject the proposal, made recently by various commentators, of raising additional revenue from individuals based on their use of the system (copayments). Instead, we recommend finding extra revenues through the tax system. Second, we look at federal–provincial tax and transfer issues and argue that additional revenues are best collected at the provincial level, rather than at the federal level, with subsequent transfer to the provinces. Third, we show that provinces can raise extra revenues most efficiently through sales taxes and that, owing to the large vertical fiscal imbalance between the two levels of government, Ottawa can afford to sacrifice some tax room. We propose that the Goods and Services Tax (GST) is more easily administered at the provincial level than is often assumed. Finally, we outline how a transfer of this tax field to the provinces might work.

Efficiency and Equity

A useful guide in the examination of public sources of health-care funding is Normand (1992, 768):

• The cost of collecting the funds should be low.
• The system should be equitable.
• The funding should be adequate and not be subject to fluctuations.
• The system should not lead to conflict with other government objectives.
• The public should be satisfied with the system.
• The system should not channel funds into low-priority programs or away from high priorities.

When we say that the cost of collecting funds should be low, we mean this in two senses. First, the system should be *efficient* in the economist's sense of the term. Almost all methods of raising public revenue impose a cost on the economy; the market economy is generally quite effective at allocating labour and capital resources to their most productive uses, and the various taxes levied by government typically change the incentives of individuals and investors such that at the margin they are directed away from their most productive use. As a result, taxes remove an amount of income out of the private economy greater than the amount of revenue actually received by government. This difference is called the efficiency loss, and an efficient tax system is one that does not cause efficiency losses beyond what is necessary, given the amount of revenue to be raised and the equity goals of the government.

Second, the cost of administering the collection of revenue should itself be low. This includes both the cost to the government of administering the revenue source and the cost to the taxpayer of complying with the system. This puts a burden on any advocates of a *new* tax to be added to the existing collection of federal, provincial, and local taxes, since the administration costs of the system would be increased, compared to an increase in the rates applied to existing taxes, which would entail no additional administrative costs.

That the system should be equitable generates many questions. There are (at least) four different concepts of equity – vertical, horizontal, and intergenerational equity and proportionality – although individual citizens are going to place very different weights on these four concepts.

The first notion is vertical equity, which holds that the financing of public health care should be based somewhat on ability to pay – i.e., the system should be 'progressive.' While this seems uncontroversial, we make two notes. First, that it is fair to have a progressive system does not imply that more progressivity always equals more fairness. There is a balance to be found between collecting revenues on the basis of ability to pay and requiring those with high incomes to bear an unfairly high burden of total revenue needs. Second, just because it is a shared value that the tax and expenditure system should be progressive does not mean that each and every one of its components needs to be progressive. For example, the best tax system is probably a combination of a progressive income tax and sales taxes that are roughly proportional in burden. The system as a whole is progressive even though the sales tax itself is not.

The second notion of equity is horizontal equity: those in similar circumstances should be treated the same way by the tax system. Again, the idea that revenue should not be collected in an arbitrary fashion is uncontroversial, but in Canada's federal system the concept of horizontal equity is at least part of the rationale for equalization transfers, meant to ensure that individuals in all provinces, regardless of the provincial tax base, have access to comparable levels of public services at comparable tax rates.

The third notion of equity is intergenerational equity. In this case, the idea is to avoid a situation where citizens of one generation pay taxes substantially higher than the benefits that they receive from the public sector as a result of their subsidizing public-sector consumption by an older or younger generation. As a hypothetical example, suppose that generation Z ran large government deficits during its working years. Further suppose that generation Z on retirement pays low taxes, perhaps because the tax system is heavily geared towards income taxes rather than towards consumption taxes, and at the same time places high demands on public expenditure through the health-care system. The generation working during generation Z's retirement years may consider the system somewhat inequitable as it struggles to finance both generation Z's health care and the government debt left by generation Z. Recent estimates by Cardarelli, Sefton, and Kotlikoff (2000) show that in most Western countries, including the United States, the generation currently over the age of 50 will receive a net benefit through the tax, transfer, and expenditure system financed by those under 50. In their estimates, Canada stands out as the only country with virtually perfect intergenerational equity. This is good news – governments in Canada can consider policies that might conceivably shift the balance without fear that they are exacerbating some pre-existing substantial inequity.

The fourth concept of equity, very controversial in health care, is proportionality: is it fair that individuals contribute to the financing of health care in a way proportional to their use of the system? As we show below, some prominent Canadians have advocated this view. However, it is a contested view. Tobin (1970) coins the phrase *specific egalitarianism* for the notion that for *some* goods, such as medical care, availability of service should not depend on income. The rationale is that equality in the distribution of a certain set of goods is necessary if all individuals are to have an equal opportunity to participate fully in society. This would include civil liberties and the justice system, at least minimum amounts of food and shelter, and necessary medical care.

Health economists have devoted considerable attention to equity in health care (Culyer and Wagstaff 1993; Pereira 1993; Hurley 2000; and Wagstaff and Van Doorslaer 2000). There are different ways in which we could choose to think about equality: equality of health, equality of health care, or equality of access, for example. In a paper on options for raising revenue, the key aspect of equity is access (which is not meant to diminish the other equity aspects). *Why* equal access matters is subject to debate. Wagstaff and Van Doorslaer (2000, 1815) stress that access is important to us because it is a means to an end – we think that equal access is crucial in health care because we think that health is a special kind of good, unlike other consumer goods – while Hurley (2000, 89) takes a different approach: 'The ethical basis for equality of access does not derive from any necessary relation with its ultimate effect on the distribution of health care or health. It is intimately linked to the notion of equal opportunity or a fair chance.'

A small copayment for health-care services, which did not apply to low-income individuals and had a cap as a proportion of income, would not eliminate availability of health care for anyone. Yet the notion that use of health-care services would become an economic decision for individuals rather than something that they simply use when they have a felt need is going to go against the grain of what has become, for good or ill, a value judgment held by many Canadians. We argue below, when we evaluate some copayment proposals, that the proponents have not provided the kind of moral argument that will be necessary to convince the public at large.

Hypothecated Taxes

General taxation, social insurance, private insurance, and payments by individuals are common options for funding health care worldwide. Hypothecated or earmarked taxes, ones whose revenues are dedicated solely to funding health care, are an option, though rarely used.

The idea has several merits. Hypothecation is a way of connecting citizens with the taxes that they pay. The current system of pooled or non-hypothecated taxes obscures the purpose of taxation. The processes by which government currently decides how to allocate revenues to given programs or areas are decided by government, out of public view. This gives the government great flexibility in what it does but promotes distrust and cynicism among taxpayers.

The concept of identifying a particular tax, or part of a tax, introduces 'transparency' into the financing of a service. There is less resistance from the public for tax increases when they are so justified (Le Grand 2000). Research done for the Fabian Society's Commission on Taxation and Citizenship in the United Kingdom on public attitudes towards taxation demonstrated that public hostility to increases in taxation drops dramatically if people are told on what the money will be spent (and if they believe what they are told). When asked if they favoured an increase of 1 percentage point in personal income tax as a contribution towards the general pool of government revenue, only 40 per cent of respondents agreed. When asked if they would favour a rise if the money was spent on the National Health Service, 80 per cent agreed.

However, there are arguments against hypothecated taxes. Departments of finance argue that it reduces their ability to control expenditure compared with funding from a general pool of revenues (Normand 1992). Also, if it is a new tax rather than a 'piggyback' on an existing tax, costs of collection and administration are high. A variant of hypothecation is that all the revenue from 'sin taxes' – i.e., taxes on tobacco, alcohol, and gambling (including lotteries) – should go to health. This has little advantage over pooling revenue from these sources with other taxes. Furthermore, the resulting revenue would probably fund only part of total health-care costs. If one wanted to earmark a single tax or part of a tax to fund health care wholly, then the only possible candidates are income tax or sales tax.

There seems to be little need for a hypothecated tax for health care in Canada. When provinces are devoting around 40 per cent of their operating budgets to health care, no single tax could come close to providing the necessary revenues on its own. As for a hypothecated tax to fund incremental spending, the taxation–expenditure link would quickly become cloudy as the government made any adjustments to other taxes or areas of spending. It would increase administrative costs in terms of trying to provide transparency in how the new tax was being devoted to the expenditure side of the budget, and this feature is necessary to the justification of a hypothecated tax in the first place.

Copayment Systems: Two Proposals

Tom Kent (2000) proposes a system of copayments for medicare that he sees as consistent with the provisions of the Canada Health Act, whereas user fees and extra-billing are not (Courchene [1994, 186–7] proposes, in passing, a similar plan). Although any system of copayments will raise questions regarding compatibility with the Canada Health Act, especially the provision on access (but also the provision on portability), the act in itself does not reveal definitively which systems of copayments would or would not be acceptable. As economists not trained in the interpretation of federal statutes, we are unable to assess Kent's claim that his proposal falls within the act's provisions, although he no doubt bases the claim at least in part on the fact that his proposal would incur no additional payments for low-income individuals.

Kent notes that medicare, as it stands, has costs and expectations that are great and rising, with patients who are generally unaware of the costs that their personal use imposes on the system (though not of the system's total cost to the taxpayer) and physicians who have little incentive to be cost-conscious. 'In short, the ideologues of market economies are right, in the sense that pressure to exceed reasonable needs is inherent in tax-financed health care. Medicare does require a way to contain its costs without breaking the principle of universal access' (Kent 2000, 11).

Kent proposes that individuals (or families) receive at the end of each year a statement of the costs of their use of the system. The statement would be in a format similar to the T4 used in the personal income tax. Medicare use up to between 5 and 10 per cent of income, depending on family size and income levels, would be treated as a taxable benefit for the purposes of federal income tax. Under current federal tax rates, the total increase in income tax should not be more than 2.9 per cent of pre-tax income for any individual. Since Kent proposes that provinces may or may not want to participate, it is not clear whether this marginal increase to federal taxes would be added to the tax base of those provinces that continue to base their personal income tax on federal tax owing (many provinces are departing from 'tax-on-tax' to 'tax-on-base'). Kent also proposes increased transfers from Ottawa to the provinces for medicare, the details of which we discuss in the next section. But there is some rationale for collecting this extra revenue at the federal level, since it is accompanied by a proposal to transfer the funds to the provinces.

The rationale for this particular method of tax increase is that: 'Few people may realize how much their own care costs, but all know that Medicare in total is expensive, that it is in some respects inefficient, sometimes abused. The ordinary sense of fairness is not offended by the idea that people should make some direct contribution to the cost of service, according to how much they use it and how much they can afford' (Kent 2000, 12). Although Kent refers to user fees and extra-billing as 'crude devices,' this is a proposal for 'progressive' user fees (indeed more progressive than the personal income tax, since the proportion of the individual use of the system that is added to taxable income is itself applied in a way that rises with income).

Aside from the federal–provincial relations aspect, dealt with below, we have two substantial concerns with Kent's proposal. First, Kent himself notes that physicians are not always the most cost-conscious users of public funds. Yet his proposal assumes that the major incentive problem facing medicare is located not with the doctor but with the patient. The vast literature on that crucial problem of health economics – supplier-induced demand – is beyond the scope of this paper, but there are significant questions about any scheme that assumes more rational use of the system if only the patient bears a direct proportion of the costs (see Barer et al. 1994; Evans, Barer, and Stoddart 1994; and Evans et al. 1994).

Second, the notion of fairness in paying for health care is subject to question. Kent claims that our notion of fairness does not object to people paying for the service based on what they use and how much they can afford. Canada's tax-financed system already funds health care on the basis of what people can afford, so the major innovation that comes with the 'taxable benefits' proposal is to have people pay according to what they use. One could *conceivably* make an argument that Kent is correct: fairness dictates that heavier users of the system should pay more, incomes being equal. The commission's interim report notes that among the four major approaches to the sustainability of medicare, at least one is that individuals should bear more financial responsibility for their use of the system (Commission 2002, 11). But Kent's claim that the 'ordinary sense of fairness' is not offended by the idea is true only for a portion of the Canadian public, and a change of attitudes is needed before this value could be used as a basis for health-care reform.

Still, Kent's paper is a valuable attempt to deal with the political and economic challenges of reforming medicare, and many of the proposed reforms, in terms of federal–provincial co-operation and harnessing the tremendous advances in information technology, are certainly worth careful consideration, although those aspects are beyond the scope of this paper.

Aba, Goodman, and Mintz (2002) propose a copayment system somewhat similar to Kent's. Key differences are that they would have the additional revenues raised directly by the provinces rather than by Ottawa, based on 40 per cent of the cost of services, to a maximum of 3 per cent of annual income above the threshold level of $10,000. They estimate that 62 per cent of families would pay the full 3 per cent. Not only would the plan raise additional revenue (by about $6.6 billion, if we judge by figures for 2000), but the incentives for individuals to economize on their use of the system would save about $6.3 billion annually (if we assume a 17 per cent drop in use by those individuals not at the 3-per cent–of-income ceiling – those at the ceiling have no disincentives on health-care use, since the marginal cost for them is the same as under the present system, i.e., zero).

Although this new payment mechanism would increase administration costs, the authors stress the positive aspect: an accounting of individuals' use of various parts of the system should increase accountability.

Like Kent, Aba, Goodman, and Mintz (2002) *assert* that there is something fair about the copayment system without providing a thorough explanation: 'Fairness is improved because individuals who consume public services contribute more to their cost' (2). 'When consumption levels of public services vary among people in otherwise similar economic circumstances, then fairness is improved if contributions are related to the cost of those services. Fairness is improved further if individuals who may assume health risks that result in greater health-care expenditures contribute more to the costs of the health care system' (5).

Evans et al. (1994) state: 'If a service is incontestably medical in intent, and is effective, and is regarded by the community as necessary, and can be provided in no other, less costly way, why would one want to impose a user charge? At that point one of the standard arguments against user charges, that they tax the sick, seems wholly justified. Such charges may be highly effective as a revenue raising devise, but why would one regard the experience of illness, and the use of effective care, as an indicator of taxable capacity or ability to pay? No answer ever seems to have been offered' (27).

The proposals by Kent and by Aba et al. each ensure that the lowest income individuals will not face additional charges. But under each proposal, the 'fairness' rationale for copayment receives no defence, and so there is insufficient reason for departing from the current system of raising revenues for core health-care services through general taxation. The remainder of this paper looks at raising additional revenues through the tax system, and the next section considers whether the additional revenues should be raised at the federal or the provincial level.

Federal–Provincial Tax and Transfer Issues

Provinces bear the burden of paying health-care providers in the medicare system. So any options for raising revenue for health care must ultimately result in an increase in funding to provincial treasuries. We group the various ways of accomplishing such an increase into three categories:

- increased block transfers from the federal government
- increased transfers from the federal government based on cost sharing
- an increase in the ability of provinces to raise own-source revenues

Block transfers from the federal government to the provinces, not tied in any way to levels of provincial funding, have two principal rationales – equalization and vertical fiscal imbalance. The first, equalization, has both equity and efficiency justifications. The equity rationale is the belief that Canadians seem to share that people across the country should be able to receive roughly comparable levels of service delivery at roughly comparable levels of taxation. Indeed, that is the reason given in the constitution for Canada's equalization system.

The efficiency rationale is less known. Canada's economy will be at its most productive if its labour force is allocated across regions and jobs so that each worker is located where his or her marginal product is highest. In general, competitive labour markets do this well, since, with equilibrium in each place of employment, wages will tend to equal marginal product. As technologies and world prices change, so do the values of workers' marginal products. Where labour has become more valuable, perhaps owing to increased demand for a particular service, wages will rise in that sector, and some workers will choose to leave the lower-productivity sector for the higher, following the higher wages. The law of diminishing returns eventually establishes equilibrium, as wages eventually equalize across sectors for any given skill level. But a complication arises when provincial governments have significantly different per-capita tax bases, since labour will allocate itself according to the *total* income that it can receive in a province – wages plus the 'net fiscal benefit,' or the difference between the government services that the individual will receive and the taxes that he or she will have to pay. In this case labour is not being allocated strictly according to productivity, and national income will fall. In a concrete context, it is a misallocation of Canadian labour if individuals move, for example, to Alberta not because wages have been rising there, but because that is the only way for them to take advantage of the benefits that flow from having public services funded by vast natural-resource revenues and only very low personal taxes.

An equalization system such as Canada's should prevent excessive migration to tax base–rich provinces by equalizing to some degree the net fiscal benefits in different provinces; see Boadway (2000) or Boadway and Hobson (1993) for a defence of the efficiency rationale for equalization. This argument is not universally held – some may wonder if it is efficient to provide the Atlantic provinces, for instance, with substantial equalization payments to prevent excessive out-migration. The United States does not have an equalization system (although some of its federal–state transfers are at least somewhat equalizing); see Courchene (1994, 107–8) for a critique of the efficiency argument.

Since the purpose of equalization is to equalize net fiscal benefits, it makes sense that the formula is based on the shortfall between a province's tax base and the average tax base of a five-province standard. It also makes sense that the equalization payments are a lump sum to be spent as a province sees fit and are not based on provincial spending.

The second rationale for block transfers is vertical fiscal imbalance (VFI). VFI arises when Ottawa has greater capacity to raise revenue through taxation than it actually needs to fund its own spending programs while provinces lack taxation capacity to fund their own programs. Much of the federal–provincial debate over health-care funding revolves around this problem, with health-care costs rising faster than other areas of government spending and provinces unable to raise revenue to fund it. The Canada Health and Social Transfer (CHST) is the primary connecting transfer, being an equal per-capita transfer to all provinces. As Hobson and St-Hilaire (2000, 160) note, the CHST is only a method of revenue transfer; it does not function as an instrument of social policy.

How large a problem is VFI? Ruggeri and Howard (2001) consider VFI through a lens that compares the future path of federal and provincial revenues and spending based on the built-in growth that would arise from the current tax and federal–provincial transfer systems. They conclude that, under current arrangements, Ottawa will see a steady increase in its budget surplus, while in general provinces will have small and somewhat precarious surpluses over the next 20 years; in other words, the problem of VFI will worsen in the absence of some sort of policy change. A significant contributor to the projected increases in VFI is the rate of increase in health-care costs, projected at 4.8 per cent annually, while total own-source revenue growth for the provinces is projected at only 3.8 per cent annually (compared to 4.3 per cent at the federal level).

Norrie and Wilson (2000) concur that VFI is likely to increase under current arrangements. In their comparison of increased transfer payments from Ottawa and greater tax capacity for the provinces, they note that increasing federal–provincial transfers might lower the marginal cost of raising tax revenue more at the federal level than at the provincial. Transfers, however, provide little guarantee of stable funding for provinces. The history of the past few decades is such that provinces will always be wary of relying even more heavily on transfers, which can be cut, sometimes in very arbitrary ways, whenever the federal government finds itself in some fiscal difficulty (also see Hobson and St-Hilaire 2000, 182–3).

There are other problems with transfers to deal with VFI. If healthcare costs are likely to continue to rise at rates higher than either other public expenditures or tax revenues under current rates, then the amount of transfer must continually be adjusted. Such circumstances, as recent history has shown, confuse the public about the two levels' accountability for decisions made on fund-raising and expenditures in health care. Current arrangements may not foster such accountability.

However, federal–provincial transfers based on cost sharing in medicare would at least help transfers keep pace with the growing cost of providing health care. But there are significant concerns with cost sharing as well.

Kent (2000) suggests that the revenue from the income tax–based copayments discussed above be distributed to provinces through a cost-sharing scheme, initially set at 20 per cent of eligible expenditure and rising as high as 25 per cent. Kent gives two rationales for cost sharing. First, 'the standard and good reason for such support is that without it Newfoundland, say, could not afford much of what Alberta can' (3). But that is a reason for equalization, not for cost sharing. Second, the Canada Health Act mandates that provinces run some very expensive programs: 'Medicare could not have begun, as a similar service for all Canadians, except as a federal–provincial partnership. It can survive only as a partnership in which shared principles are backed by shared costs' (3). But again, this ensures that provinces can pay for federally mandated public health care, something which can be achieved through either a lump-sum transfer or an (equalized) increase in the capacity of provinces to raise own-source revenues. Kent has in mind perhaps Ottawa's using its financial contribution to enforce, through the threat of withholding funds, the Canada Health Act. The National Forum on Health (1996) speculated that as much as the federal government might use its powers of 'moral suasion' to persuade the provinces to uphold the existing principles of medicare, 'unless it is backed by some financial or regulatory clout, there is no reason to believe this would be an effective strategy.'

The CHST is the culmination of a long federal withdrawal from cost sharing for medicare, welfare, and postsecondary education. The rationale for cost sharing at the time was that Ottawa wanted to encourage provinces to expand service provision beyond what they would provide under a lump-sum transfer of equivalent value. In other words, the aim was a 'substitution effect' – a change in the relative prices of goods to encourage a particular activity, namely particular government programs – as well as an 'income effect' – the effect on provincial budgetary decision making resulting from a lump-sum transfer with no changes in the relative costs of programs. But why would we want to give provinces an incentive to allocate more of their budgets to health care, at the expense of other programs, than they would in the absence of a shared-cost program? Normally economists justify cost sharing through a significant interprovincial externality arising from expenditure in a particular program. But there is no evidence for such an externality in health care, certainly not enough to justify a 25 per cent subsidy.

Cost-shared programs produce other problems. First, are they to be open- or closed-ended? In open-ended programs, Ottawa came to resent funding a program while having no control over spending. If programs were closed-ended, then at the margin the desired substitution effect, if it initially justified cost sharing, disappeared as provinces became responsible for all spending at the margin. Second, cost sharing can cause an inefficient allocation of resources across policy areas, as provinces devote too many resources to cost-sharing programs at the expense of other programs that may achieve wider policy goals. For example, officials in provincial departments of social services report much greater willingness today to experiment with programs in human services, integrating training, employment, and income supplements, in ways that were not done under the cost-sharing Canada Assistance Plan, which provided 50 per cent cost sharing to a limited selection of welfare programs. Given governments' vast range of policy instruments to improve population health, there should not be artificial incentives to focus on some instruments rather than others purely because of cost sharing.

The third option for increasing the resources in provincial treasuries so as to allow greater expenditure on health care is to provide provinces with increased capacity to raise own-source revenues. To preserve horizontal equity across Canada, any new revenue source must be fully included in equalization.

The critical problem with increasing provincial revenue capacity is that Canada possesses an unusual tax structure for a federation, with all major tax fields occupied by both Ottawa and the provinces. Economists have often remarked on this fact, and despite differences of opinion on some details, there seems to be a broad, three-part consensus – first, corporate income taxes are an inefficient way for provinces to raise own-source revenue and are probably best left to Ottawa; second, sales taxes are most efficiently left at the provincial level, with a federal presence in the field not really necessary; and third, personal income taxes are such a substantial source of revenue at both levels that sharing them makes sense.

In an oft-cited review of the issues, Richard Musgrave (1983) asks about who in a federal system should tax, what, and where. The standard answer from the theory of federal public finance is that those taxes that progressively redistribute income, as well as those that apply to highly mobile bases, should be federal. Provincial governments are best suited for taxing less-mobile bases and will be limited in the degree to which they can pursue income redistribution. From this analysis, observers suggest that Ottawa should handle corporate income taxes, since their base is highly mobile. Although the tax base for corporate income for firms operating in more than one province is allocated by a simple averaging of total payroll and total sales in the province as a share of national levels, a recent empirical study by Mintz and Smart (2001), confirming prior work by other researchers, found substantial shifting of corporate tax across Canada in response to variations in provincial rates of corporate tax.

If there are problems with corporate taxation at the provincial level, and indeed even internationally as capital becomes more mobile, then increasing provincial personal income taxes or sales taxes becomes the best option.

But since Ottawa occupies both taxes in a significant way, provinces can increase tax rates in either area only if Ottawa creates some 'tax room.' The case for this move can certainly be made in revenue terms, given the evidence of an increasing VFI in favour of Ottawa over the next few decades. But we recognize the substantial political issues involved in having the federal government being willing to cede a substantial revenue source.

Our recommendation is for a transfer of sales tax room from Ottawa to the provinces; the GST should become a provincial tax. The next section outlines a method for administering the GST at the provincial level, which amounts to Canada-wide adoption of the Quebec 'zero-rating' system. Increased sales taxes by the provinces are the most efficient means for them to collect revenue. Indeed, the GST will prove even more efficient than existing provincial sales taxes. We also show that the proposal would not entail large administration costs.

The proposal is not a radical one. Giving the sales tax field to the provinces was recommended by the Rowell–Sirois Commission and the Carter Commission, and is supported, although the specifics vary, by Boadway and Hobson (1993, 154) and by Ip and Mintz (1992). However, since many observers wonder whether such an arrangement is administratively feasible (Bird 1994), we set out the details clearly.

Increasing Provincial Tax Revenues: A Proposal

Our proposal for transferring the GST to the provinces was first set out in Hill and Rushton (1993) and draws on the recent experience in the European Union (EU) with value-added taxes (VAT) that resemble the GST. We refer readers to the original reference for detailed exposition – we give a brief outline of the proposed system and some of its implications.

The Europeans faced the following problem. Each country in the EU administered a VAT. Rates differed across countries, as did the base; for example, in some countries basic groceries were subject to the tax, and in others they were not. Into such a system came the initiative to end border controls within the EU on goods and services. The European problem was how to administer a system of VATs without border controls.

Achieving an administratively simple method for running the GST as a provincial tax involves the same problem as the Europeans faced, albeit from a different path. Canada already has a system of interprovincial trade without border controls, and the question is how to organize provincial VATs that might differ in rate and tax base. Some commentators thought it impossible except with a single national rate and base (Bird 1994; Boadway and Hobson 1993, 154, who argue that provinces alone should occupy the sales tax field, resign themselves to the current system of provincial retail sales taxes, on the assumption that a VAT could exist interprovincially only with a single rate and base). Negotiations on harmonizing sales taxes in the early 1990s broke down probably when provinces refused to accommodate the federal request for a single national rate and base. But Europe has achieved a method of solving the problem, and it can be applied to Canada.

The GST is run on the 'credit-invoice' method: firms pay GST on their purchases and remit the receipts for a fully refundable credit. Firms collect no GST on foreign exports; in this sense it is a 'destination-based' tax, applying to Canadian *consumption* rather than to Canadian *production*. In the end, the entire burden of the 7 per cent tax falls on Canadian consumers. There are no hidden and carried-forward sales taxes from the production and distribution process, since any GST paid at those levels has also been refunded (production by firms so small that they need not register for the GST does not affect the essence of the plan). The incidence of the GST differs from that of non-harmonized provincial retail sales taxes.

While much of the retail sales tax is collected from Canadian consumers, there are also non-refundable taxes paid on business inputs. The incidence of these taxes is complex:

- For goods retailed in Canada where there is competition from imports, the tax on business inputs cannot be shifted forward to consumers and so is shifted backwards and borne by the less-mobile factors of production – i.e., labour and land, rather than capital.
- For goods retailed in Canada where there is lack of import competition, the tax can be shifted forward to consumers.
- For goods exported abroad, for which there is almost always competition, the tax cannot be shifted forward to foreign consumers and so is borne by domestic producers, again especially by labour and land. Firms do not collect provincial retail sales taxes on exports, even if they move only out of province.

Since retail sales taxes are borne at least partly by producers, they may cause inefficiencies in the choice of location of production; such inefficiencies do not arise with the GST.

Existing provincial retail sales taxes do not affect out-of-province exports; like the GST, they are meant to be destination based. But the *importer* is expected to pay sales tax in his or her province. Provinces monitor interprovincial shipments with regular exchanges of information, sometimes formal and sometimes informal; the administrative machinery for interprovincial trade and sales taxes already exists. Under our proposal, firms shipping interprovincially would continue to collect no sales tax on the sale. The importer would pay no tax on the import but simply declare the value of the shipment and the tax that ordinarily would be owing, along with the claim for credit that it would normally file for within-province purchases.

Such a system allows different provinces to levy different rates of VAT, or even, as Alberta might choose to do, no sales tax at all. No tax revenues from this provincial VAT system would need to flow across provincial boundaries, and so there is no need for any sort of central clearing-house of payments across Canada. Further, provinces could have a different final tax base. Under the scheme, if, for example, Manitoba decided to tax children's clothing but Saskatchewan chose not to, no administrative complications would arise.

The proposed system would be more efficient than Boadway and Hobson's (1993) proposal simply to continue with retail sales taxes. It is simpler than Bird and Mintz's (2000) proposal for harmonizing the provincial sales taxes with a continuing federal GST (their proposal for harmonization is very similar to ours; see 280) and further adding a new tax for provinces and municipalities – a 'business value tax' that is similar to a VAT except origin based rather than destination based and applying to the income generated by each firm (its 'value-added') rather than to the final value of consumption. (Note that Bird and Mintz propose an origin-based tax because provinces will want to tax business income somehow, especially if, as Bird and Mintz recommend, responsibility for corporate income tax shifts to Ottawa. They justify provincial and local taxation of business income as a 'benefit tax' – when the public sector is providing valuable inputs to the production process, users of those inputs should pay some of the price.)

Our proposal for shifting the GST to the provinces transfers one of the most efficient taxes available, which would not exacerbate interprovincial competition like the corporate tax, or even the personal income tax, has, especially when provinces attempt to make the income tax relatively progressive. It does not entail creation of a new tax and would probably lead to elimination of an old one – the retail sales tax. So administrative costs are reasonable. And even though the GST is more a proportional tax than a progressive one, recall our earlier comment that what matters is that the overall system be progressive, not each and every component. Unlike new federal taxes that could subsequently be transferred to provinces, the sales tax proposal allows individual provinces more flexibility in choosing a tax mix for their residents, rather than a uniform federal tax (although Zeckhauser [1994] proposes a federal VAT in the United States to pay for a proposed Canadian-style health-care system). Finally, as opposed to a new hypothecated tax or a new copayment mechanism, our proposal does not presuppose that Canadians need to pay more in taxes – it allows for increased revenues without insisting on them.

Conclusion

As Bird and Mintz (2000) note, the exchange of tax fields between the federal and provincial governments requires a lot of co-operation and transitional funding for any province that looks to lose thereby. It is also critical that equalization continue to be applied effectively. Given the acrimonious debates during the past decade over federal 'off-loading' and inadequate federal–provincial transfers, we are not so naïve as to think that Ottawa would easily transfer a major revenue source without some kind of trade-off, and that jeopardizes our main goal – more funds for provincial treasuries. But since it has not been established that the Canadian system of public finance as a whole is underfunded, and indeed with large and growing federal surpluses predicted, we believe that Canadians' interests are best served by a reallocation of public funds between levels of government, rather than by addition of new revenue sources. There is simply not a strong enough case for a hypothecated tax or for treating a portion of medicare use as a taxable benefit through the personal income tax.

Implementation of the plan would need strong leadership at both levels of government: in Ottawa, to be willing to give away a significant source of revenue, and in the provinces, to work with a tax that had been rejected as an option when first introduced (though rejected in the context of federal insistence on a national uniform tax rate and base). But, despite this political hurdle, transferring the GST is surely preferable to the *continuous* debates that come from federal–provincial transfers (Hobson and St-Hilaire 2000; Norrie and Wilson 2000). A transfer of GST also avoids the problem that is often at the root of VFI – superior federal ability to collect taxes – since a destination-based consumption tax such as the GST minimizes interprovincial distortions.

There are no politically straightforward ways of increasing provincial funds, and so we look to a solution that is at least efficient and administratively reasonable, does not shift the equity in taxation in the combined federal–provincial system, and lowers the potential for future political disputes.

REFERENCES

Aba, Shay, Wolfe D. Goodman, and Jack M. Mintz. 2002. *Funding Public Provision of Private Health: The Case for Copayment Contribution through the Tax System.* Toronto: C.D. Howe Institute.

Barer, Morris L., et al. 1994. *The Remarkable Tenacity of User Charges.* Toronto: Premier's Council on Health, Well-Being and Social Justice.

Bird, Richard M. 1994. 'A Comparative Perspective on Federal Finance.' In Keith G. Banting, Douglas M. Brown and Thomas J. Courchene, eds., *The Future of Fiscal Federalism.* Kingston: School of Policy Studies, Institute of Intergovernmental Relations, Queen's University, 293–322.

Bird, Richard M., and Jack M. Mintz. 2000. 'Tax Assignment in Canada: A Modest Proposal.' In Harvey Lazar, ed., *Toward a New Mission Statement for Canadian Fiscal Federalism.* Montreal: McGill-Queen's University Press, 263–92.

Boadway, Robin. 1992. *The Constitutional Division of Powers: An Economic Perspective.* Economic Council of Canada. Ottawa: Supply and Services Canada.

– 2000. 'Recent Developments in the Economics of Federalism.' In Harvey Lazar, ed., *Toward a New Mission Statement for Canadian Fiscal Federalism.* Montreal: McGill-Queen's University Press, 41–78.

Boadway, Robin, and Paul A.R. Hobson. 1993. *Intergovernmental Fiscal Relations in Canada.* Canadian Tax Paper No. 96. Toronto: Canadian Tax Foundation.

Boase, Joan Price. 2001. 'Federalism and the Health Facility Fees Challenge.' In Duane Adams, ed., *Federalism, Democracy and Health Policy in Canada.* Montreal: McGill-Queen's University Press, 179–206.

Cardarelli, Roberto, James Sefton, and Laurence J. Kotlikoff. 2000. 'Generational Accounting in the UK.' *Economic Journal* 110: F547–74.

Commission on the Future of Health Care in Canada. 2002. *Shape the Future of Health Care.* Interim Report. Saskatoon: The Commission.

Courchene, Thomas J. 1994. *Social Canada in the Millennium.* Toronto: C.D. Howe Institute.

Culyer, A.J., and Adam Wagstaff. 1993. 'Equity and Equality in Health and Health Care.' *Journal of Health Economics* 12, 431–57.

Evans, Robert G., et al. 1994. *It's Not the Money, It's the Principle: Why User Charges for Some Services and Not Others?* Toronto: Premier's Council on Health, Well-Being and Social Justice.

Evans, Robert G., Morris L. Barer, and Greg L. Stoddart. 1994. *Charging Peter to Pay Paul: Accounting for the Financial Effects of User Charges.* Toronto: Premier's Council on Health, Well-Being and Social Justice.

Hill, Roderick, and Michael Rushton. 1993. 'Harmonizing Provincial Sales Taxes with the GST: The Problem of Interprovincial Trade.' *Canadian Tax Journal* 41, no. 1: 101–22.

Hobson, Paul A.R., and France St-Hilaire. 2000. 'The Evolution of Federal–Provincial Fiscal Arrangements: Putting Humpty Together Again.' In Harvey Lazar, ed., *Toward a New Mission Statement for Canadian Fiscal Federalism.* Montreal: McGill-Queen's University Press, 159–88.

Hurley, Jeremiah. 2000. 'An Overview of the Normative Economics of the Health Sector.' In A.J. Culyer and J.P. Newhouse, eds., *Handbook of Health Economics, Volume 1.* Amsterdam: Elsevier, 56–118.

Ip, Irene K., and Jack M. Mintz. 1992. *Dividing the Spoils: The Federal–Provincial Allocation of Taxing Powers.* Toronto: C.D. Howe Institute.

Jack, William. 1999. *Principles of Health Economics for Developing Countries.* Washington, DC: The World Bank.

Kent, Tom. 2000. *What Should Be Done about Medicare.* Ottawa: Caledon Institute of Social Policy.

Le Grand, Julian. 2000. 'Should the NHS Be Funded by a Hypothecated Tax?' *Fabian Review* (winter), 8.

Marzouk, M.S. 1991. 'Aging, Age-Specific Health Care Costs and the Future Health Care Burden in Canada.' *Canadian Public Policy* 17, no. 4: 490–506.

Mintz, Jack, and Michael Smart. 2001. 'Income Shifting, Investment, and Tax Competition: Theory and Evidence from Provincial Taxation in Canada.' Working Paper No. 554. Munich: Centre for Economic Studies and Ifo Institute for Economic Research (CESifo).

Musgrave, Richard. 1983. 'Who Should Tax, Where, and What?' In Charles E. McLure, Jr, ed., *Tax Assignment in Federal Countries.* Canberra: ANU Press, 2–19.

National Forum on Health. 1996. 'Maintaining a National Health Care System: a Question of Principle(s) ... and Money.' wwwnfh.hc-sc.gc.ca/publicat/maintain/intro.htm, 29 April 2002.

Normand, Charles. 1992. 'Funding Health Care in the United Kingdom,' *BMJ* 304: 768–70.

Norrie, Kenneth, and L.S. Wilson. 2000. 'On Re-Balancing Canadian Fiscal Federalism.' In Harvey Lazar, ed., *Toward a New Mission Statement for Canadian Fiscal Federalism.* Montreal: McGill-Queen's University Press, 79–98.

Pereira, Joao. 1993. 'What Does Equity in Health Mean?' *Journal of Social Policy* 22: 19–48.

Ruggeri, G.C., and R. Howard. 2001. 'On the Concept and Measurement of Vertical Fiscal Imbalances.' Public Policy Paper No. 6. Regina: Saskatchewan Institute for Public Policy.

Tobin, James. 1970. 'On Limiting the Domain of Inequality.' *Journal of Law and Economics* 13: 263–77.

Wagstaff, Adam, and Eddy Van Doorslaer. 2000. 'Equity in Health Care Finance and Delivery.' In A.J. Culyer and J.P. Newhouse, eds., *Handbook of Health Economics, Volume 1*. Amsterdam: Elsevier, 804–62.

Zeckhauser, Richard. 1994. 'Public Finance Principles and National Health Care Reform.' *Journal of Economic Perspectives* 8, no. 3: 55–60.

9 The Changing Political and Economic Environment of Health Care

GERARD W. BOYCHUK

Public health care in Canada is portrayed with increasing frequency and urgency as unsustainable. The desire to eliminate government deficits, reduce the debt load, and lower taxes appears to have come in conflict with the desire to sustain a comprehensive, universal, and publicly administered health-care system. Both the federal and provincial governments have had to struggle with conflicting demands from the public (and some organized interests) for lower taxes and balanced budgets while maintaining a high-quality, publicly administered, and publicly funded health-care system. This conflict has raised questions about the sustainability of the current system of health care, which in turn has provoked related questions: Is the crisis a fiscal reality driven by a changing economy? Is it caused by the changing political context? Is it temporary and linked to the transition to a post-deficit era? Does the 'new' political economy mean permanent changes to Canada's health systems?

A fiscal crisis in health care is not evident in current expenditure patterns. While the tension between health care as a large public-expenditure program and neoliberal fiscal pressures for balanced budgets, debt retirement, and tax reduction seems relatively obvious, this relationship is not so straightforward. Rather, the link between the two issues is both political and institutional, with the political fragility of health care being neither the automatic nor the necessary result of a neoliberal political environment. Yet public belief in a fiscal crisis is real. For now, the sustainability of public health care is fundamentally a political rather than simply a fiscal question. How and why has this link between health-care spending and fiscal issues – captured by the term *sustainability* – become so firmly embedded in Canadian policy debates? Understanding this link becomes all the more pressing as a neoliberal context oriented towards balanced budgets, deficit/debt reduction, and reduced taxes appears likely to magnify the impact of this link.

The fiscal crisis in health care is not merely an ideological construct. The real crisis lies in a paradox: the system's institutional underpinnings – especially federal–provincial relations – undermine rather than bolster public support for the system. Its political weakness is the result of nearly a decade of federal–provincial wrangling over funding in an era of fiscal restraint. These incentives and resulting patterns of interaction have led members of the elite and the broader public to believe that health care is of rapidly declining quality, wracked by a funding crisis, unable to control costs, and, ultimately fiscally unsustainable.

Because the current perception is rooted in the system's institutional framework, pressures have not eased and will probably not do so as fiscal pressures abate or as mechanisms to control future cost pressures are implemented. Making the system more politically sustainable requires serious rethinking of federal and provincial roles and responsibilities in the funding and delivery of public health care and of the resulting incentives and public perceptions.

The first section of the paper examines provincial health-care expenditures during the 1990s. It suggests that current expenditure patterns provide few indications that the system is fiscally unsustainable. Such claims must be based either on forecasts of cost escalation above and beyond cost increases caused by population growth, ageing, and moderate cost increases in services now offered or on the belief that current levels of tax are unsustainable. The conclusion of the section addresses the sustainability of current provincial tax levels in the face of increasing global and continental economic integration.

Even though provincial health expenditures relative to gross domestic product (GDP) are the same as they were in the early 1990s, there is now a widespread perception of a fiscal crisis in public health care. The second section of the paper argues that this perception springs from the institutional underpinnings of health care – especially federal–provincial fiscal arrangements. While they appeared to work well enough in a period of expansion, these arrangements, in an era of more generalized restraint, began to create dynamics that have undermined public support for the current system. First, the illusion of a rapid growth in the overall fiscal burden represented by health expenditures (relative to the economy) is an artefact of federal–provincial financing arrangements. Second, the manipulation of the fiscal system to move the burden of government debts and deficits primarily to the provinces has strongly reinforced the link in public debates between health-care spending and the issue of deficits and debt. Finally, in a context of federal transfer restraint, current fiscal arrangements provide provinces with strong incentives to emphasize the failings of their health-care system and its fiscal unsustainability.

The third section examines the effects of government responses to the negative incentives outlined above on public perceptions of health care. People now question the quality of health care, often despite positive personal experiences. Many people believe that the system is experiencing a major financial crisis and that increased funding is crucial. Finally, public confidence in federal and provincial handling of health-care issues is decreasing, and more and more Canadians think that governments are falling further and further behind vis-à-vis the problems facing health care.

In its conclusion, the paper argues for a definition of *sustainability* that incorporates the political – rather than just the fiscal – sustainability of the health-care system. In the absence of reform, the dysfunctional incentives built into the federal–provincial institutional structure are likely to keep undermining the political sustainability of public health care.

Fiscal Sustainability

Sustainability, in current debates, has been understood primarily in fiscal terms. This section examines fiscal sustainability and claims that current patterns of expenditure, on their own, are not sufficient to demonstrate unsustainability.

Assessing Current Patterns

There are two approaches that generally support the alleged fiscal unsustainability of health care. The first extrapolates future health-care costs from current spending patterns (primarily since 1996), and the second extrapolates current trends in these expenditures expressed as

Figure 9.1
Annual provincial health expenditures versus 1992 expenditure (adjusted for
population growth), Canada, 1992–2001

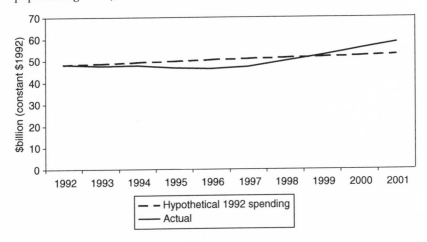

a proportion of total provincial program expenditure. However, both
approaches are highly problematic. First, they fail to identify the
appropriate time frame on which to base extrapolations. Extrapolations of health-care costs based on the late 1990s ignore the fact that
expenditure restraint in mid-decade probably helped create pent-up
demand, which was reflected in higher annual spending levels later in
the decade. Second, expressing health-care expenditures as a proportion of total provincial program spending is an inappropriate measure
of the fiscal sustainability of health-care expenditures.

Expenditure Restraint and Pent-Up Demand
One of the difficulties encountered in extrapolating from current
trends in health-care expenditure is judging the 'drivers' underlying
recent increases. The report of the provincial and territorial ministers
of health (2000) on health-care costs notes the 'severe restraint directed
toward health care in the early-to-mid 1990s [which] produced a very
low annual average growth rate' (3.17). The report notes that 'since
1996, provinces and territories have been reinvesting, partly to make
up for the restraint applied in the early years of the decade' (3.17).
    Annual provincial health expenditures (see Figure 9.1) did increase
significantly after 1996.[1] However, from 1993 to 1996, actual provincial

Figure 9.2
Cumulative provincial health expenditures versus 1992 expenditures (adjusted for population growth), Canada, 1992–2001

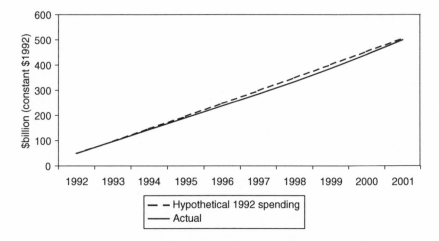

expenditures were lower than they would have been if public health expenditures per capita had been simply maintained at 1992 levels. By 1997, actual provincial expenditures were cumulatively over $13 billion (in constant 1992 dollars) less than they would have been if provinces had simply maintained their per-capita expenditures at 1992 levels. As provinces began to reinvest in health care after 1996, actual cumulative provincial expenditures by 2001 reached *almost* the amount that provinces would have spent in the 1992–2001 period if they had simply maintained per-capita expenditures at 1992 levels. (See Figure 9.2.)

Thus the crucial issue is delineating expenditure increases that resulted from discretionary choices to enhance or expand health services, those that were responses to pent-up demand created by expenditure restraint in the early and mid-1990s, and those necessitated by other cost pressures. Each element has different implications for future expenditure patterns. Discretionary enhancement or expansion of services is more amenable to restraint than other non-discretionary cost pressures. Cost expansion driven by pent-up demand is likely to abate. Neither element suggests inevitable future cost increases. It is only the third element that is germane to inevitable fiscal unsustainability. Therefore, extrapolating from current expenditure patterns without demarcating underlying drivers of cost escalation and their future

Figure 9.3
Provincial health expenditures, various measures, indexed (1991 = 1.00),
1991–2001

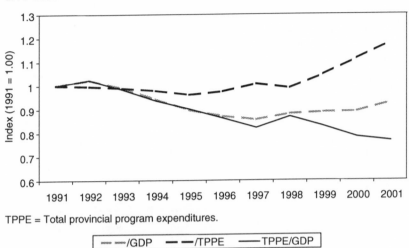

TPPE = Total provincial program expenditures.

| ⟳⟳/GDP | — —/TPPE | ——TPPE/GDP |

implications is not an appropriate method for forecasting future expenditure patterns.

Health Expenditures as a Relative Measure

The barometer of provincial health spending in recent public debates is health expenditure as a proportion of total provincial program expenditures. This measure is significant, but not as a measure of the fiscal burden of health-care spending or as an indicator of the overall fiscal sustainability of current patterns of health-care expenditure.

Provincial expenditures on public health fell relative to provincial gross domestic product (GDP) from 1993 to 1997. (See Figure 9.3.) While expenditures have increased since 1997, provincial health expenditures as a proportion of GDP are still lower than they were over a decade ago. At the same time, they have increased relative to total provincial program spending. The explanation for this apparent discrepancy is that the latter remained static from 1991 to 2000 in real-dollar terms and have dropped to 78 per cent of their 1991 levels relative to GDP. Thus provincial expenditures on health rose as a propor-

Figure 9.4
Provincial health expenditures, as percentage of total revenues and of
provincial own-source revenues, 1991–2001

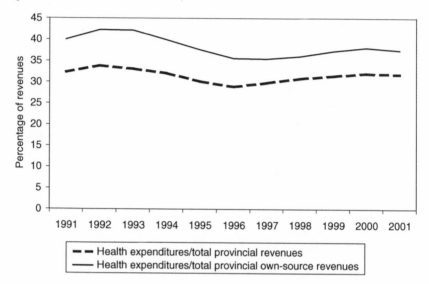

tion of total provincial program expenditures while remaining static
relative to GDP.

A more appropriate measure of fiscal burden and fiscal sustainability is provincial public-health expenditure relative to total provincial
revenues. In 2001, provincial health expenditures (measured relative to
total provincial revenues) were the same as they were in 1991 and
slightly lower than they were throughout the early 1990s. (See Figure
9.4.) Relative to fiscal resources, there has been no increase in the fiscal
burden represented by provincial health-care expenditures. Changes
in the fiscal burden posed by them have been neither masked nor
exaggerated by changes in overall provincial own-source revenues as
a percentage of GDP, which remained constant through the 1990s. (See
Figure 9.5.) At the same time, the overall federal contribution to provincial total revenues has declined.[2]

Thus restraint in federal transfers has meant that an increasing proportion of the growth in provincial own-source revenues is going to
health care rather than to other provincial programs or to provincial def-

Figure 9.5
Federal transfers and provincial own-source revenues, 1991–2001

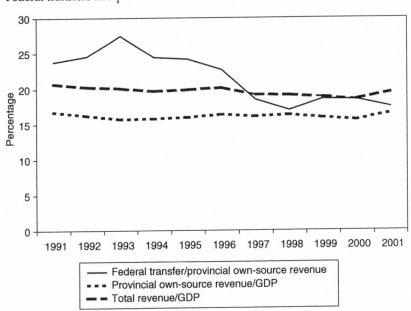

icit reduction/debt retirement. To this extent, health care is crowding out the provision of other public goods. Clearly, this is a serious problem from the provincial perspective. It says nothing, however, about the unsustainability of the overall fiscal burden of health care relative to the overall ability of Canadian governments to bear this burden.

Thus the overall picture that emerges is that restraint in federal transfers has meant that an increasing proportion of *the growth* in provincial own source revenues is going to health care rather than to other provincial programs or provincial deficit reduction/debt retirement. To this extent, health care is crowding out the provision of other public goods. In this sense, the fiscal sustainability of health care expenditures is a very real problem *from the provincial perspective*. It is *not*, however, indicative of the unsustainability of the overall fiscal burden of health care relative to the overall ability of Canadian governments to bear this burden.

Assessing Future Fiscal Sustainability

In the current circumstances, the sustainability of the overall fiscal bur-den of health care relative to the ability of government (as opposed to individual governments) to bear that burden is not in question. How-ever, in the longer term, fiscal sustainability becomes a serious issue under two scenarios: first, rapidly accelerating health costs or, second, the erosion of current provincial fiscal revenues or of the ability of pro-vincial governments to maintain current levels of taxation.

Growth in Spending

In the absence of cost acceleration, other cost factors such as age-ing will not increase the burden of the health system relative to the economy in the foreseeable future. The report of the Provincial and Territorial Ministers of Health (2000), *Understanding Health Care Costs*, presents a detailed forecast of health care costs to 2026–27. Including the effects of population growth, ageing, inflation, and a 1 per cent per year increase to reflect 'other' health-care service needs, the report con-cludes that 'the base scenario gives rise to health operating expendi-tures that remain fairly consistent as a share of GDP over the period' (31). The report does not outline the source of the GDP forecasts, although it notes that 'nominal GDP growth rates will moderate from 6.5 percent for 2000 to 4.8 percent for 2002, and more slowly thereafter to 4.0 percent in 2026' (31). (The average annual growth rate in GDP (expenditure-based at market prices) for the 1990s was 4.4 per cent.) Using conservative economic growth rates based on expectations of a long-term secular decline in GDP growth, and adding in a 1 per cent per year increase for expenditure growth on top of ageing, inflation, and population growth, give health-care costs that will not pose a greater burden over the next quarter-century than is the case today or was so a decade ago.

However, questions of fiscal sustainability emerge if costs accelerate above and beyond those caused by ageing, population growth, and modest cost increases in the services currently provided. There are compelling reasons to expect considerable future cost pressures – a topic outside the scope of this paper. The fact that current patterns of expenditure are not unsustainable does not mean that affordability poses no threat or that fiscal restraint is unnecessary. However, it raises different questions than the claim that current expenditure patterns

Figure 9.6
Provincial own-source revenues, as percentage of GDP and standard deviation
(as percentage of average), 1989–2001

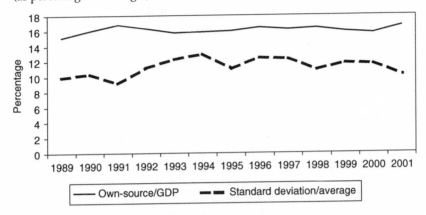

demonstrate the system's fiscal unsustainability. First, and most important, is unsustainable acceleration of costs inevitable? This question involves provincial willingness to attempt to control health-care costs in the face of powerful political pressures for expansion. Secondly, can governments control health-care costs even if they are determined to do so? If provinces are unable to control spending in the long term, the system will eventually become fiscally unsustainable – a serious concern vis-à-vis overall sustainability.

The Sustainability of Provincial Taxation Efforts
Alternatively, increasing health-care costs may become fiscally unsustainable if overall current provincial levels of taxation are unsustainable. Provincial own-source revenues as a percentage of GDP remained constant through the 1990s. (See Figure 9.6.) Evidence of an erosion of provincial capacity to maintain current levels of taxation has not yet emerged. There has not been any convergence among provinces in own-source revenue as a proportion of GDP, and therefore there is no evidence of a downward harmonization of fiscal efforts.

At the same time, downward pressure on provinces' taxation rates and on their ability to maintain fiscal efforts may build as a result of increasing global and continental economic integration.[3] Such pressures will be felt probably earlier and more acutely at the provincial than at the federal level. Provincial governments are arguably more sensitive to the competitive pressures generated by cross-border economic integration and competition. According to Courchene, provinces will increasingly tailor their public policies – including taxation – to the patterns prevailing in the U.S. states with which they are increasingly integrating and competing (Courchene and Telmer 1998, 289–91).

There is now a substantial body of literature that is sceptical of the general proposition that globalization is generating convergence in social policy or in taxation regimes across OECD countries. Few governments can escape the pressure to adjust their social-policy regimes to the new economic order, but differences in national politics still condition the way in which countries react, mediating the impact of economic pressures on the social contract. As a result, there is no reason to presume that social-policy or taxation regimes will converge on a single approach to the social needs of citizens. Banting (forthcoming) has pointed out that social spending as a proportion of GDP in OECD members continues to inch upwards and that there is no overall pattern of convergence in the proportion of national resources devoted to social programs. Olewiler's (1999) detailed analysis of taxation trends and Garrett's (1998) study of both taxation and public expenditures similarly find no evidence of significant OECD convergence. These themes recur in a variety of studies (Krugman 1996; Martin 1996; Esping-Andersen 1996; Swank 1998, 2001; Iversen 2001). Conclusions that emerge from considerations of policy in Canada and the United States echo findings elsewhere. There is also increasing scepticism regarding arguments (predominant early in the free-trade period) that Canada will ultimately be unable to maintain higher tax rates than to the United States. (Brown 2000; Kesselman 2001; Skogstad 2000).

These conclusions are nevertheless open to challenge. The 'lagged effect' argument contends that the full logic of economic integration is still unfolding and that a pervasive pattern of convergence between Canadian and U.S. policy systems is sure to emerge over time. There are two forms of this argument – economic and cultural. The economic version postulates a natural sequencing in adjustments to integration, with the first wave emerging in industrial structures and building pressure over time to narrow tax and expenditure differentials. The cultural version holds that economic integration will inevitably produce greater cultural integration, as media and other links steadily pull Canadian attitudes more firmly towards American norms. In this scenario, Canadians will start to bring more American values to their own politics, including an increasingly limited tolerance for differential taxation rates. This objection is impossible to counter fully, since evidence of continuing policy divergence can always be dismissed on the grounds that the anticipated lag is simply longer and that convergence remains just around the corner. However, downward pressure on provinces' overall revenue-generating ability is not yet evident.

Federal–Provincial Dynamics in Health Care

Even though provincial health expenditures relative to GDP are the same as they were in 1990, there is now a widespread perception of a fiscal crisis in public health care. This perception is rooted in the institutional underpinning of health care – especially in federal–provincial fiscal arrangements. While these arrangements appeared to work well enough in a period of expansion, in an era of more generalized restraint they began to create dynamics that undermined public support for the current system.

Both levels of government play a role in health care, although most of the jurisdictional responsibility lies with provincial governments. (For a general overview, see Maioni 2002.) Ottawa pays for part of provincial medicare, administers health protection (for example, regulates drugs), funds health care to Aboriginals on reserves, and shares health promotion and education with the provinces. The federal role in sharing the costs of provincially provided health services falls within the rubric of the Canada Health and Social Transfer (CHST) under terms governed by the Canada Health Act (CHA).

The CHA governs federal transfers to provinces for the provision of public insurance for hospital care and for physicians' services. There are five federally defined principles[4] comprising the core of the CHA, which is the legislative basis for the Canadian health-care system:

- *Public administration*. Each provincial plan must be run by a non-profit, public authority accountable to the provincial government.
- *Comprehensiveness*. Provinces must provide coverage for all necessary physician and hospital services.
- *Universality*. Insured services must be universally available to all residents of the province under uniform terms and conditions, with waiting periods for new entrants limited to a maximum of three months.
- *Portability*. Each provincial plan must be portable, so that eligible residents are covered while they are temporarily out of the province.
- *Accessibility*. Reasonable access to insured services is not to be

impaired by financial or other barriers, and reasonable compensation must be made to physicians for providing insured services.

The CHA mandates dollar-for-dollar reductions of federal transfers for funds collected by a province through user fees and extra billing. In contrast, application of penalties for violation of the five federally defined principles is discretionary, and no province has ever been penalized for violation of any of them, even though a number of provinces have been and continue to be in clear violation of various principles.[5]

Given this division of responsibility, the dynamics of federal–provincial relations in regard to health are relatively straightforward. Ottawa strives to minimize its fiscal commitment while ensuring its visibility in health and its ability to claim credit for enforcing the CHA. Provincial governments seek to maximize federal fiscal commitments while preserving room to manoeuvre vis-à-vis constraints imposed directly or indirectly through public pressure as a result of the CHA.

The significance of federal–provincial fiscal arrangements did not become fully evident so long as federal transfers were expanding. Pressures began to build as growth in Established Programs Financing (EPF) transfers was restricted (indexed to GNP growth minus 2 per cent in 1986, which was changed to GNP growth minus 3 per cent in 1989) and frozen in the early 1990s. However, the shift from EPF to the CHST in 1996 signalled the full extent of federal withdrawal from financial commitments to public health care. The shift saw transfers drop by $2.5 billion in 1996–97 and by $4.5 billion in 1997–98. Ottawa pushed the 'restraint envelope' to the point that the CHA principles appeared to be imperiled, and many observers wondered how those principles could be enforced against a recalcitrant provincial government, as the cash component of the CHST was programmed to phase out of existence. Federal implementation of a floor on the cash component of the CHST transfers was an attempt to balance between minimizing fiscal contributions and maintaining federal ability to claim credit for the politically popular aspects of medicare.

There are three crucial effects generated out of this situation. The first is the illusion of health care as a rapidly growing fiscal burden relative to the ability of government to bear this burden, which contributes to concerns regarding its sustainability. Public expenditures on health care do not constitute a higher proportion of GDP than they did a decade ago. Yet, as a result of federal transfer restraints, provincial governments now make a compelling case that public health care as it currently exists is no longer affordable. This argument appears compelling and, from the provincial perspective, is real, regardless of whether or not federal–provincial fiscal arrangements are to blame.

Second, in part as a result of its transfer retrenchment, Ottawa's overall fiscal position is disproportionately brighter than the provinces'. A situation with surpluses at the federal level (which has limited direct involvement in the delivery of health care) and deficits or near-deficits at the provincial level (whose most important single program responsibility is for health care) contributes to the political construction of a strong link between health care and the issues of balanced budgets and reducing debts and deficits. The goals of providing public health care and reducing debt/deficits appear in sharp political competition as a result of the fiscal imbalance, exacerbated by fiscal arrangements for funding health care.

Finally, these fiscal arrangements have generated perverse incentives for provincial governments. The provincial strategy in reaction to reduced federal transfers was to generate public pressure on Ottawa to increase the cash component of transfers. As a result, provinces face limited incentives to combat forcefully public perceptions regarding the declining quality of health care and sensationalist media coverage, which strongly reinforces such perceptions. Provinces have incentives to leverage their demands for greater federal funding by allowing such perceptions to flourish – if not actually encouraging them – so long as they can shift some of the blame to the federal government. Provinces also have a similar incentive to focus disproportionately on the funding of health care and to emphasize the perception that lack of financial resources is a crucial problem. Finally, as part of their blame-shifting strategy, provinces have an incentive to claim that the CHA is a straitjacket that does not allow for serious innovation to health care and limits their ability to respond to the problems themselves. Not surprisingly, a national newspaper recently called for the CHA 'to be scrapped, given the intolerable "constraints" it imposes on provinces' freedom to innovate' (Coyne 2002).

The line of argument that provincial governments have developed in response to in-built incentives has culminated – predictably – in provincial claims that the current system is unsustainable. In concluding a meeting of premiers in Victoria, Premier Gordon Campbell of British Columbia noted: 'We all agree as premiers that health care under the current situation is not sustainable' (*Globe and Mail*, 25 Jan. 2002). The *National Post* reported comments by Don Mazankowski: 'Public health

care in Canada will soon collapse unless bold reforms are introduced'
(Kennedy 2002). These responses simply represent the provincial cal-
culation of a rational response to the incentives structured into current
fiscal arrangements.

These various effects combine to form a vicious circle. Federal shifting of part of its debt burden to the provinces through transfer restraint
has created incentives for provinces to emphasize the failings of the
public health-care system in Canada. At the same time, the shift has
encouraged linking of debt and deficits to health care, thereby exacerbating the image of the fiscal unsustainability of the system. To the
degree that the federal fiscal situation is now relatively brighter than
that of the provinces, provinces face increased incentives to attempt to
extract larger transfers through the kinds of strategies outlined above.
The more that Ottawa now responds by enriching transfers, the more
successful the strategy appears to the provinces.

The Effects on Public Opinion

Public perceptions regarding health care that otherwise might seem
puzzling become more explicable in the light of the political dynamic
emerging out of federal–provincial fiscal arrangements operating in a
period of fiscal restraint. While there are very good reasons to be highly
sceptical regarding the reliability and interpretation of public-opinion
polling on public policy, this section examines three relatively stable
and well-documented trends in public opinion that appear likely to be
related to federal–provincial jockeying over health-care funding.

*1. A belief that the system is in crisis and that the quality of health care is
declining, despite personal experiences to the contrary.* The increase in the
perception among Canadians that health care is the highest priority
facing the country is nothing short of astounding. During the 1990s,
health care shifted from being a non-issue to being far and away the
highest priority among Canadians. (For an overview, see Vail 2001,
1–2.) While interest in other, more perennial issues such as the economy has waxed and waned, health care emerged out of nowhere to
become in less than five years the top issue of concern. It has become
such an important issue partly because of growing perceptions that the
system is in crisis – a belief now held by nearly four out of five survey
respondents (Vail 2001, 1).

This increase in the salience of health care is related to public perceptions of declining quality of health care provision in Canada. The erosion of public confidence did not take place gradually; rather, it emerged in the early 1990s and accelerated significantly in the mid-1990s (Vail 2001, 8). The predominance of the popular perception of decline has remained stable since 1997, even though provinces have begun to reinvest in health care. When asked if Canadians generally are receiving quality care, the proportion of respondents agreeing dropped from 67 per cent in 1999 to 49 per cent in 2001 (Health Care in Canada 2001, 6). This is a staggering decline in positive perceptions in such a short period.

These stark trends require explanation. The most obvious would be that the system *is* in crisis. To the degree that what Canadians know about health care stems primarily from their contact with it – which has been overwhelmingly positive – the image of crisis must lie elsewhere. There is little evidence of decline in positive personal experiences, and individual perceptions are strikingly favourable. For example, respondents who experience a hospital stay or have a family member who has done so reported an 80 per cent satisfaction rate, and those visiting an emergency room had a 70 per cent satisfaction rate (Vail 2001, 17). Similarly, Canadians are much more sanguine about the system's ability to meet their own personal health needs and those of their families than about its ability to meet the needs of the population as a whole. Vail speculates that the consistent discrepancy between levels of confidence in health care at the system level and those at the individual level may reflect a problem of communication (2001, 17). However, this discrepancy is more plausibly explained by media reporting of many stories depicting the stresses and strains in the system. While these problems are certainly not imaginary, they are not representative of the norm and are exaggerated by virtue of being generalized. As we saw above, key to this process is apparent provincial willingness to allow and sometimes even encourage such perceptions. This behaviour is perhaps a reaction to built-in incentives rather than simply a failure to communicate effectively.

2. A belief that there is now a major funding crisis and that the system needs more resources. There is a widespread belief either that the system is currently short of funds or that such a crisis is imminent. These public perceptions are not surprising given ongoing provincial efforts to demonstrate the existence of such a crisis. No wonder four out of five Canadians believe that too little is being spent on health care. Certainly, while most citizens do not maintain that funding alone is the answer, most are also sceptical about improvements without increased funding: the 'conviction that the system needs more resources is an increasingly held view' (Compas Inc. 2001, 13). While Canadians may not be convinced that simply adding more money is the complete answer, they do not suppose that the system can be 'fixed' without the addition of resources and 'are more and more resistant to the idea that the system can be improved without more money. They no longer believe that there remain more efficiencies to be extracted from the system' (Compas Inc. 2001, 13). Nor is it surprising that a majority prefer to deal with rising costs by increased spending rather than by allowing private services or limiting services. Thus 'increasing public funding was Canadians' preferred option for relieving pressure on the health-care system' (Vail 2001, 21).

3. *A striking decline in public approval ratings for how both federal and provincial governments are handling health care and a belief that governments are losing ground in solving the problems facing it.* Public satisfaction with both federal and provincial handling of health care reached a peak in the early 1990s. After 1992, public approval ratings for both governments began a precipitous and long-term decline that has not recovered much beyond the lowest points of the late 1990s. Again, as with many of the trends described here, the picture is not one of slow and steady erosion of support, but rather of sudden and rapid decline. This trend is hardly a surprise, considering general perceptions of a system in crisis and declining quality of health care. It seems likely that it has been exacerbated by intergovernmental strategies in which both levels, in an effort to avoid accepting public blame for problems, attempt to shift blame.

Conclusion: Political Sustainability?

The sustainability of the health-care system has been increasingly portrayed as primarily a fiscal issue arising from the inherent tension between public demands for lower taxes, debt reduction, and balanced budgets and for accessible, high-quality, and primarily publicly funded health care. Sustainability needs also to be considered from a political vantage point. As we saw above, there is no *immediate* threat to the fiscal sustainability of the system – the threat lies in potential patterns of future cost acceleration. However, the conflation in public debates of the notions of existing and potential fiscal crisis points to serious problems in the political sustainability of health care. Political sustainability requires ensuring the system's ongoing ability to maintain sufficient popular and elite support to guarantee that there are incentives for governments to fund and provide public health-care services. Fiscal sustainability is a moot issue if the system is politically unsustainable, and vice versa. Reforms that address only one of these components are likely to founder.

Political sustainability will be no easier to address than fiscal sustainability. The most simplistic solution is to suggest that Ottawa and the provinces simply 'get their act together and fix health care.' Certainly, the public is unlikely to disagree with this motherhood prescription. While the failure of both orders of government to collaborate effectively has fuelled public cynicism, to suggest that they simply work together without rethinking the incentives that they each face under current institutional arrangements will merely raise public expectations without increasing the likelihood that governments will deliver. It is a prescription that entails greater risk than promise.

In the absence of appropriate institutional change, a continuing and not easily reversible decline in public perceptions of both the quality and the sustainability of public health care in Canada seems likely. It is there that the real potential for crisis lies.

NOTES

1 All data on provincial health expenditures come from Canadian Institute for Health Information 2001b. All other data (provincial revenues, total federal transfers, and so on) come from CANSIM II.
2 All major federal transfers to the provinces (equalization, CHST) go directly into consolidated revenue, so to identify particular transfers for health (as is often attempted) is simply not relevant to the overall fiscal sustainability of provincial health-care expenditures. At the same time, the issue of federal contributions to health is extremely important vis-à-vis the legitimacy of the conditional nature of specific transfers.
3 The following four paragraphs draw from Gerard W. Boychuk and Keith G. Banting (forthcoming).
4 Drawn from Robert Chernomas and Ardeshir Sepheri, eds., 1998.
5 Colleen Flood, presentation to Ontario Health Coalition public forum 'Does Medicare Work?' Toronto, 3 April 2002.

REFERENCES

Adams, Duane. 2001a. 'Canadian Federalism and the Development of National Health Goals and Objectives.' In Duane Adams, ed., *Federalism, Democracy and Health Policy in Canada*. Montreal: McGill-Queen's University Press, 61–106.
– 2001b. 'Social Union Study of the Canadian Health System: Introduction and Overview.' In Duane Adams, ed., *Federalism, Democracy and Health Policy in Canada*. Montreal: McGill-Queen's University Press, 1–26.
Alberta. Premier's Advisory Council on Health for Albertans. 2001. *A Framework for Reform: A Report of the Premier's Advisory Council on Health for Albertans*. Edmonton, Dec.
Banting, Keith G. Forthcoming. 'What's a Country For? The Social Contract in the Global Era.' In R. Roberge and D. Wolfish, eds., *Reinstating the Line: The Canada–US Border*. Ottawa: University of Ottawa Press.
Boychuk, Gerard W., and Keith G. Banting. Forthcoming. 'The Paradox of Convergence: National versus Sub-National Patterns of Convergence in Canadian and American Income Maintenance Policy.' In Richard G. Harris, ed., *North American Linkages: Opportunities and Challenges for Canada*. Calgary: University of Calgary Press.
Brown, Robert D. 2000. 'The Impact of the US on Canada's Tax Strategy.' *ISUMA* 1, no. 1 (spring): 71–8.
Canadian Institute for Health Information (CIHI). 2000. *Health Care in Canada 2000: A First Annual Report*. Ottawa: CIHI.
– 2001a. *Health Care in Canada 2001*. Ottawa: CIHI.
– 2001b. *National Health Expenditure Trends, 1975–2001*. Ottawa: CIHI.
Chernomas, Robert, and Ardeshir Sepheri, eds. 1998. *How to Choose? A Comparison of the US and Canadian Health Care Systems*. Amityville, NY: Baywood.
Compas Inc. 2001. *Muddled Mandate: Ambivalence, Conflict, Frustration and Other Plaints of Public Opinion on Health Care Policy*. Toronto: Compas, Dec.
Courchene, Thomas, with Colin Telmer. 1998. *From Heartland to North American Region State*. Toronto: Centre for Public Management, Faculty of Management, University of Toronto.
Coyne, Andrew. 2002. 'Maz Proves Medicare Can Be Reformed.' *National Post* (on-line edition), 11 Jan.
Esping-Andersen, Gosta, ed. 1996. *Welfare States in Transition: National Adaptations in Global Economies*. London: Sage.
Fierlbeck, Katherine. 2001. 'Cost Containment in Health Care: The Federalism Context.' In Duane Adams, ed., *Federalism, Democracy and Health Policy in Canada*. Montreal: McGill-Queen's University Press, 131–78.
Garrett, Geoffrey. 1998. 'Global Markets and National Politics: Collision Course or Virtuous Circle?' *International Organization*. 52: 787–824.

Health Care in Canada. 2001. *Health Care in Canada Survey 2001: A National Survey of Health Care Providers, Managers and the Public*. http://mediresource.sympatico.ca/images/hcics/hcic.pdf

Iversen, Thorben. 2001. 'The Dynamics of Welfare State Expansion: Trade Openness, De-industrialization, and Partisan Politics.' In Paul Pierson, ed., *The Politics of the Welfare State*. Oxford: Oxford University Press, 45–79.

Kennedy, Mark. 2002. 'Health Care Report Sets Stage for Showdown: "System Is Not Sustainable."' *National Post*, 5 Jan.

Kesselman, Jonathan R. 2001. 'Policies to Stem the Brain Drain – without Americanizing Canada.' *Canadian Public Policy* 27, no. 1 (March): 77–93.

Krugman, Paul. 1996. *Pop Internationalism*. Cambridge, Mass.: MIT Press.

Maoini, Antonia. 2002. 'Federalism and Health Care in Canada.' In Keith G. Banting and Stan Corbett, eds., *Health Policy and Federalism: A Comparative Perspective on Multi-Level Governance*. Montreal: McGill-Queen's University Press, 173–99.

Martin, Andrew. 1996. 'What Does Globalization Have to Do with the Erosion of the Welfare State? Sorting Out the Ideas.' ARENA Working Paper, No. 17.

Olewiler, Nancy. 1999. 'National Tax Policy for an International Economy: Divergence in a Converging Word.' In Thomas Courchene, ed., *Room for Manoeuvre? Globalization and Policy Convergence*. Kingston: John Deutsch Institute for the Study of Economic Policy, Queen's University.

O'Reilly, Patricia. 2001. 'The Canadian Health System Landscape.' In Duane Adams, ed., *Federalism, Democracy and Health Policy in Canada*. Montreal: McGill-Queen's University Press, 17–60.

Provincial and Territorial Ministers of Health. 2000. *Understanding Canada's Health Care Costs: Final Report*. www.gov.on.ca/health/english/pub/ministry/ptcd/ptcd_doc_e.pdf

Skogstad, Grace. 2000. 'Globalization and Public Policy: Situating Canadian Analyses.' *Canadian Journal of Political Science* 33, no. 4: 805–28.

Swank, Duane. 1998. 'Funding the Welfare State: Globalization and the Taxation of Business in Advanced Market Economies.' *Political Studies* 46, no. 4: 671–92.

– 2001. 'Political Institutions and Welfare State Restructuring: The Impact of Institutions on Social Policy Change in Developed Democracies.' In Paul Pierson, ed., *The New Politics of the Welfare State*. Oxford: Oxford University Press, 197–237.

Vail, Stephen. 2001. *Canadians' Values and Attitudes on Canada's Health Care System: A Synthesis of Survey Results*. Ottawa: Conference Board of Canada, Jan.

10 Paying to Play?
Government Financing and
Health Care Agenda Setting

KATHERINE FIERLBECK

> If health care itself is not – yet – in deep trouble, its governance is. The mechanism of government partnership and collaboration – that of federal-provincial – has become totally dysfunctional.
>
> – Hon. Monique Bégin (2002)

Two overarching questions inform the relationship between governments regarding health care. First, what kind of change is desirable? Second, how is it possible politically to achieve such change? The objective of Canadian public health care is of course the health of the Canadian public: yet patients are also taxpayers and citizens and as such often have contradictory expectations. Thus to say simply that government must be responsive to the voice of the people is not particularly useful, for democracy is a cacophony. The question of *whose* voices register is the very heart of democratic politics and may not provide a clear basis for public policy.

Moreover, any change in the relationship must be limited. First, any change must conform to the Canadian constitution. Second, political convention as well as constitutional requirement must be acknowledged. Third, any discussion of health care must take into account financial constraints and economic efficiency: given governments' emphasis on cost containment and 'sound fiscal management,' any potential solutions must be 'affordable.' And, finally, the proper distribution of roles also depends on governments' willingness to embrace change. In health care, particularly, autonomous political jurisdictions do exist (both de facto and de jure), and the motivation for change must ultimately come from within each unit.

This paper holds that change in federal–provincial relations regarding health care is necessary, that it is timely, and that each level of government can be persuaded to make these changes. It also argues for a balance between federal involvement and provincial autonomy. Change is necessary because of the current cost of health care, because of the complexity of maintaining a modern health care 'system,' and because of the awareness and expectations of the very people to whom it is directed. This paper argues that there exists a 'window of opportunity' to improve intergovernmental relations in health. The challenge is to harness the flexibility and innovation possible in a federal system without succumbing to beggar-thy-neighbour dynamics. Neither 'greater federal involvement' nor 'more provincial autonomy' is a helpful way of rethinking roles. Rather, Ottawa ought explicitly to accept the provinces as equal partners in health care and enter into binding regulations regarding long-term funding and administration. The provinces should explicitly accept some formal and consistent federal presence in health care. In this way, they can achieve stability and predictability in funding, dispute resolution, and federal accountability, while Ottawa can better achieve adherence to the principles of the Canada Health Act as well as provincial accountability.

The first section of the paper discusses the constitutional division of powers constraining intergovernmental relations in health care and then explains how federal spending in the field has evolved since the establishment of medicare from about 1966 to 1972. The second section discusses how to achieve both predictability and accountability within a highly politicized intergovernmental context. The third section considers what role, if any, regional or municipal governments ought to play.

Federal Spending in Health Care: Fiscal Powers and History

Three distinct types of constitutional powers in Canada together form the fiscal relationship that determines and circumscribes public policy: these are regulatory, expenditure, and taxation powers. In health care, the Constitution Act, 1867, clearly gives the provinces regulatory power over hospitals (section 92.7) and 'local and private matters' (92.16). However, the federal expenditure power (the 'spending power') refers specifically to 'the power of Parliament to make payments to people, institutions, or provincial governments for purposes on which Parliament does not necessarily have the power to legislate, for example, in areas of exclusive provincial legislative jurisdiction' (Watts 1999, 1). Although this spending power is not explicitly articulated in the Constitution Act, 1867, the courts have interpreted other sections of the constitution to mean that the federal government may spend in any area as long as it does not amount to a 'regulatory scheme' within an area of normal provincial jurisdiction. That the spending power is not in the constitution is an important factor in negotiations over delegation of roles in health care.

Third, both senior levels of government enjoy the power of taxation. As Watts (1999) and Brown (2002) have pointed out, Canada is quite distinct among federal states in the provinces' wide-ranging ability to garner money for expenditure within their own jurisdictions. This gives provinces much greater independence from the federal government, even though, somewhat paradoxically, both levels of government must work more closely together to harmonize their systems of taxation. The present arrangement allows both for greater decentralization (the increased capacity for provinces to raise taxes) *and* for greater centralization (the de facto recognition, and sustained exercise, of the federal spending power, as well as the federal commitment to minimize regional disparity). Ottawa also enjoys indirect and/or obscure pieces of legislation (such as the 'Peace, Order and Good Government' provision) that it can in principle invoke, but they cannot ground new and overarching health-care provisions (as opposed to very specific legislation in very specific areas).

How important is the federal spending power? And can it help restructure health care? Evaluations vary, although the answer seems to depend largely on the economic and political realities of the day. Some commentations, such as Muszynski, argue that the spending power has become 'significantly eroded as a result of economic conditions, the deficit and debt, and the emergence of more conservative attitudes toward social policy' (Muszynski 1995, 289). Yet others have the same conditions as conducive to federal control, given the wider federal fiscal powers; as Campbell writes, 'If a neo-conservative orientation to economic policy persists – with market goals, inflation control, and deficit spending in the forefront – then the federal government will remain in the economic management driver's seat' (1995, 209). Ottawa's direct influence on the structure of national health care depends primarily on two factors: how much money it has to spend and any specific limitations to this power negotiated by provincial and federal governments (as in, for example, the ill-fated Meech Lake Accord and the Charlottetown Agreement, and in the current Social Union Accord). I discussed this matter in greater detail below.

The evolution of federal spending in health care falls roughly into five periods, each launched by major federal legislation: the Hospital Insurance and Diagnostic Services Act, 1957 (HIDSA); Established Programs Financing, 1977 (EPF); the Canada Health Act, 1984 (CHA); the Canada Health and Social Transfer, 1996 (CHST); and the Social Union Framework Accord, 1999 (SUFA). With each piece of legislation, the focus oscillates from the nature of health care itself (HIDSA, CHA, and SUFA) to cost containment (EPF and CHST).

The initial period of conditional, shared-cost grants gave way in 1977 to a model of block grants distributed to province on an equal per-capita basis (EPF). Funding increases according to this formula were based no longer on provincial expenditure, but on the growth rate of the gross national product (GNP). This measure not only decreased federal costs but also allowed Ottawa to remove itself from a situation where its own spending was determined by the provinces' policy decisions. But the EPF ultimately created even more friction between governments (Maslove 1992, 59). Moreover, its lack of any mechanism obliging provinces to spend in specific areas was exacerbated by social and economic circumstances, and, largely at the instigation of the New Democratic Party (NDP), Ottawa was increasingly pushed from 1979 on to address the 'erosion of Medicare' (Bégin 2002, 2). In 1984 it tabled Bill C-3 (later the Canada Health Act) to eliminate (or at least discourage) extra-billing by physicians and user fees by penalizing provinces dollar for dollar for the levying of such fees. Provincial adherence was voluntary, but full federal funding was conditional on provinces' observing these principles. By 1987, the practice of extra-billing and the imposition of user fees had largely ceased.

Yet EPF was still highly problematic. Provinces objected that the federal government was not pulling its share of the load, while Ottawa recognized keenly that its transfer of tax points meant increased provincial revenues and a decreased residual federal cash transfer: no longer paying the piper, it was unable to call the tune. Moreover, it was dissatisfied with the minimal visibility it received for the monies that it expended, while the provinces resented the fact that Ottawa's spending power undermined the long-term stability and predictability of funding for health and post-secondary education, two of the most expensive provincial programs (Bégin 2002, 61).

Ottawa replaced EPF unilaterally, and without intergovernmental consultation, with the CHST in April 1995. Conceived by the Department of Finance, the CHST was generally acknowledged as a strategy to reduce federal expenditures and deficits. But while it achieved its primary objective – alleviating fiscal pressure on Ottawa – it failed to address the substantive problem evident in the EPF: it did not give the federal government enough financial clout to compel compliance to the principles of the CHA.

The final period of evolution began in February 1999, with partial ratification of the Social Union Framework Agreement. Specifically, the SUFA required Ottawa to consult with the provinces regarding any changes to conditional block grants or shared-cost programs and to build 'due notice' into any new social transfers, to permit a form of 'opting out' of national jointly funded initiatives with the support of a majority of provinces, and to give at least three months' notice to (and to offer to consult with) the provinces regarding direct transfers. It also calls for mechanisms to ensure broad public access and public consultation, establishes support for the existing principles of medicare, addresses the need for joint fact-finding, and articulates the need for dispute-avoidance and -resolution mechanisms.

Evaluation of the SUFA is mixed. Maioni, for example, argues that the SUFA 'has done little to encourage a focus on the real political debate over two unresolved but crucial issues on the health agenda: Who should make the rules in health care? And what should the rules look like?'(2000, 39). Lazar, however, is more cautiously optimistic: if the political will exists to work within the agreement, he writes, 'the Framework Agreement could turn out to be a major innovation in the workings of the federation, heralding a new era of collaboration, mutual respect among the orders of government and a more coherent and systematic approach to policy-making' (2000a,100).

While we can plot the trajectory of federal–provincial funding with relative ease, the roles that governments have played (or been expected to play) have lacked that sort of clarity. If clarity is determined by Occam's razor, then the period represented by the HIDSA (1957) and the Medicare Care Insurance Act (1966) is overwhelmingly clear in its simplicity. The federal government would cover half the costs of provincial medical insurance plans, as long as the provinces adhered to the conditions of comprehensibility, universality, portability, and public administration (accessibility was added in 1984). However, the political nature of health care became emphasized over time: not only did the actual costs of its provision increase, but the field became – especially for Ottawa – a form of political capital, in which federal financial support for medicare was a form of political leverage over provincial governments. This tendency confronted the fiscal trend experienced by the provinces, which were by 2000 devoting at least one-third of their total expenditures to health care (Ontario, for example, spent almost 40 per cent of its total expenditure in 1999 on health: see CIHI 1999, Table B.4.4). As the political stakes rose, both levels of government wanted more from their respective roles (viz., maximizing their influence and minimizing their costs). Thus, increasingly detailed documents (CHA and SUFA) have attempted to explicate the roles of each: if clarity refers to the amount of detail rather than to the level of simplicity, the current regime best exemplifies the rights and obligations of each government.

Have changes in the federal role over the past thirty years been consistent with changes in cost-sharing and other fiscal arrangements? On the surface, no: the current federal funding levels of 14–16 per cent contrasts quite dramatically with the 50 per cent that it gave to the provinces for the major health-care services (doctors and hospitals) when the system of national health care was established. And yet over the past two decades Ottawa has become more, not less, concerned with its role in maintaining the principles of the CHA. The EPF was largely responsible for this imbalance, for it not only cut federal funding levels to the provinces, but also transferred tax points to them. In retrospect, writes Monique Bégin, the EPF was in a sense 'a mistake, maybe an unavoidable one in that decade of provincial autonomy.' But, she adds, 'tax points transfers are a taxation capacity lost forever and they carry no enforcement power whatsoever. So let us stop talking of them' (Bégin 2002, 5). The EPF was enacted well before Ottawa realized the (long-forgotten) political capital to be found as protector of a national medicare system. But this imbalance has forced the federal government to hone its influence more precisely and surgically, rather than depending on its broad economic clout. And there is certainly more room for this approach (see below).

Ottawa now recognizes both that there is a great deal of public support for its position as protector of medicare (no party in the last federal election argued for eliminating the CHA) and that enforcing adherence to the CHA cannot rest purely on an economic approach. The current strategy is therefore one of legislative horse trading, with Ottawa somewhat willing to blunt the force of its federal spending power in exchange for achieving specific policy objectives (such as agreement on the CHA). While changes in the federal role since the early 1970s have not been at all consistent with shifts in cost sharing, today's more sophisticated and nuanced approaches depend less on economic influence and more on a strategic political give and take. This I discuss more fully below.

One of the best accounts of Ottawa's various roles in setting health-care policy appears in the interim report of the fourth volume of the Standing Senate Committee on Social Affairs, Science, and Technology (2001), known also as the Kirby Report. The report lists (chapter 3) five distinct federal roles in health and health care:

1 *financing*, which covers the transfer of funds for the provision of health services administered by the provinces and territories
2 *research and evaluation*, which includes funding innovative health research and evaluating innovative pilot projects
3 *infrastructure*, which addresses support for the health-care infrastructure and the health infostructure, including human resources
4 *population health*, which focuses on protecting health, promoting health and wellness, preventing illness, and improving population health
5 *service delivery*, which targets the direct provision of health services to specific population groups

Though not addressed by the report, the provincial roles in health and health care can fit into the same groupings, though with scope and nature differing among provinces and often quite distinct from the federal role. The report's breakdown of roles can remind us that direct funding to the provinces (and territories) is not the only federal role. Ottawa's influence is indeed limited by the amount of funding that it directs to health care per se; there is, however, some room regarding the precise allocation of these funds.

Suggestions for Change: Seeking Predictability and Accountability

To figure out what health-system objectives might be served by changes in the roles of the senior governments, one must first determine which objectives ought to be promoted. The mandate of the Commission of the Future of Health Care in Canada perhaps best reflects the dominant opinion in Canada: to 'ensure over the long term the sustainability of a universally accessible, publicly funded health system, that offers quality services to Canadians and strikes an appropriate balance between investments in prevention and health maintenance and those directed to care and treatment.'

There are two ways of achieving this goal from an intergovernmental perspective. First, greater stability and predictability are crucial for this system of national standards noted above. A number of the current problems result not from the specific organization of health policies as much as from the federal political context in which they occur. If a greater sense of common purpose and trust emerged between governments, it is likely that the first set of objectives could be more readily achieved. But these conditions will not arise simply through sustained exhortation: they require institutional changes. Second, promoting and protecting such a system are possible only through the development of substantial and evident accountability between governments (as well as within the system). Not only are accountability and transparency manifestly democratic qualities, but they help achieve a sense of common purpose – it is easier to trust other parties when their actions are transparent and predictable.

How then to achieve such objectives? Intergovernmental roles are characterized by institutional divisions of power. Simple governmental fiat cannot solve problems; it has in fact been the cause of much recent intergovernmental dispute. Compromise and trade-offs are essential; any attempt to move forward may dissatisfy all parties. 'If workable solutions in policy terms create untenable intergovernmental tensions that spill over into other relationships or clearly violate the constitutional division of power or marginalize the oversight roles of legislators and citizens, then the very ability of social policy to weave and

strengthen the ties that bind Canadians to each other is compromised'
(Adams 2001b, 6).

Towards Predictability

The most important component of a stable and predictable working
relationship between governments, either nationally or internationally,
is a set of clear procedural rules (as well as understood consequence
for failure to comply). The SUFA is a major step in this direction
because of its emphasis on procedure. Trust is essential to reaching a
co-operative system of administration: as Lazar comments, 'with trust,
SUFA will survive the periodic hurricanes that come from changing
government, prickly personalities and external shocks. Without trust,
SUFA will be a footnote in Canadian history' (2000b, 12). This change
in the governance of health care must come cautiously and consensu-
ally. Thus is a difficult strategy for people who want comprehensive
solutions and feel that political give-and-take simply produces
watered-down compromise. However, as Adams (2001a) reminds us,
in intergovernmental relations compromise is essential, and, as Kennett (1998) and others have argued, autonomous policy making in
health policy is inefficient and possibly obsolete.

Thus, regardless of the temptations to seek wholesale change, the
best-considered strategy here is one of evolutionary change, of delicate
surgery rather than of wielding blunt instruments. If improvements
require long-term consensus and stability, horse trading trumps political muscle. The federal government has been generally quite unwilling
to commit itself in this way, because such undertakings limit its flexibility in policy making writ large. But governments do engage in such
agreements internationally, hoping for greater gains despite constraints on flexibility (notably, recent agreements limiting state sover-
eignty in the European Union); and the same seems true for intergovernmental agreements. Given its desire to maintain some say over a set
of national standards in health care, and given its unwillingness simply to use its pocketbook extensively for this purpose, Ottawa must
accept some constraints on its flexibility to achieve these ends.

In general terms, the quid pro quo is this: Ottawa explicitly accepts
provincial governments as equal partners by entering binding procedural rules for the long-term administration and funding of health
care. It gives up some flexibility but wins greater recognition for its
spending power, and, importantly, it can maintain some control over

national standards while spending less on health than provincial governments do (and far less, proportionately, than it once did). The provinces accept some (lasting) federal presence in health care but achieve stability and predictability in funding, dispute resolution, and, not least, clearer limits on federal actions.

The SUFA is an appropriate blueprint. 'It contemplates both orders of government agreeing on Canada-wide objectives, the federal government transferring some funds to the provinces to assist them in pursuing the objectives, provinces then designing and delivering their own programs to achieve the objectives and public accountability for the results' (Lazar 2000a, 122). SUFA secured for the provinces federal agreement to consult with them on 'significant changes in existing social transfers' and to 'build due notice provisions into any new social transfers'; to offer provinces a de facto opting-out provision; and to promise due notice and consultation regarding new direct federal spending. These measures were in large part due to Ottawa's unilateral drive to put its own financial house in order throughout the 1990s, which led in turn to resentment by the provincial and territorial governments, which bore the brunt of this federal housekeeping. As Maslove points out, the level of federal–provincial fiscal harmonization that actually exists is quite impressive: none the less, 'the consequence of one government's being forced to react to major revenue (or expenditure) shocks resulting from the unilateral decisions of another causes strains to the fiscal system' (1996, 296).

The primary component of stability is the predictability built into federal CHST funding under section 5 of SUFA, which again calls for federal–provincial consultation on 'significant changes in existing social transfers' and 'due provision' regarding any new social transfers. And, while this stipulation does not prevent drastic federal spending changes (such as the CHST), the provinces' ability to plan for the consequences of such programs well in advance increases policy coherence and improves intergovernmental relations. To the extent that health care is experiencing a sea change from an emphasis on acute care to a focus on health promotion and disease prevention, and from isolated 'stovepipe' programs to greater consolidation between programs, provinces are reconfiguring their own systems to serve better a modern population. Predictability of funding is essential to this reconfiguration. The essential starting-point is simply to maintain consultation and due process, as articulated in section 5 of the SUFA.

The next steps are more provocative. These are, first, an acceptable 'opting-out' formula regarding both transfer and direct funding programs and, second, formalized federal spending power. SUFA came into being through concerted provincial negotiations in response to implementation of the CHST. These negotiations, eventually joined by Quebec, proposed a formal opting-out provision that was later dropped when Ottawa agreed to adjust its position on issues including public accountability and dispute settlement in return for the provinces' modifying their position on the federal spending power. Quebec then refused to sign the accord (Lazar 2000a, 110).

The discussion of an opting-out option is not new. Such a measure was established in 1964 for the administration of a separate pension plan for Quebec and has since been raised with reference to constitutional change. The Meech Lake Accord, for example, would have allowed the federal government 'to provide reasonable compensation to the government of a province that chooses not to participate in a national shared-cost program that is established by the Government of Canada after the coming into force of this section in an area of exclusive provincial jurisdiction, *if the province carries on a program or initiative that is compatible with the national objectives.*' The SUFA is similar, permitting Ottawa to establish new initiatives with the support of any six provinces, and stipulates that any dissenting province could then receive federal compensation for its own program as long as it meets the agreed objectives of the national program. However, as Lazar points out, SUFA goes further in accommodating provinces: first, by permitting those that do 'not require the total transfer to fulfill the agreed objectives' to 'reinvest any funds not required for those objectives in the same or a related priority area'; and, second, by applying this formula not only to shared-cost programs but also to jointly financed programs that are not based on cost sharing (Lazar 2000a, 111). In Lazar's view, SUFA is at least as flexible for the provinces as the provisions of the Charlottetown and Meech Lake accords, although its stipulations are implicit rather than explicit (2000b, 10).

This point speaks to the wider problem of Quebec's position within the federation and relates not only to health policy but to federalism more generally. But even if the opting-out provision were accepted with an eye to satisfying Quebec, it is arguable whether this would pose a threat to the national standards of Canadian health care; for example, Quebec's more idiosyncratic policies in health care have actually been more innovative and up-to-date – including community health-care centres, early-childhood centres, and public provision of long-term care – than those in much of Canada (Vaillancourt 2002).

Most commentators agree that any federal–provincial arrangement on health policy cannot function well without the participation of Quebec. Some critics hold that the SUFA's failure to secure Quebec's signature 'confirmed and further deepened the Canada–Quebec impasse' and also demonstrates the 'significant bias' against Quebec 'and its particular concerns' (Dufour 2002, 8, 9). During the annual Premiers' Conference in 1998 in Saskatoon, observes Alain Noël, Quebec compromised on three conditions: 'It left aside unsolved constitutional difficulties to join a bargaining process that did not make the opting-out formula unconditional; it accepted much of the inter-provincial – and pan-Canadian – discourse on the social union; and it recognized implicitly a legitimate role for the federal government in social policy' (2000, 8). The other provinces agreed to a formal opting-out formula as a bargaining position – a stance that resulted in a limited and informal opting-out condition.

Others, however, object that Quebec refuses to participate in such a collaborative measure – and would potentially refuse to collaborate on any but the most lucrative agreements – because its position of non-participation is advantageous from a game-theoretical perspective, wherein 'Quebec will either get transfer money without having had to agree to broad rules of engagement vis-à-vis Canadians in other provinces, or the federal government will deny Quebec money that the other provinces are receiving' (Robson and Schwanen 1999, 5), thereby playing into the separatist agenda of the Parti Québécois government (see also Gibbins 1999).

Two points emerge from the above. First, for larger political reasons as well as for more specific policy reasons, Quebec cannot be left out of any social-policy agreement on health care. Second, as Dufour maintains, 'Quebec cannot remain on the sidelines of Canadian intergovernmental relations in the field of social policy,' for its *own* benefit (2002, 7). Harvey Lazar argues that a formal opting-out provision 'would explicitly acknowledge that opting out is possible without making it a right. In effect it would leave room for considering opting out on a case-by-case basis, which is consistent with practice during the years of building the post World War Two welfare state' (Lazar 2000b, 10). Lazar stipulates four characteristics of such a possible compromise: first, the opting-out provision would be explicit, rather than implicit; second, any province opting out would publicly acknowledge

Ottawa's financial contribution; third, the province would use the funds either in a way that was 'broadly compatible with the purposes of the new program' or, if it already had a program that met Canada-wide objectives, in the same or in a related priority area. Finally, to ensure the possibility of Quebec's agreeing with 'Canada-wide priorities,' national consensus would be measured by agreement by seven provinces with at least half the population, rather than simply by any six provinces (Lazar 2000a, 117–18).

Except for people who object to asymmetrical federalism on principle, however, the issue here for most is not what Quebec will do with any opting-out provision: its commitment to a public health-care system is clearly on record (Vaillancourt 2002). The real concern is Alberta, with its stated intention to use private health-care resources more fully. Nevertheless this formula could be applied only in cases where a province's existing programs were 'broadly compatible with the purposes of the new program,' or else, where existing programs already were achieving such objectives, it could use the funds in a related priority area. The more political concern might be that Ottawa would tailor its objectives to make them more consonant with Quebec's in order to avoid political disputes (Lazar 2000a, 116, 118), thereby skewing health policy in general toward Quebec's. This may be a valid concern, but Quebec's health policy is much more in line with CHA principles than is Alberta's potential blueprint, so any such informal tinkering should not threaten CHA standards. Problems from implementing an explicit opting-out clause would also be mitigated by the concurrent formalization of the federal spending power. Would Ottawa agree to this? It persuaded the provinces to sign the initial SUFA largely by offering extra money; thus, unless it is willing to pay, either in cash or in tax points, for an enhanced agreement on health care, it will have to share political power.

Like the principle of opting out, the federal spending power is more implicit than explicit, although the SUFA 'institutionalizes' recognition of this power. Hamish Telford argues that 'the federal spending power, at best, can only be *inferred* from the constitution; the JCPC ruled that the spending power was *ultra vires*; the gift-giving argument is tenuous; and justifying the spending power as in the national interest is highly problematic in a multinational federation,' for that power limits Quebecers' 'freedom to determine their own social and cultural policies' (Telford n.d., 11).

However, one can respond with three arguments. First, decades of practice (as well as the Supreme Court's recent decision regarding the cap on CAP) have embedded the principle of federal spending into the fabric of intergovernmental relations. Recognizing the power explicitly may be a relatively cheap way for provinces to achieve other objectives (including a formal opting-out clause or a binding dispute-resolution mechanism). Second, the federal spending power is important from a *policy* point of view – it is still Ottawa's most potent instrument for corralling disparate points of view into a workable national health plan, and it will be essential in balancing out some of the provisions allowing for greater provincial influence in national health policy. Third, explicit recognition may be helpful in persuading Ottawa to accept some formal restrictions on it; having it legitimized may be worth the cost of some clear limitations on it. Explicit recognition of the federal spending power is partially symbolic, but it holds a great deal of political potential. Again, its force is counterfactual and thus difficult to evaluate: in essence, provinces simply could not challenge federal spending on broad constitutional grounds. This is of small import if Ottawa has little inclination (or money) for health services; but Ottawa would have a great deal of added political and moral clout were it desirous of doing so.

It is also imperative that both levels of government articulate a consonance of direction, which would help provinces to alter the way in which they focus health-service delivery in the medium- to long-term future and would assist in federal attempts to reconsider its nonfinancing roles in health care. Governments are collaborating in health information: a national infostructure system, the development of common data standards, and health reports to Canadians. The federal government, which has contributed to the Canadian Health Infostructure program since 1997, committed $500 million in September 2000 'to accelerate the adoption of modern information technologies to provide better health care' (Senate Standing Committee 2001, chap. 10). Another collaborative strategy should address the issue of health human resources (generally, doctors and nurses). Although the training and provision of health personnel are under clear provincial jurisdiction, issues of professional mobility (including the practice of better-funded provinces 'poaching' health-care personnel from poorer provinces) ideally need a national rather than a regional perspective.

As Adams (2001a, 278) observes, there is evidence to support 'the use of a more collaborative intergovernmental regime in certain circumstances,' including development of health programs with a country-wide impact, new program initiatives, and common political problems (such as reinvigorating the blood-collection service). Given a clear assignment of major roles to the senior levels of government, especially on funding levels, funding formulas, and dispute resolution, the two levels can address more specific programmatic issues collaboratively. As Lazar notes, federal and provincial line ministries such as health are much more likely to have common purposes and viewpoints (2000b, 8–9); sorting out of long-term funding patterns (usually by the respective departments of finance) can ease intergovernmental co-operation on specific policy questions. Thus the specific type of body to handle such collaboration would be a Canada Health Council (discussed at length by Adams 2001b, 282–7).

Perhaps the federal government has the most independence in research and evaluation. This role is crucial, with health reform and evidence-based medicine the focus of much governmental activity. The Health Transition Fund (1997–2001) and the Canada Health Info-structure Partnerships Program (2000–02) are two such examples of national health-evaluation programs involving federal funds. Given the importance of health research, federal funding must increase in this area. The pharmaceutical industry has for almost a decade been the leading source of funding for Canadian health research (Senate Standing Committee 2001, chap. 9), which troubles those concerned with independent research. Federal funding for health research should again rise to at least 25 per cent of total expenditure on health research (from its low of 16 per cent in 1998 – see Senate Standing Committee 2001, sec. 9.1.1), to balance the strength of the drug industry in Canada. Another aspect of Ottawa's research and evaluation role, albeit one that would require co-ordination with the provinces, is support for innovative pilot projects in the delivery of health services. This emphasis on federal funding of innovative programs also supports the 'experimental laboratory' model of federalism espoused by those defending provincial jurisdiction over health care.

Towards Accountability

Section 3 of the SUFA promises to increase the scope of democratic government by keeping Canadians informed on the progress of social programs, by engaging in ongoing dialogue, and by providing a procedure for appeals on administrative decisions. Greater accountability can facilitate intergovernmental relations in health-care funding and expenditure; accountability to the public allows governments to hold each other accountable.

The values of democratic governance, including transparency and accountability, are held to be self-evident. But efficiency and the ability to get things done are also highly valued in a complex and contradictory environment. And, as Lazar states, 'the more successful the social union turns out to be from an executive federalism perspective, the greater the risks that it will increase the size of the democratic deficit' (2000a, 110). For the health system, accountability ensures that funds reach their intended destination. The most publicized bad example is the $1 billion fund for medical equipment that Ottawa set up during the first ministers' conference of September 2000. Instead of paying for high-technology equipment such as dialysis machines, MRIs, and computer tomography (CT) scanners, some of the money went for lawn tractors, dishwashers, floor scrubbers, paper shredders, and fax machines (Priest 2002, A1). The provinces were to provide a public accounting of how they spent the funds, but, because federal money (including CHST funds) goes directly into provinces' general revenues, it is extremely difficult to determine their ultimate use. The issue is not the lack of accountability per se: the provinces (subject to the CHA) must account to their constituents regarding their use of health-care funds. But when one or both levels of government engage in cost containment, each level can blame the other for the cutbacks that result, with both refusing to take primary responsibility (Fierlbeck 2001).

Political motivations shape governments' advocacy of any form of accountability. As Susan Phillips recounts, during SUFA negotiations the provinces supported a form of accountability based on individual provinces' stipulation of indicators (thus preserving provincial autonomy) in order systematically to show the effects of future potential federal cutbacks on their health-care systems. Ottawa wanted to be able indirectly to press 'underperforming provinces to direct spending towards social programs and to design more effective programs' (Phillips 2001, 18). Even though its transfers are formally unconditional beyond CHA restrictions, it can use public pressure (or, more specifically, public censure) to goad provinces into certain types or levels of spending.

Despite protestations citing autonomy and jurisdiction, accountability and transparency should be augmented and strengthened. Both levels of government should report formally to their constituents and to each other regarding both outcomes and activities, using a set of standardized processes and indicators. There has been some progress at recent premiers' meetings; but provinces still resist losing the autonomy to determine the standards of measurement and having to measure outcomes of health programs (although this situation is improving). Governments have in the past two decades shown some willingness to put political ends before health-care objectives; if, as the rhetoric would imply, both levels desire sincerely to protect these objectives, they should regularize this commitment. Governments' becoming more accountable to each other rather than simply using 'the public' as a watchdog is important because, as Phillips notes, 'outcome measurement of social policies has proven to be much more complex in practice than in concept, and citizens and voluntary organizations are extremely limited in their ability to be effective watchdogs' (2001, 23).

Provincial governments may argue that they have the constitutional jurisdiction and thus the ultimate responsibility for health spending and that they should thus be able to account for these funds as they see fit. But, as federal transfers involve taxpayers' money, Ottawa too has a responsibility to inform its constituents of how its funds are used. The principle of 'ultimate provincial jurisdiction' also evokes little sympathy from the broader public, which, as public-opinion surveys show, sees both levels of government as appropriate watchdogs for the other's activity (Centre for Research and Information on Canada 1997). Moreover, as Phillips observes, now that federal transfers have returned to earlier levels, 'the idea of public reporting and rendering of accounts for the modification of existing programs and their funding, coupled with commitments to clearly state the roles and responsibilities of each order of government,' becomes less attractive to the provinces (2001, 22). Although provinces may well object to more stringent accountability, they should do whatever they can to ensure the long-term stability of federal funding.

The measurement and comparison of outcomes will require sustained and vigorous development, and Canadians should not expect useful results in the short term. Perhaps a health commissioner (along the lines of the auditor general) could report on dubious or inefficient allocations of health funds but would be no panacea (see, for example, Kroeger 2000, Sutherland 2001). Such a mechanism could oblige governments to account for their activities simply by opening existing practices to public scrutiny (and thereby keep the *other* party in check). Finally, a jointly appointed ministerial council could develop a national framework for public accountability, facilitate co-ordination between governments at the sectoral level, serve as a neutral fact-finding body for intergovernmental disputes, and report back to governments and the public (see Adams 2001a, 283).

Involving Other Levels of Government?

Intertwined with the discussion on the roles of federal, provincial, and territorial governments is the debate on the place of municipal government and regional health authorities (RHAs) in the provision of health care. Roger Gibbins, for example, suggests that because so much creative policy making occurs at the local level, we can expect 'an intensified campaign for greater legislative scope, financial powers, and constitutional recognition' (Gibbins 1999, 210). This is indeed the crux of the problem: while local governments and RHAs design and implement the details of health care (and take responsibility for their policy choices), they have little to no tax base or constitutional authority. This imbalance of responsibility and power has allowed provincial governments to offload politically unpopular decisions to local bodies, echoing federal strategy throughout the 1990s (see, for example, Fierlbeck 1997).

Large municipalities are trying to increase both their legislative power and their financial capacity. In a brief to the Prime Minister's Caucus Task Force on Urban Issues, the Federation of Canadian Municipalities (2002, 6) argued that 'Canadian politics is defined principally by a divisive federal/provincial dynamic driven heavily by partisan issues. Structural realities dictate that the federal/provincial equation will never be easy. But when partisan interest is added, this natural tension can become debilitating conflict and confrontation. In contrast, municipal governments are non-partisan, focused generally on practical outcomes and the delivery of services to citizens.' The 'big city' mayors have proposed a charter that would give cities 'powers and resources that match their responsibilities' (Canada's Cities 2001, 1) but have not related their campaign to health policy. Andrew Sancton finds insufficient political support at the municipal level to challenge provincial policy makers and believes that, as long as this state continues, 'municipalities will remain minor actors in the drama of Canadian federalism' (2002, 275).

Is there a good case for shifting responsibility for health towards the local level in Canada? We just do not know. As most observers concur, in health care local governance varies 'considerably in terms of structure and responsibilities; thus 'it is very difficult to generalize about them' (Rasmussen 2001, 250). Analytical conclusions are also very difficult. First, competing ideological visions underlie decentralization. One side sees decentralization and regionalization as routes to inclusive and participatory public policy by facilitating individuals' involvement. Proponents of market-oriented delivery also view decentralization and regionalization approvingly (for more on this debate see Fierlbeck 1997; Taft and Steward 2000; Tomblin 2002). Second, in the matter of accountability: should health-care governance structures be responsible ultimately to a local population or to national standards? Third, as Tomblin notes, regionalization was never designed to deal with adjacent components of the health-care system (such as the professional medical colleges), which operated relatively autonomously: 'the jury is still out,' states Tomblin, 'on whether regionalization was ever intended or designed to challenge the old bio-medical model' (2002, 19).

Moreover, the functions of regionalization are varied and potentially contradictory. It has, for example, an *integrative* function, which focuses moving health-care delivery away from the traditional 'stovepipe,' design and towards a more comprehensive system of provision (Rasmussen 2001). Its *economic* function attempts greater economies of scale in services (for example, the Council of Atlantic Premiers: see Tomblin 2002, 20). Its *political* element (either explicit or implicit) debates the respective roles of the population, the market, and the state (Rocher and Rouillard, for example, argue that the move towards decentralization in Canadian federalism veils 'another approach that seeks less to reform intergovernmental relations than to instill in the institutional framework a desire to see the State (provincial and federal) disengage from economic and social regulatory mechanisms' [1998, 233].)

There is no clear conception of regionalization, its functions, its operations, and its implications. More formal information gathering could illuminate the nature and potential of local and regional forms of government. Although the number of phenomena that 'ought to be studied' in Canadian health care is high, information-gathering mechanisms are already in place. A substantial comparative study of the qualitative and quantitative dynamics of health-care regionalization is essential before policy proposals can with confidence be articulated. Pilot projects under provincial jurisdiction could then test perceived options in the light of evidence collected in the larger survey.

Conclusion: A Sizeable Step Forward?

The discussion of senior governments' roles in formulating health policy is bound most directly by constitutional jurisdiction but must recognize policy objectives, what governments are willing to do, and their motivations. A clear assignment of roles in terms of health objectives would facilitate accountability. It would hamper 'buck passing,' finger-pointing, or gainsaying vis-à-vis policy failures, funding cuts, or simple mismanagement. Given the political and constitutional context of the Canadian health system, however, autonomy could also result in highly disparate provincial systems (if provinces received more capacity to tax) or in unpredictable financing and greater acrimony (if Ottawa funded provinces more on its own terms). Mutual co-operation, in contrast, facilitates greater communication over policy objectives and strategy. This approach, however, can lead to beggar-thy-neighbour practices or blame shifting unless mechanisms exist to mitigate differences of opinion or conflicting policy directions.

Canada may be entering what Tuohy (1999) calls a 'window of opportunity' in health-policy formulation, where the actors are either willing to change the rules of the game or simply have no preferable alternatives. Changes in the federal role have clearly not been consistent with shifts in cost sharing; relative levels of federal funding have dropped while Ottawa has become more enthusiastic about protecting national standards. It is unwilling to pay for this role, but it seems equally unwilling to relinquish it.

This paper has argued that one way forward may be balancing the clear assignment of responsibility with mutual co-operation, thereby securing both accountability and stability. If Ottawa does not wish to pay to enforce the CHA to its satisfaction, it must use its legislative powers as its capital. It can agree to limit its autonomous spending power in terms of both scope and application in exchange for a formal and ongoing presence in health policy making. It gains not only greater political control for less economic outlay, but also wins formal recognition for a power never formally constitutionalized. Provinces may be amenable because of explicit and predictable limits on federal activity combined with funding for similar-but-distinct programs under a justiciable opting-out option.

This solution does, however, depend on certain assumptions (that, for example, provincial objectives are largely consonant), which may rightfully be queried. It is also contingent on political dynamics (such as the relationship between departments of health and finance within discrete jurisdictions) external to intergovernmental relations. It depends, most profoundly, on the judgment of those who have the power to grasp such an opportunity and the acuity to recognize that such a distribution of roles, although it may not permit the best of all possible worlds, may at the very least avoid the worst.

That such a trade-off builds on the logic of the SUFA makes its possible implementation slightly more likely, as the basic form of the compromise is already set out. Perhaps it is also too dependent on the health of SUFA? The accord is coming to the end of its three-year agreement and is currently being evaluated by governments. Some governments are sceptical about its usefulness, and about the willingness of others to observe its spirit; if it is all about trust and collaboration, some might ask, then why did it take a year and a half to get a dispute-resolution mechanism in place? SUFA is somewhat of a counterfactual safeguard: for example, the provinces *would* be informed *were* Ottawa to introduce radical new changes to programs. Ottawa has not done so; and thus the utility of SUFA in its safeguard function is largely undetermined. Moreover, SUFA is relatively silent on the federal use of one-off, targeted funding initiatives: for instance, some provinces have not received money from the Primary Healthcare Fund set up in 2000 September because of federal–provincial disputes over conditions. Thus provinces dislike targeted funding because it is too conditional and too 'short term' (again undermining the predictability of long-term health funding), while the federal government prefers it because of its high public profile, limited financial liability, and detailed conditionality.

These are serious reservations, but they are not conclusive evidence that a compromise could not work. The proposal suggested here is merely a possibility, not a foregone conclusion (nor even an easy sell). The demise of SUFA would surely make such a trade-off less likely, as it would lessen even further the trust or goodwill between parties and increase the perception that nothing but hard-nosed political realism can work in intergovernmental relations. But the idea of an explicitly recognized federal spending power could be broached again, whether SUFA survives or not; the desire for predictable funding patterns will continue (especially in difficult economic times); and the public will probably keep pressing for intergovernmental accountability and transparency. Thus the elements of such a compromise will be with us for some time, even if SUFA is not.

Some might observe that the suggestions noted here are largely institutional and give short shrift to a more sustained social and political analysis. Does this mean that the right institutional solution could end intergovernmental disputes? Absolutely not. However, there are better and worse institutional contexts, and one that minimizes confrontation goes a long way in easing intergovernmental conflict. As the focus here must of necessity be very narrow, such measured social and political analysis must be found elsewhere (for example, Maioni 1998, O'Reilly 2001, Tuohy 1999).

Finally, one must (paradoxically) be wary also of successful intergovernmental collaboration, a.k.a. executive federalism – a form of decision making that involves in-camera negotiations and decisions made by government officials. That approach, as Smiley (1979) argued, sacrifices transparency and accountability to the wider public in order to facilitate collaboration between governments. At this point, however, an overly cosy intergovernmental relationship is not one of the most pressing issues facing Canadian health care.

In sum, the institutional and policy changes suggested here are premised both on the need to ensure the long-term sustainability of a universally accessible, publicly funded health system and on the recognition that governments make decisions with an eye to whether measures strengthen or disadvantage them vis-à-vis other political actors. Trade-offs may have to be made, however unpalatable they may be to participants or to those preferring a model unsullied by political concessions. Compromise is a hallmark of politics writ large, not only of federalism; and if the only way forward is with a few sidesteps, it is preferable to an unproductive status quo.

REFERENCES

Adams, Duane. 2001a. Conclusions: Proposals for Advancing Federalism, Democracy, and Governance of the Canadian Health System.' In Duane Adams, ed., *Federalism, Democracy, and Health Policy in Canada*. Montreal: McGill-Queen's University Press, 271–306.
– 2001b. 'Social Union Study of the Canadian Health System: Introduction and Overview.' In Duane Adams, ed., *Federalism, Democracy, and Health Policy in Canada*. Montreal: McGill-Queen's University Press, 1–16.
Alberta. 2002. *The Premier's Advisory Council on Health* (Mazankowki Report). Jan.

Bégin, Monique. 2002. *Revisiting the Canada Health Act (1984): Impediment to Change?* Speech presented to the Institute for Research on Public Policy, Ottawa, 20 Feb.

Boadway, Robin, and Paul Hobson. 1993. *Intergovernmental Fiscal Relations in Canada.* Canadian Tax Paper No. 96. Toronto: Canadian Tax Foundation.

Brown, Douglas. 2002. 'Fiscal Federalism: The New Equilibrium between Equity and Efficiency.' In Herman Bakvis and Grace Skogstad, eds., *Canadian Federalism.* Don Mills, Ont.: Oxford University Press, 59–84.

Campbell, Robert. 1995. 'Federalism and Economic Policy.' In François Rocher and Miriam Smith, eds., *New Trends in Canadian Federalism.* Peterborough, Ont.: Broadview Press, 187–210.

Canada's Cities. 2001. 'Canada's Big City Mayors Launch Campaign to Give Urban Canada "21st Century" Powers.' www.canadascities.ca/news.htm, 18 April 2002.

Canadian Institute of Health Information. (CIHI). 1999. *National Health Expenditure Trends, 1975–1999.*

Centre for Research and Information on Canada. 1997. *Opinions on Social Programs* (Dec.–July).

Courchene, Thomas. 1994. *Social Canada in the Millennium: Reform Imperatives and Restructuring Principles.* Toronto: C.D. Howe Institute.

– 1997. 'ACCESS: A Convention on the Canadian Economic and Social Systems.' In *Assessing ACCESS: Towards a New Social Union.* Kingston, Ont.: Institute of Intergovernmental Relations, 77–112.

Dufour, Christian. 2002. Restoring the Federal Principle: The Place of Quebec in the Social Union. *Policy Matters* 3, no. 1: 1–26.

Federation of Canadian Municipalities (FCM). 2002. Brief to the Prime Minister's Caucus Task Force on Urban Issues. www.fcm.ca/english/communications/presbrief.htm, 4 April 2002.

Fierlbeck, Katherine. 1997. 'Canadian Health Reform and the Politics of Decentralization.' In C.W. Altenstetter and J.W. Bjorkman, eds., *Health Policy Reform, National Variations, and Globalization.* London: Macmillan, 17–38.

– 2001. 'Cost Containment in Health Care: The Federalism Context.' In Duane Adams, ed., *Federalism, Democracy, and Health Policy in Canada.* Montreal: McGill-Queen's University Press, 131–78.

Gagnon, Alain-G., and Can Erk. 2002. 'Legitimacy, Effectiveness, and Federalism: On the Benefits of Ambiguity.' In Herman Bakvis and Grace Skogstad, eds., *Canadian Federalism.* Don Mills, Ont.: Oxford University Press, 317–30.

Gibbins, Roger. 1997. 'Democratic Reservations about the ACCESS Models.' In *Assessing ACCESS: Towards a New Social Union.* Kingston, Ont.: Institute of International Relations, 41–4.

- 1999. 'Taking Stock: Canadian Federalism and Its Constitutional Framework.' In Leslie Pal, ed., *How Ottawa Spends 1999–2000*. Toronto: Oxford University Press, 197–220.

Kennett, Steven. 1998. *Securing the Social Union: A Commentary on the Decentralized Approach*. Kingston, Ont.: Institute of Intergovernmental Relations.

Kroeger, Arthur. 2000. *The HRD Affair: Reflections on Accountability in Government*. Speech to the Canadian Club of Ottawa, 12 Dec.

Laghi, Brian. 2002. 'Premiers Threaten to Act Alone on Health' *Globe and Mail*, 25 Jan. A1.

Lazar, Harvey. 2000a. 'The Social Union Framework Agreement and the Future of Fiscal Federalism.' In Lazar, ed., *Canada – The State of the Federation 1999–2000: In Search of a New Mission Statement for Canadian Fiscal Federalism*. Kingston, Ont.: Institute of Intergovernmental Relations.

- 2000b. *The Social Union Framework Agreement: Lost Opportunity or New Beginning?* Queen's University Working Paper 3, Kingston, Ont.

Maioni, Antonia. 1998. *Parting at the Crossroads: The Emergence of Health Insurance in the United States and Canada*. Princeton, NJ: Princeton University Press.

- 2000. 'Assessing the Social Union Framework Agreement.' *Policy Options*, April, 39–41.

- 2002. 'Health Care in the New Millennium.' In Herman Bakvis and Grace Skogstad, eds., *Canadian Federalism*. Don Mills, Ont.: Oxford University Press, 87–104.

Maslove, Allan. 1992. 'Reconstructing Fiscal Federalism.' In Frances Abele, ed., *How Ottawa Spends 1992–93: The Politics of Competitiveness*. Ottawa: Carleton University Press, 57–73.

- 1996. 'The Canada Health and Social Transfer: Forcing Issues.' In Gene Swimmer, ed., *How Ottawa Spends 1996–1997*. Ottawa: Carleton University Press, 283–301.

Mendelsohn, Matthew, and John McLean. 2000. 'SUFA's Double Vision: Citizen Engagement and Intergovernmental Collaboration.' *Policy Options*, 23 April 43–4.

Muszynski, Leon. 1995. 'Social Policy and Canadian Federalism: What Are the Pressures for Change?' In François Rocher and Miriam Smith, eds., *New Trends in Canadian Federalism*. Peterborough, Ont.: Broadview Press, 288–318.

Noël, Alain. 2000. 'Without Quebec: Collaborative Federalism with a Footnote?' *Policy Matters* 1, no. 2: 1–26.

O'Reilly, Patricia. 2001. 'The Canadian Health System Landscape.' In Duane Adams, ed., *Federalism, Democracy, and Health Policy in Canada*. Montreal: McGill-Queen's University Press, 17–59.

Phillips, Susan. 2001. SUFA and Citizen Engagement: Fake or Genuine Master-piece? *Policy Matters* 2, no. 7: 1–36.

Priest, Lisa. 2002. 'Fund for Medical Machines Buys Lawn Tractors.' *Globe and Mail*, 4 April, A1.

Rasmussen, Ken. 2001. 'Regionalization and Collaborative Government: A New Direction for Health System Governance.' In Duane Adams, ed., *Federalism, Democracy, and Health Policy in Canada*. Montreal: McGill-Queen's University Press, 239–70.

Robson, William, and Daniel Schwanen. 1999. 'The Social Union Agreement: Too Flawed to Last.' *C.D. Howe Institute Backgrounder*, 8 Feb. 1999, 1–5.

Rocher, François, and Christian Rouillard. 1998. 'Décentralisation, subsidiarité et néo-liberalisme au Canada: Lorsque l'arbre cache la forêt.' *Canadian Public Policy* 24, no. 2: 233–58.

Sancton, Andrew. 2002. 'Municipalities, Cities, and Globalization: Implications for Canadian Federalism.' In Herman Bakvis and Grace Skogstad, eds., *Canadian Federalism*. Don Mills, Ont.: Oxford University Press, 261–77.

Smiley, D.V. 1979. 'An Outsider's Observations of Intergovernmental Relations among Consenting Adults.' In R. Simeon, ed., *Consultation or Collaboration: Intergovernmental Relations in Canada Today.* Toronto: Institute of Public Administration.

Smith, Jennifer. 2002. 'Informal Constitutional Development: Change by Other Means.' In Herman Bakvis and Grace Skogstad, eds., *Canadian Federalism*. Don Mills, Ont.: Oxford University Press, 40–58.

Snoddon, Tracy. 1998. The Impact of the CHST on Interprovincial Redistribution in Canada. *Canadian Public Policy* 24, no. 1: 49–70.

Sutherland, Sharon. 2001. *Biggest Scandal in Canadian History: HRDC Audit Starts Probity War*. Working Paper 23. Queen's University School of Policy Studies, Kingston, Ont.

Standing Senate Committee on Social Affairs, Science, and Technology. 2001. *The Health of Canadians: The Federal Role*, 4 Vol. 4 – *Issues and Options* (Kirby Report). Ottawa: Senate of Canada, Sept.

Taft, Kevin, and Gillian Steward. 2000. *Clear Answers: The Economics and Politics of For-Profit Medicine*. Edmonton: University of Alberta Press.

Telford, Hamish. N.d. *The Federal Spending Power in Canada: Nation-Building or Nation-Destroying?* Institute of Intergovernmental Relations Working Paper, Queen's University, Kingston, Ont.

Tomblin, Stephen. 2002. 'Regionalization: Does It Really Matter?' Paper presented to the Dalhousie Law School, 1 March.

Tuohy, Carolyn Hughes. 1999. *Accidental Logics: The Dynamics of Change in the*

Health Care Arena in the United States, Britain, and Canada. New York: Oxford University Press.
Vaillancourt, Yves. 2002. 'Le modèle québécois de politiques sociales et ses interfaces avec l'union sociale canadienne.' IRPP Policy Matters Working Paper, Jan.
Watts, R.L. 1999. *The Spending Power in Federal Systems*. Kingston, Ont.: Institute of Intergovernmental Relations.

PART FOUR

INTERNATIONAL TRADE REGIMES

11 International Trade Agreements and Canadian Health Care

JON R. JOHNSON

Canada has been a party to multilateral trade agreements since 1948, when the General Agreement on Tariffs and Trade (now known as GATT 1947) entered into force. GATT 1947, along with agreements elaborating certain of its provisions achieved in successive rounds of GATT negotiations from 1948 to 1980, had a minimal effect on the organization of Canada's health-care system.

Since those earlier GATT rounds, Canada has entered into trade liberalizing agreements that impose obligations that constrain governments' ability to organize the delivery of services. The Canada–United States Free Trade Agreement (FTA), which became effective on 1 January 1989, imposed obligations respecting services, investment, and the designation of monopolies. The North American Free Trade Agreement (NAFTA), which superseded the FTA on 1 January 1994 and added Mexico as a party, elaborated on the obligations respecting monopolies, expanded those on services and investment, and imposed new ones respecting intellectual property.

Contemporaneously with the negotiation of the FTA and NAFTA, the Uruguay Round of GATT negotiations ended. It culminated in the Marrakesh Agreement Establishing the World Trade Organization (WTO Agreement), which came into effect on 1 January 1995. The annexes to that document carry forward GATT 1947 as the General Agreement on Tariffs and Trade 1994 (GATT 1994) and set out other agreements affecting trade in goods. The annexes also set out entirely new agreements on trade in services and on intellectual property and establish a formal dispute-resolution process within the WTO.

Canada's Public Health Care System

While prime responsibility for health care in Canada is provincial, the basic structure of the Canadian system is set out in the Canada Health Act (CHA) of 1984. The act establishes five criteria that must be satisfied for a province to qualify for a full cash contribution as part of the Canada Health and Social Transfer (CHST):

- *Public administration.* The province must establish a health-care insurance plan administered by a public authority that it appoints or designates.
- *Comprehensiveness.* The insurance plan must cover all insured health services provided by hospitals, medical practitioners, or dentists. The act defines these services as 'hospital services,' 'physician services,' and 'surgical-dental services.'
- *Universality.* A provincial plan must entitle all of the insured persons in the province to these services on uniform terms and conditions.
- *Portability.* The plan cannot impose any minimum period of residence or waiting period in excess of three months and must provide coverage for temporary absences.
- *Accessibility.* Payment must be in accordance with a tariff or system of payment authorized by provincial law. The plan must provide for reasonable compensation for all insured health services rendered by medical practitioners or dentists and for payment of amounts to hospitals. There are deductions from the federal cash transfer if the province permits extra-billing for insured health services by medical practitioners or dentists. Extra-billing is billing over and above the amount provided for the insured service under the plan.

The health insurance plans established in all the provinces follow this format.

The Canadian public health-care system requires the establishment of a monopoly in each province to cover payment for all insured health services delivered within the province. Such services must be covered by a health-insurance plan administered by a public authority designated by the province. That authority must pay for all insured services. The funding for payment can come wholly from public revenues or partly from premiums charged by the public authority, but user fees are prohibited. Whether by law or as a practical matter, insured services are not covered by plans administered by private insurers.[1]

Canada's health-care system is public, in that a public authority in each province pays for insured services. However, there is nothing in the Canada Health Act that prevents the supply of insured services by private firms, whether non-profit or for-profit (Flood 1999, 31), and insured services are usually delivered by private individuals or firms. Most medical practitioners and dentists are self-employed people who usually operate for profit on a fee-for-service basis (31). While hospitals frequently receive most funding from public sources, they are rarely government owned. Most 'public' hospitals are owned by non-profit firms (36).

While private individuals and firms deliver insured services, providers may not contract with patients for the price of the service and can receive only the price for each insured service fixed by provincial law. Service providers usually bill the public authority directly. If a provider bills a patient, the bill must be for the amount prescribed by the public authority, and the patient receives reimbursement from that source.

The insured health services defined in the CHA and elaborated on in provincial legislation do not cover all health services. For example, the only insured dental services are surgical–dental procedures performed by a dentist in a hospital. Insured services include the cost of drugs provided in hospitals, but not drugs provided elsewhere. Non-necessary medical procedures, such as cosmetic surgery, are not insured. Private insurers offer coverage for these services, and private firms, including for-profit firms, provide non-covered services.

Objectives of the Trade Agreements

The agreements liberalizing trade relate to goods and services and to the protection of direct foreign investment and of intellectual property rights. They achieve these objectives by placing limits on governmental action. The limits take the form of non-discrimination requirements and, in some instances, the establishment of norms to which government measures must conform. The agreements generally favour market-based as opposed to government-administered structures in the areas where they impose obligations. However, they expressly permit the designation of monopolies and recognize, subject to qualifications, the right of governments to regulate.

Those agreements most affecting the organization and structure of the Canadian health-care system are NAFTA[2] and several agreements set out in the annexes of the WTO Agreement – most notably, the General Agreement on Trade in Services (GATS).[3]

The agreements generally require that Canada's federal government ensure compliance by provincial and local governments. NAFTA's Article 105 requires each NAFTA party to ensure implementation of NAFTA provisions, including (except where otherwise provided) their observance by provincial governments. A number of WTO agreements, notably GATS and GATT 1994,[4] require that member countries ensure compliance by regional governments.

Provincial compliance is the general rule under both NAFTA and the WTO agreements, but with exceptions. This paper identifies, for each agreement, application to provincial measures.

Four provisions of the agreements affect Canadian health care. First, as we saw above, the Canadian health-care system establishes a government monopoly in each province for payment of insured health services. Both NAFTA's Chapter Fifteen and GATS set out requirements for the designation and maintenance of monopolies.[5]

Second, Chapters Eleven and Twelve of NAFTA set out obligations respecting investment and cross-border trade in services. The health-care system affects the delivery of services and the investments of firms that deliver them. GATS also imposes obligations respecting trade in services.

Third, both NAFTA's Chapter Seventeen and the Agreement Respecting Trade-Related Aspects of Intellectual Property Rights (TRIPS Agreement, or TRIPS)[6] impose extensive requirements respecting intellectual property rights, including patents. Many prescription drugs are subject to patents. Both NAFTA's Chapter Seventeen and TRIPS restrict the extent to which the health-care system may use cheaper generic drugs.

Fourth, the trade-in-goods provisions of the agreements permit countervailing duties against imported goods that are subsidized and impose other disciplines on subsidization. Canada's health-care system is based upon the payment of subsidies.

Monopolies

Article 1502 of NAFTA sets out obligations respecting monopolies. Chapter Fifteen defines a 'monopoly' as follows: 'monopoly means an entity, including a consortium or government agency, that in any relevant market in the territory of a Party, is designated as the sole provider or purchaser of a good or service.' The public authority established by each province to pay for insured health services is clearly the sole provider of insurance services in respect of the health services covered because private insurers, either by law or as a practical matter, are excluded from that market. Also, the public authority is arguably the sole purchaser of those services because no one else may pay for them.

Article 1502(1) provides that nothing in NAFTA prevents the designation of a monopoly. Article 1502(2) sets out requirements that must be observed if a party (including a provincial government) intends to designate a monopoly. It must give prior notice to other NAFTA parties and must introduce conditions on the operation of the monopoly that will minimize or eliminate nullification and impairment of certain NAFTA provisions, including Chapter Twelve (Cross-Border Trade in Services) but not Chapter Eleven (Investment). This provision is not relevant to existing provincial public authorities because these were designated many years ago. Article 1502(2) would be relevant if a province expanded the public component of its health-care system by increasing the number of insured services subject to the exclusive coverage of its health-insurance plan. Of much greater relevance there, however, is Article 1110 (Expropriation and Compensation), discussed below.

Article 1502(3) sets out a number of requirements that a party must observe respecting any monopoly that it designates. However, it applies only to privately owned monopolies and federal monopolies. Provincial monopolies are not subject to these requirements. While the CHA is a federal statute, it merely sets out certain requirements that provinces must satisfy to receive grants. The public authorities that pay for insured health services are clearly provincial, not federal.

These provisions respecting monopolies did not exist when Canada's public health-care system was established. They have minimal impact on provincial ability to maintain a health-care system and would not impede an expansion of the public component of the system. However, NAFTA Article 1110 (Expropriation and Compensation), discussed below, significantly inhibits expansion of that public component.

GATS Article VIII sets out requirements that members must observe vis-à-vis their monopoly suppliers of services. As these obligations are closely tied to other GATS obligations, they are described below.

The rest of this paper examines the impact of the trade-liberalizing agreements on Canada's health-care system – specifically, the effects of Chapters Eleven and Twelve of NAFTA, of GATS, of other provisions in the agreements, and of dispute resolution under the WTO and

NAFTA. A conclusion assesses the strengths and weaknesses of these agreements in terms of heath care in Canada and suggests future options.

Health Care and NAFTA Chapters Eleven and Twelve

NAFTA's Chapters Eleven (Investment) and Twelve (Cross-border Trade in Services) clearly have a potential impact on Canada's ability to maintain a public health-care system. Subject to certain reservations described below, the obligations that they impose apply to provincial as well as to federal measures. The investor/state procedures described below apply only to breaches of Chapter Eleven, not to breaches of Chapter Twelve.

Chapter Eleven covers measures relating to U.S. and Mexican investors and their investments within Canada. The expression 'investment' is broadly defined and includes a subsidiary of a U.S. or Mexican investor as well as a wide range of other property interests.

Chapter Twelve applies to measures relating to the cross-border trade in services – the provision of a service from the United States or Mexico into Canada, in Canada by a Canadian national or firm to a person in the United States or Mexico, or by a U.S. or Mexican national in Canada.

Federal or provincial measures relating to a company in Canada owned by U.S. investors that provides services to consumers in Canada are covered by Chapter Eleven, not by Chapter Twelve. Federal or provincial measures relating to a company in the United States providing services from the United States to consumers in Canada are covered by Chapter Twelve, not by Chapter Eleven.

The obligations under Chapters Eleven and Twelve are general in their application but are subject to some general exceptions for particular sectors not considered in this paper.[7]

Certain obligations under both Chapters Eleven and Twelve are subject to two important categories of reservations. First, a reservation under NAFTA's Annex I for provincial measures grandfathers all such measures in effect on 1 January 1994. Second, a sectoral reservation under Annex II covers social services, including health. There are other significant obligations under Chapter Eleven that are not subject to any reservations.

This paper first considers the Chapter Eleven and Chapter Twelve obligations that are subject to reservations, because the reservations significantly shield Canada's health-care system from these obligations. It then looks at the obligations that are *not* subject to reservations and hence may affect health care.

Obligations under Chapters Eleven and Twelve Subject to Reservations

The following obligations under NAFTA's Chapters Eleven and Twelve are subject to reservations:

- national treatment (Articles 1102 and 1202)
- most-favoured-nation (MFN) treatment (Articles 1103 and 1203)
- performance requirements (Article 1106)
- senior management and boards of directors (Article 1107)
- local presence requirements (Article 1205)

The national-treatment obligations are by far the most important for Canada's health-care system

National Treatment
The combined effect of Articles 1102(1) and (2) is to require that the federal government and each province accord to U.S. and Mexican investors and their investments treatment no less favourable than it accords, in like circumstances, to its own investors and their investments with respect to the establishment, acquisition, expansion, management, conduct, operation, and sale or other disposition of investments. Article 1202(1) sets out a similarly worded obligation respecting U.S. and Mexican cross-border service providers.

Article 1102(3) establishes a special rule when applying Article 1102(1) and 1102(2) to provincial measures that requires treatment no less favourable than the most favourable treatment accorded by the province, in like circumstances, to Canadian investors and to their investments. Article 1202(2) sets out a similar rule respecting cross-border services.

Article 1102(4)(a) prohibits minimum equity requirements, and 1102(4)(b) prohibits requiring an investor of another party, by reason of its nationality, to sell or otherwise dispose of an investment.

Under both GATT and WTO jurisprudence, a measure need not be overtly discriminatory to breach a non-discrimination obligation. A measure can be neutral on its face but can be found to have a discriminatory effect (de facto discrimination). While the concept has existed for a long time under GATT, findings of de facto discrimination have been made case by case, with few if any general principles to act as a guide. The concept has been carried over into Chapter Eleven jurisprudence, with even less clarity than exists under the GATT and WTO jurisprudence.

Articles 1102 and 1202 address situations in which U.S. or Mexican investors and their investments, or U.S. or Mexican cross-border service providers, are treated differently and less favourably than their Canadian counterparts. Case law respecting national treatment under other trade agreements such as GATT 1947, GATT 1994, and GATS has equated 'no less favourable treatment' with 'equality of competitive opportunities.'

The concept of 'no less favourable treatment' has been complicated rather than clarified by jurisprudence on NAFTA's Chapter Eleven. The Chapter Eleven tribunal in *Pope & Talbot Inc. and The Government of Canada (Pope & Talbot)*[8] interpreted Articles 1102(1) and (2) as imposing a best-in-jurisdiction treatment obligation. Under this interpretation, if a single U.S. investment is treated less favourably than a single domestic investment, there is a potential de facto violation, even if the measures do not discriminate on their face unless the circumstances are not 'like.' While the finding is arguably wrong and is not binding on other tribunals, it has established an unhelpful precedent.

As we saw above, the less favourable treatment must be accorded 'in like circumstances' in order for there to be a violation. The meaning of 'in like circumstances' under Articles 1102 and 1202 is as yet uncertain. Investors have argued in Chapter Eleven cases that investments in the same business sector are 'in like circumstances,' regardless of any other circumstances. The *Pope & Talbot* tribunal rejected this view, adopted an expansive view of 'in like circumstances,' and found that any difference in treatment linked to a rational government policy not motivated by discrimination created a situation of unlike circumstances. However, the NAFTA Chapter Twenty panel in *In the Matter of Cross-Border Trucking Services (Trucking Services)*[9] considering Article 1202 interpreted 'in like circumstances' narrowly and treated it as an exception.

Application to Canadian Health Care. The essential characteristic of Canada's health-care system is that a public authority in each province pays for all insured health services within that province, thereby excluding private insurers from the business of insuring those services. This essential characteristic does not raise a national-treatment issue.

Canadian insurers are excluded to the same extent as U.S. or Mexican insurers, whether seeking to provide insurance services through Canadian subsidiaries (and therefore subject to Chapter Eleven) or on a cross-border basis (and therefore subject to Chapter Twelve). Article 1502(1) clearly permits both the federal and provincial governments to establish and maintain monopolies, and Articles 1102 and 1202 cannot be interpreted so as to frustrate this right.

There is no inherent problem under Articles 1102 or 1202 with the requirement that insured health services be supplied at rates that are established by the province or that prevent suppliers from contracting with patients for the price of those services. Canadian suppliers are subject to the same constraints.

Articles 1102 and 1202 are problematic to the extent that Canada's health-care system treats Canadian firms more favourably than U.S. or Mexican firms. A measure that excludes or severely limits the extent to which a U.S. or Mexican firm can engage in an activity connected with the health-care system, when compared to its Canadian counterparts, can cause a potential violation of Articles 1102 or 1202. This circumstance could arise with measures that exclude for-profit firms from certain activities and limit participation to non-profit firms. A U.S. owner of a for-profit firm could argue that such limiting of participation in effect reserves the activity to Canadians, because non-profit U.S. firms do not operate in Canada. Contrary arguments can be made that for-profit firms and non-profit firms are not 'in like circumstances.' However, the potential for a violation remains.

One question that arises regarding the NAFTA obligations of national treatment as applied to provinces is the extent, if any, to which treatment by one province can set a standard of treatment that must be observed by other provinces. Suppose that one province departs from the principles of the CHA and permits private insurers, including U.S.-owned insurers, to pay for insured health services. Does this province, in permitting private insurers to carry on a business from which insurers were formerly excluded, set a new standard, so that a breach of Article 1102 occurs because the other provinces do not permit private insurers to carry on that business? The answer is that it does not. When Articles 1102(1) and (2) are read together with Article 1102(3), it is clear that the comparison of the treatments accorded to U.S. versus domestic insurers is the treatment by 'that province,' not the treatment accorded by some other province. The province departing from the CHA's principles would have to treat U.S. insurers no less favourably than domestic insurers. However, the treatment by the departing province would not constitute the treatment benchmark for any other province.

The Other Obligations under Chapters Eleven and Twelve Subject to Reservations

Articles 1103 and 1203 also impose no-less-favourable-treatment requirements, but the obligation relates to U.S. or Mexican investors and their investments or to U.S. or Mexican cross-border service providers vis-à-vis each other or their counterparts from other countries. There does not appear to be any attribute of Canada's health-care system that necessitates treating one set of foreign investors or their investments or foreign service providers less favourably than another.

Article 1106(1) prohibits a government from imposing or enforcing certain requirements in connection with the establishment, acquisition, expansion, management, conduct, or operation of the Canadian investment of a U.S. or Mexican investor. One such requirement is 'to purchase, use or accord a preference to goods produced or services provided in its territory, or to purchase goods or services from persons in its territory.'[10] Subject to the reservations described below, a provincial government would trigger a breach of Article 1106 if it required a U.S.-owned Canadian company providing health services to purchase goods or services within Canada. Article 1106(3) sets out similar but narrower obligations respecting conditions for receipt of advantages such as subsidies.

Article 1107 prohibits measures that require that an investor of another party appoint to senior management positions individuals of any particular nationality. This obligation has no effect on Canada's ability to maintain public health care.

Article 1205 prohibits the federal government or a province from requiring cross-border service providers to establish or maintain a representative office or any form of enterprise or to be resident in Canada or the province. While this requirement may affect certain health-related issues, it has no impact on the ability of Canada to maintain its public health-care system.

The foregoing obligations under NAFTA Chapters Eleven and Twelve are subject to reservations under NAFTA Annexes I and II. Articles 1108(1) and 1206(1) permitted each NAFTA party to exempt from the application of Articles 1102, 1103, 1106, 1107, 1202, 1203, and 1205 any non-conforming measure that existed on 1 January 1994. It claimed the exemption by listing the measures in its Schedule in Annex I. The federal governments of the NAFTA parties prepared their schedules before the agreement came into effect. The Canadian government did not list the CHA, but the CHA is not 'non-conforming.'

Provinces were allowed until 1 January 1996 to list their non-conforming measures. While lists were prepared and exchanged, in the end provinces were allowed to claim the reservation for all non-conforming measures existing on 1 January 1994. Therefore each and every measure of every province affecting the Canadian health-care system that existed on that date is exempt from all the obligations listed above.

The exemption applies to any renewal of such measures and to amendments to such measures that do not make them more non-conforming. However, if a non-conforming measure is repealed or made less non-conforming, it cannot subsequently be reinstated or made more non-conforming.

The Annex I reservation establishes a safe haven that shields all provincial measures implementing the Canadian health-care system existing on 1 January 1994 that do not conform to the foregoing NAFTA provisions. However, the shield is static. While amendments to measures that do not make them more non-conforming are covered by grandfathering, there is always room for debate as to the effect of the amendment. As time goes by and the system evolves and laws change, the safe haven afforded by Annex I becomes less secure.

NAFTA Articles 1108(3) and 1206(3) permitted each NAFTA party to exempt sectors from the application of the foregoing NAFTA articles by listing the sectors in its schedule to Annex II. Unlike Annex I reservations, which do not permit future changes that increase non-conformity, Annex II reservations are absolute. As long as a new measure is covered by the reservation, the new measure can increase the degree of non-conformity with these NAFTA articles.

Canada listed a reservation for social services as follows: 'Canada reserves the right to adopt or maintain any measure with respect to the provision of public law enforcement and correctional services, and the following services to the extent that they are social services established or maintained for a public purpose: income security or insurance, social security or insurance, social welfare, public education, public training, health and child care.'

The United States and Mexico have taken similar reservations. The NAFTA parties accept that the Annex II reservations apply to provincial and state as well as to federal measures.

While the social-services reservation has not been tested, its plain wording is sufficiently broad to cover the purely public component of the health-care system in each province – i.e., payment for insured health services by a provincial public authority. While the services covered are called 'insured' health services, they are paid for directly by the provincial governments or by direct reimbursement to the consumer. Health services are 'social services,' and the 'public purpose' is to ensure universal access to health care. However, how far the Annex II reservation extends beyond this is debatable. It may cover the provision of health services exclusively by non-profit organizations, but it is questionable whether it covers a situation where health services are provided by for-profit entities or by a mix of for-profit and not-for-profit entities.[11]

None of the obligations discussed above existed when the Canadian health-care system was established. All these obligations apply to provincial as well as to federal measures. The obligations under Chapter Eleven have the potential for greater impact than those under Chapter Twelve because of the availability to U.S. and Mexican investors of investor/state dispute procedures described below.

While not affecting the essential characteristics of Canadian health care, the non-discrimination requirements of the national-treatment obligations may affect any aspect of the system that treats U.S. or Mexican firms less favourably than their Canadian counterparts. The other NAFTA obligations discussed above have much less potential effect. The Annex I and Annex II reservations reduce substantially the potential impact of all these obligations. The Annex I reservations provide a safe haven, but one that will erode as the system evolves. The Annex II reservation completely shields the purely public component of Canada's health-care system.

Obligations under Chapters Eleven and Twelve Not Subject to Reservations

The obligations under Chapters Eleven and Twelve of NAFTA that are not subject to reservations are:

- expropriation and compensation (Article 1110)
- minimum standard of treatment (Article 1105)
- transfers (Article 1109)
- licensing and certification (Article 1210)

Of the foregoing, the obligation respecting expropriation and compensation (Article 1110) is by far the most important.

Expropriation and Compensation
NAFTA's Article 1110(1) provides as follows: 'No party may directly or indirectly nationalize or expropriate an investment of an investor of another party in its territory or take a measure tantamount to nationalization or expropriation of such an investment ('expropriation'), except: (a) for a public purpose; (b) on a non-discriminatory basis; (c) in accordance with due process of law and Article 1105(1); and (d) on payment of compensation in accordance with paragraphs 2 through 6.' Paragraphs 2–6 set out rules for calculating compensation.

Article 1110 has the effect of codifying the international-law standard on expropriation. Customary international law requires that states provide compensation to aliens for expropriated property. Several NAFTA Chapter Eleven tribunals have found that the concept of expropriation under Article 1110 is not more expansive than that under international law. The notion of 'tantamount' merely carries into NAFTA the concept of creeping expropriation in customary international law that occurs when a state does not take property outright but applies measures that have the same effect.

That being said, there are difficulties with Article 1110. The domestic law in both the United States and Canada recognizes that many actions taken by the state adversely affect property rights but should none the less not be treated as compensable. The power to regulate without having to compensate is sometimes referred to as the 'police power.' The police power exists under international law. However, unlike in the United States and Canada, where ample jurisprudence defining the police power exists, the notion is poorly developed in international law. Most international jurisprudence, such as that of the Iran–United States Claims Tribunal, has addressed expropriation in circumstances, such as revolution, where regulation of public interest was not an issue.

Substantial interference with business interests has been held by international tribunals and by the NAFTA Chapter Eleven tribunal in

Metalclad Corp. v. The United Mexican States[12] to constitute an expropriation. In the *Metalclad* case the interference obliterated the value of the
investment. Unfortunately, the measure in question was an ecological
decree, and so *Metalclad* has been incorrectly characterized as an
assault on environmental regulation.

Substantial interference could occur in health care in Canada if the
public component of the system were expanded in a way that
increased the exclusion of private firms. For example, suppose that the
decision was taken to include all dental services as 'insured health services,' not just those provided in hospitals. The effect would be that
insurers providing dental coverage would be forced to exit that business. While the decision would have been taken to fulfil the public
purpose of ensuring increased accessibility for those who could not
afford dental coverage or dentist's fees, it is likely that a Chapter
Eleven tribunal would treat this as an expropriation and require the
payment of compensation. The same applies to other health services
such as home care.

Article 1110 does not prohibit expropriation. A provincial government may expropriate so long as the expropriation is for a public purpose (which expanding the public component of health care would
clearly be), is non-discriminatory (which would apply because *all* private insurers are excluded), and is in accordance with due process and
Article 1105 (which would preclude statutory limits on rights to judicial relief), *and* provided that compensation is paid. The fact that Article 1110 does not prohibit expropriation but merely sets conditions on
it means that the article does not prevent the designation of a monopoly. This has a negative consequence, because Article 1110 cannot be
construed as being inconsistent with Article 1502(1), which permits the
designation of a monopoly, because Article 1110 does not prevent the
designation of a monopoly. However, Article 1110 can make the designation of a monopoly much more expensive if private firms that are
excluded from businesses that they formerly carried on have to be
compensated.

Other Obligations

NAFTA's Article 1105(1), on minimum standard of treatment, reads as
follows: 'Each Party shall accord to investments of investors of another
Party treatment in accordance with international law, including fair
and equitable treatment and full protection and security.'

This provision has created considerable interpretive difficulties. On 31 July 2001, the NAFTA Free Trade Commission (NAFTA Commission) adopted an agreed interpretation that construed Article 1105 as applying the minimum standard of treatment under international law and ruled that the references to 'fair and equitable treatment' and 'full protection and security' did not expand on this standard. Article 1131(2) provides that agreed interpretations are binding on Chapter Eleven tribunals.[13]

The minimum standard of treatment under international law is an elusive, imprecise concept. However, Article 1105(1) is not likely to have any impact on the Canadian health-care system as currently structured. A breach of it could be triggered if a decision were taken to extend the public component of the system, such as through the establishment of a universal national home-care program, and affected private firms were expressly denied legal recourse through a privative clause. A denial of access to the court system could constitute a denial of justice, which would constitute a breach of the minimum international-law standard.

Article 1109 prohibits restrictions on repatriation of profits, dividends, and various other payments. It has no effect whatsoever on Canada's ability to maintain its public health-care system.

Article 1210 sets out certain requirements for the licensing of nationals of other NAFTA countries. While the professional service providers referred to in the article include health-care professionals, the article has no impact on Canada's ability to maintain public health care.

The obligations imposed by Article 1110 and 1105 codify international-law standards that existed when Canada set up its health-care system. However, they have far greater impact now because of the NAFTA investor/state procedures described below. Under international law, an investor whose property in another country had been expropriated would have to convince its government to commence proceedings in the International Court of Justice. The proceedings could take many years and would not necessarily ever result in compensation. Under NAFTA, an investor whose property in another NAFTA country is expropriated can commence a Chapter Eleven proceeding against the federal government of the country where the expropriation took place, without the permission or involvement of its own government, and receive compensation.

The obligations imposed by Articles 1109 and 1210 did not exist at the time Canada's public health-care system was established but have no effect on it. The obligations imposed by Articles 1110, 1105, 1109, and 1210 apply to provincial as well as to federal measures. Article 1110 should have no effect on Canadian health care as constituted but would have a major impact if the public component of the system were expanded in any way that hurt private firms. Article 1110 does not prevent the expansion of the system but could make it very expensive.

Similarly Article 1105 should have no impact on public health care as now constituted. However, it would affect any expansion that is coupled with a denial of recourse to the courts by private firms.

GATS and Trade in Services

GATS applies to measures of WTO members affecting trade in services. It defines 'services' broadly and includes any service in any sector except those supplied in the exercise of governmental authority. According to Article I:3(c), 'service supplied in the exercise of governmental authority' means any 'service which is supplied neither on a commercial basis nor in competition with one or more service suppliers.' This definition applies to the purely public component of the Canadian health-care system – i.e., to payment under provincial health-insurance plans for 'insured health services.' Under each provincial plan, the government is acting as an insurer but does not supply such 'insurance' services on a commercial basis because it charges no premiums, or any premiums that are charged are unrelated to risk. The government does not compete with private insurers, which, either by law or as a practical matter, are excluded from this market. The extent to which the GATS 'carve-out' for services supplied in the exercise of governmental authority extends further is debatable. For example, Sinclair and Grieshaber-Otto (2002, 20) question how the carve-out would be applied to situations involving a mix of governmental, private for-profit, and private not-for-profit delivery.[14]

Using the United States and a U.S. service supplier as an example, we see that GATS applies to services supplied by the U.S. supplier from the United States into Canada, in the United States by the U.S. supplier to a Canadian service consumer, by the U.S. supplier through a commercial presence in Canada such as a subsidiary corporation, and by the U.S. supplier through the presence of a U.S. national in Canada. The scope of GATS is broader than NAFTA's Chapter Twelve because GATS covers provision of services from within Canada by a subsidiary of the U.S. service supplier, as well as the cross-border provision of services. However, Chapter Eleven would cover this situation.

Significant GATS Obligations

Schedule of Commitments
Each GATS member, including Canada, completed a schedule of commitments in which it identified the service sectors respecting which it was willing to undertake commitments. Each schedule identifies the sector and lists limitations on market access and national treatment that the member wishes to retain for that sector. Canada has included in its list of sectors 'Life, accident and *health* insurance services' (emphasis added).[15] It lists a number of limitations on market access and national treatment vis-à-vis this sector, but the limitations do not refer to provincial health-insurance plans. Canada has not listed other services relating directly to health care.[16] Some commentators have pointed out that hospital support services such as food, laundry, and janitorial services may be covered by GATS obligations. However, inclusion of such services should have virtually no effect on Canada's ability to maintain public health care.

Market Access and National Treatment
Article XVI requires that each member accord service suppliers of other members, through the modes of supply described above, treatment no less favourable than that specified in its schedule of commitments. Article XVI also prohibits (unless specified in the schedule) certain limitations such as those on the number of service suppliers, or on the value of services or service operations, or on numbers of natural persons employed, or on the form of legal entity or the participation of foreign capital. However, these prohibitions do not include price controls or government-established tariffs of fees for services such as those required by the CHA for insured health services.

Subject to the limitations specified in the schedule of commitments, Article XVII requires for each listed sector that each member shall accord to services and service suppliers of any other member in regard to measures affecting the supply of services treatment no less favourable than it accords to its own like services and service suppliers. This means that the Canadian subsidiary of a U.S.-owned insurance company providing health insurance must be treated no less favourably than its Canadian-owned counterpart.

Most-Favoured-Nation Treatment

Article II requires in connection with measures covered by GATS that each member accord, immediately and unconditionally, to services and service suppliers of any other member, treatment no less favourable than it accords to like services and service suppliers of any other country. Members were permitted to list exemptions, but none of Canada's applies to health care.

As with the most-favoured-nation obligations under NAFTA Articles 1103 and 1203, this obligation has minimal effect on Canada's health-care system, as the measures essential to its continuance do not depend on according more favourable treatment to service and services suppliers of one country as compared to those of other countries.

Monopolies

GATS clearly permits the establishment of monopolies, because Article VIII:1 requires each member to ensure that a monopoly supplier of a service act consistently with the member's obligations under Article II (most-favoured-nation) and its specific commitments. As well, Article VIII:2 provides that a member must ensure that a monopoly supplier does not abuse its non-monopoly position in services outside the scope of its monopoly that are covered by specific commitments. A provincial health-insurance plan could not unfairly compete with private, foreign-owned insurers in the health-insurance market for services outside the scope of 'insured health services.' This GATS provision should not create difficulties: provincial health-insurance plans (which pay for insured health services but not for non-insured services) do not compete with private health insurers, because they serve different markets.

Canada could expand the monopoly rights of the provincial insurance plans by increasing the range of insured health services to include services such as home care. However, since Canada has made a specific commitment on health insurance, its government would have to negotiate a compensatory adjustment with any affected member. The adjustment would take the form of liberalizing commitments in other service sectors and should not be confused with compensation of the sort required under NAFTA Article 1110(1) for expropriation. How onerous this exercise would be would depend on the extent to which the expansion of the monopoly displaced private-sector entities from the market. In the absence of such entities with real economic interest, the obligation to compensate is a purely theoretical concern.

GATS is an entirely new agreement that came into existence on 1 January 1995 and did not exist when Canada's health-care system was created. It covers provincial as well as federal measures.

The exclusion of 'a service supplied in the exercise of governmental authority' from the services covered by GATS is significant, because such exclusion covers the activities of the provincial health-insurance plans in paying for 'insured health services.' The impact of GATS is also muted by the fact that it permits monopoly service suppliers. To the extent, if any, that the health-insurance plans are not excluded by the 'government authority' carve-out, the provincial plans would be subject to the monopoly requirements but none the less permitted. It is unlikely that any provincial plan would have an interest in competing, fairly or unfairly, in the private insurance market.

The market-access and national-treatment provisions under GATS impose obligations vis-à-vis any health service concerning which Canada assumes commitments. So far, its commitments on direct delivery of health services (as distinct from health insurance) are minimal or non-existent. This could change in subsequent negotiating rounds. Canada should carefully assess the impact on the health-care system of each and every health-related commitment that it undertakes in future negotiations.

Other Provisions of the Trade-Liberalizing Agreements with Some Potential Impacts

Provisions with Potential Impact

As we saw above, there are other provisions of the trade-liberalizing agreements that may affect Canadian health care. These relate to intellectual property and subsidies.

Intellectual Property

Both TRIPS and NAFTA Chapter Seventeen set out extensive obligations towards intellectual property rights, including patents. TRIPS establishes a minimum term of protection of twenty years from the date of filing a patent application. Patent owners must be able to prevent third parties from making, using, offering for sale, selling, or importing the patented product during the term of protection. Compulsory licensing, while permitted under limited circumstances, has been significantly curtailed.

Some flexibility is provided through limited-exception provisions. In *Canada – Patent Protection for Pharmaceutical Products*,[17] a WTO panel upheld a provision of Canada's patent legislation challenged by the European Union that permits generic drug producers to make patented drugs for the purposes of testing the generic version before the patent has expired that is of critical importance to Canada's generic-drug industry.[18]

The intellectual-property obligations under TRIPS and NAFTA Chapter Seventeen did not exist when Canada launched its health-care system. The intellectual-property conventions in force at the time, such as the Paris Convention for the Protection of Industrial Property,[19] did not impose hard obligations respecting patents such as exist under TRIPS and NAFTA Chapter Seventeen.

The question of application to provincial governments is irrelevant because the matters covered by TRIPS and Chapter Seventeen, unlike most aspects of the health-care system, fall within exclusive areas of federal jurisdiction.

TRIPS and Chapter Seventeen have no direct impact on Canada's ability to maintain public health care. However, the obligations imposed have an indirect effect on drug prices, through the patent rights enjoyed by brand drug producers and through the limitations placed on compulsory licensing.

Subsidies

GATT 1994 and the Agreement on Subsidies and Countervailing Measures (SCM Agreement)[20] impose disciplines on the granting of subsidies and permit members to impose countervailing duties to offset the effect of subsidized imports that cause material injury to domestic industries. The Canadian health-care system provides a significant advantage to companies with unionized workforces (such as automotive assemblers) in Canada, because those firms do not have to provide health benefits that are a part of the collective agreements of their U.S. counterparts. If public health care is a 'subsidy' under the SCM Agreement, it is unequivocally available widely and not 'specific' within the meaning of the agreement. Countervailing duties may be imposed only against subsidies that are 'specific' as described in the SCM Agreement. Furthermore, subsidies that are not specific are 'non-actionable' and not subject to any of the proceedings that may be taken against 'actionable' subsidies.

Export subsidies, and subsidies that are contingent on the use of domestic over imported goods, violate the SCM Agreement. While the prohibition on export subsidies is irrelevant to Canada's health-care system, any government measure under the system that favoured local over imported goods would be a prohibited subsidy under the SCM Agreement.

While the provisions in GATT 1994 on countervailing duties existed at the time that public health care started in Canada, the SCM Agreement came into existence only in 1995, replacing an earlier, Tokyo Round subsidies code. The agreement is significant for the health-care system in the positive sense that it defines subsidies and the circumstances in which they are actionable, whether through the application of countervailing duties or by invoking dispute-settlement procedures. It is clear that if Canada's system constitutes a subsidy at all, it is non-actionable because non-specific. The provisions in the SCM Agreement on prohibited subsidies are unlikely to be violated by any measure adopted for Canada's health-care system.

Provisions with Minimal Effect

The trade-liberalizing agreements contain many other provisions not discussed above that should have minimal impact on Canada's maintenance of its public health care. These relate to trade in goods, standards, and government procurement.

Trade in Goods

GATT 1994 imposes obligations respecting trade in goods that include most-favoured-nation (MFN) and national treatment, tariff bindings and prohibitions of quotas, and other forms of import and export restrictions. Obligations under GATT 1994 are subject to a number of exceptions, including those relating to health and conservation issues that have been the subject of extensive jurisprudence and on which there are conflicting views.

NAFTA Chapter Three also sets out obligations towards trade in goods. It provides for the elimination of tariffs and imposes certain other obligations. However, the obligations imposed based largely on incorporated provisions of GATT 1994, including its exceptions. NAFTA Chapter Three imposes some conditions on export restrictions in addition to the requirements of GATT 1994.

GATT 1994 carries forward the obligations set out in GATT 1947, before creation of Canada's health-care system. The trade-in-goods provisions in NAFTA did not exist when Canada established public health care, except to the extent that they consisted of incorporated GATT provisions. Both sets of obligations apply to provincial as well as to federal measures. While the trade-in-goods provisions in GATT 1994 and NAFTA may affect health care, including the ability to protect health or the environment through trade-restricting measures, they have virtually no impact on Canada's ability to maintain its health-care system.

Standards

Chapter Nine of NAFTA imposes obligations affecting the establishment of standards for goods and services, and Section B of Chapter Seven establishes obligations towards sanitary and phytosanitary (SPS) measures. These provisions have counterparts in the WTO Agreement. The Agreement on Technical Barriers to Trade (TBT Agreement)[21] imposes obligations concerning technical regulations, standards, and conformity-assessment procedures. The Agreement on Sanitary and Phytosanitary Measures (SPS Agreement)[22] imposes obligations about SPS measures similar to those in NAFTA's Chapter Seven.

SPS measures include measures dealing with contaminants in food and pest control that certainly relate to human health. Both the SPS Agreement and NAFTA's Chapter Seven require a scientific basis for measures and impose least-trade restrictive requirements that worry non-governmental organizations (NGOs) concerned with issues such as genetically modified foods.

The SPS Agreement, the TBT Agreement, and the NAFTA obligations on standards all came into effect after Canada launched public health care. There was an earlier, Tokyo Round agreement on technical barriers to trade, but Canada's health-care system was virtually in place before it took effect.

NAFTA Chapter Nine contains only a best-efforts provision regarding compliance by provincial governments. However, subject to a few exceptions, Section B of NAFTA's Chapter Seven is subject to the provision in NAFTA Article 105 about provincial observance. For the most part, the SPS Agreement and the TBT Agreement apply to regional (i.e., provincial) as well as national measures.

The obligations towards standards imposed by these agreements clearly concern health-related issues, such as those respecting contaminants in food or those that prohibit or prescribe strict rules for handling hazardous materials. However, these obligations have no impact on Canada's ability to maintain its public health-care system.

Government Procurement

The Agreement on Government Procurement (GPA)[23] and Chapter Ten of NAFTA impose obligations respecting government procurement by certain federal (but not provincial) departments and entities that do not affect maintenance of its public health care. Canada was subject to an earlier and less comprehensive Tokyo Round agreement on government procurement, after it launched medicare. Even if payment for insured services by provincial authorities does constitute 'government procurement,' this critical feature of public health care would not be subject to GPA or NAFTA obligations and would be exempt from certain provisions under NAFTA Chapters Eleven and Twelve. However, government procurement for these purposes would probably be interpreted as meaning procurement for government consumption. While insured health services are paid for by provincial authorities, they are consumed by patients.

Dispute Resolution

The impact of the trade-liberalizing agreements on Canadian governments' ability to maintain public health care is affected by the method of dispute resolution under these agreements, which provide the means for challenging non-conforming measures. The more effective the procedures, the greater the potential impact of a successful challenge. This section looks in turn at dispute resolution under the WTO Agreement and under NAFTA.

WTO Agreement

Disputes under the WTO Agreement are resolved through the dispute-settlement procedures set out in the Understanding on Rules and Procedures Governing the Settlement of Disputes (DSU).[24] These are purely state-to-state proceedings. The complaining member country or countries, and the member against which the complaint is made, are the principal parties in these proceedings. Other members have limited rights as third parties. No other entity (including provincial governments, non-governmental organizations, or private firms) has any standing. Disputes are heard by ad hoc panels of three, chosen by the director general of the WTO in consultation with the parties. Panel decisions may be appealed to a standing Appellate Body. Reports of panel and Appellate Body decisions are adopted by the Dispute Settlement Body (DSB) established under the DSU. Unlike under GATT 1947, the member whose measures have been found inconsistent with WTO obligations cannot block adoption of the report. Once the report is adopted, the member country whose measures have been found to be inconsistent with WTO obligations has a 'reasonable period of time' to comply, which can be fixed by arbitration. The DSU permits compensation in lieu of bringing measures into conformity with WTO obligations in limited circumstances. It sets out procedures for determining whether a member has complied with DSB requirements. If a member does not comply, the complaining member can retaliate by withdrawing WTO concessions, but must do so only in accordance with the procedures set out in the DSU. The practical effect of the DSU is that a member whose measures have been found to be inconsistent with WTO requirements has the option of accepting retaliation in lieu of complying.

WTO agreements are interpreted in accordance with the rules of the Vienna Convention on the Law of Treaties (VCLT). The principal rule of interpretation is set out in article 31: a 'treaty shall be interpreted in good faith in accordance with the ordinary meaning to be given to the terms of the treaty in their context and in the light of its object and purpose.' The approach that has been taken by the Appellate Body is strongly textual, with context and object and purpose generally being used to support an interpretation based on text. It tends to favour market-based solutions but has expressed support for the ability of members to adopt certain public-interest measures, such as those protecting the environment.[25] However, if faced with a case involving Canada's health-care system, it is unlikely to be influenced at all by the fact that many Canadians regard the system as a defining national characteristic.

The burden of proof is on the complaining party to establish a prima facie case of violation. The burden then shifts to the other party to establish that a violation has not occurred. The reverse applies to exceptions, with the party claiming the benefit of the exception having to establish that it applies. Exceptions tend to be construed narrowly.

WTO jurisprudence is extensive and reasonably consistent, which is the result of panels being assisted in their deliberations by the staff of the WTO Secretariat and of the Appellate Body.

NAFTA: Chapters Twenty and Eleven

Chapter Twenty of NAFTA provides for state-to-state dispute resolution for virtually all provisions of NAFTA.[26] Its provisions are similar in concept to those in the DSU, but there are differences in detail. Panels, which are ad hoc, consist of five members, with a reverse selection process (i.e., a disputing party selects citizens of the other or another disputing party rather than its own citizens). Panel decisions are final, with no appeal. Compensation is an option in lieu of implementation, and the complaining party may suspend NAFTA benefits. Unlike the DSU, which requires review of retaliatory measures before they are imposed, Chapter Twenty provides only for review after imposition. As under the DSU, only federal governments have standing.

Subject to a few exceptions, a NAFTA party with a complaint about measures of another party can choose between NAFTA and the WTO Agreement. A party will invariably choose the agreement whose dispute-resolution process is most favourable to its case.[27]

NAFTA's Chapter Eleven makes provision for investor/state dispute settlement that supplements the procedures of Chapter Twenty. An investor of a party who has incurred loss or damage, by reason of a breach by another party of an obligation under Chapter Eleven,[28] may initiate arbitral proceedings against the federal government of the party committing the breach, which can lead to an award of monetary damages payable by the federal government.[29] Proceedings may involve provincial measures, but the federal government is liable for the damages. Provincial governments have no standing. An investor can also initiate arbitral proceedings on behalf of an enterprise that it controls of the party committing the breach (for example, a U.S. investor commencing proceedings against Canada on behalf of its Canadian subsidiary) that has incurred damage as the result of a breach. The investor may choose between the Arbitration Rules of the United Nations Commission on International Trade Law (UNCITRAL) and the Additional Facility Rules of the International Centre for the Settlement of Investment Disputes (ICSID).[30] Cases are decided by tribunals of three members, one chosen by the investor, one by the party complained against, and the third (presiding member) by agreement or by the ICSID's secretary. NAFTA Chapter Eleven does not provide for appeal but does not preclude judicial review in the domestic court system.

Like the WTO agreements, NAFTA is interpreted in accordance with the VCLT. However, NAFTA Article 102 sets out expansive objectives that both Chapter Twenty panels and Chapter Eleven tribunals have characterized as 'trade liberalizing.' Panels and tribunals have sometimes used Article 102 as a route to a more 'trade liberalizing' resolution of a dispute than the text would justify.

The approach to burden of proof is similar to that under the DSU, and exceptions tend to be construed narrowly. However, in investor/ state proceedings under NAFTA Chapter Eleven, there is a special rule for determining the applicability of the reservations in the NAFTA annexes. The NAFTA party asserting the reservation as a defence may request an interpretation from the NAFTA Commission as to whether the reservation applies. For example, if Canada asserted that the social-services reservation in Annex II provided a defence, it could request an interpretation from the NAFTA Commission that, if issued within 60 days of the request, would be binding on the tribunal. The position that a U.S. member of the NAFTA Commission would adopt in such a circumstance is difficult to predict. A number of commentators have noted that statements made by the United States Trade Representative shortly after NAFTA was signed indicate a view of the social-services reservation that was much narrower than the Canadian view at the time. However, the positions of all three NAFTA governments since then have hardened against NAFTA Chapter Eleven, and all three NAFTA parties have tended to support each other's positions, including the party whose investor is making a claim.

Such NAFTA jurisprudence as there is has a decidedly ad hoc quality to it. While there is a NAFTA Secretariat, it is skeletal, and panels and tribunals function pretty much on their own. As we saw above, unlike the DSU, NAFTA has no standing Appellate Body. To date, there have been only three Chapter Twenty panel decisions, so it is difficult to predict future actions. Chapter Eleven tribunals have made more decisions. While some themes are developing, the Chapter Eleven decisions are uneven in quality, and, as with Chapter Twenty, it is difficult to make predictions.

The dispute-settlement procedures set up by the DSU did not exist when Canada's public health-care system was established. These procedures are much more effective than those under GATT 1947. The country losing a case can no longer block the adoption of a report, as was the case under GATT 1947. NAFTA Chapter Twenty also provides for reasonably effective dispute-settlement procedures.

The investor/state procedures under NAFTA Chapter Eleven represent a real departure, giving control over whether to initiate a claim to an investor, not to a government.

The existence of effective procedures for settling disputes heightens the impact of these trade-liberalizing agreements. While they clearly do not have the status of domestic law, non-compliance has more immediate consequences than was the case under earlier international agreements.

Yet the trade-liberalizing agreements do not have the same status as a constitution. In Canada, neither the federal government nor a province is required to change any measure just because a WTO or NAFTA panel or tribunal finds a breach. Retaliation under the DSU or NAFTA Chapter Twenty must be proportional to the economic interests affected,[31] and will not have a significant impact unless the economic interests affected are substantial. While the consequences of a damages award under Chapter Eleven are more immediate, only substantial economic interests would generate an award of major concern.

As well, it is not easy for private interests to convince a government to initiate dispute-settlement proceedings. Government agendas do not correspond to private-sector aspirations, and all governments, including the American, have limited capability of pursuing such claims.

While an investor does not need government concurrence to initiate a claim under NAFTA Chapter Eleven, these processes are very expensive. While serving a Notice of Intent to Submit a Claim is easy enough, a proceeding may go through multiple phases and entail several hearings with arbitrators who charge high hourly rates. The amount of money involved must be considerable to make this worthwhile.

Conclusion

The trade-liberalizing agreements described in this paper have established a comprehensive set of norms with which federal and most provincial laws must conform. These norms limit the measures that governments can adopt to protect the public interest. Most of them did not exist when Canada launched public health care. Some that did exist, such as the obligation under customary international law to provide compensation in the event of expropriation, have become much more significant because of effective means of dispute resolution under NAFTA and the WTO. This conclusion examines probable negative effects, likely positive effects, options, and future possibilities.

Negative Potential Impact

The single provision in all the agreements that has the most negative potential impact on Canada's public health care is NAFTA Article 1110 (Expropriation and Compensation). If this provision and the accompanying investor/state dispute-settlement procedures had existed in the 1960s, the system in its present form would never have come into existence. While Article 1110 does not affect the system as it now exists, the requirement to compensate, enforceable through investor/state procedures, makes expansion of the public component impracticable. Article 1110 also makes reduction of the public component irreversible. Once private firms acquire economic interests as the result of deregulation, returning to the status quo ante is possible only on payment of compensation.

The next most significant provisions with negative potential are the requirements of national treatment and market access under NAFTA and GATS. To the extent that these obligations apply, they preclude treating foreign service providers (either within Canada or cross-border) less favourably than their Canadian-owned counterparts. While they may not affect the core of public health care – namely, the payment by provincial health-insurance plans of insured health services – these provisions certainly affect ancillary aspects, especially those that may favour non-profit over for-profit suppliers.

NAFTA's Annex I (grandfathering) reservation and its Annex II (social services) reservation largely shield Canada's health-care system from these NAFTA obligations. However, the Annex I reservation is a one-way street and will erode over time. The Annex II reservation certainly covers the purely public component of health care, but probably not other aspects of the system.

Positive Potential Impact

The potential influence of the trade-liberalizing agreements is not wholly negative for health care. Most provisions have little or no effect, and several have a positive impact.

Notwithstanding the market bias of these agreements, both NAFTA and GATS contain clear statements that parties/member countries may designate and maintain monopolies. The obligations imposed are not onerous, particularly regarding provincial monopolies. The only caveat is that the ability to expand existing monopolies is, for all practical purposes, limited by the obligation to compensate in the event of an expropriation.

The clear definition of subsidies in the SCM Agreement removes once and for all any concern that Canada's health-care system constitutes a countervailable subsidy. U.S. law on countervailing duties historically provided that non-specific subsidies were not countervailable, but its substance and application have been notoriously subject to manipulation by interest groups, and GATT 1947 did not define what constituted a countervailable subsidy. Potential U.S. countervail of Canada's health-care system was a major concern during FTA negotiations. The SCM Agreement has eliminated that issue.

Challenges

The trade-liberalizing agreements present more challenges than opportunities. The opportunities come from trade liberalization in other countries, not within Canada. Trade liberalization in the provision of health-care products and services in other countries may present opportunities to Canadian entrepreneurs in those lines of business, as well as to Canadian private insurance companies looking for foreign markets. However, the regulation of Canada's health-care system is a domestic matter, and the international trading system, as modified by the new agreements, does present some challenges.

As indicated above, any decision to expand the public component of health care (i.e., insured health services being paid for solely by provincial insurance plans) will face the challenge of establishing that the expansion is not an expropriation.

There is considerable pressure on provincial governments to reduce the public component of health care – i.e., to reduce the number of insured health services that must be paid for through a provincial plan. Any province that responds to these pressures should carefully consider the impact of any such reduction, because returning to the public status quo ante could be difficult and expensive.

There is also pressure on provincial governments to open up the public component of health care by allowing patients to arrange their own coverage for insured health services. Under this model, provincial health-insurance plans would pay for insured services for some people, while other people would arrange for coverage through private insurers of these same services. Both NAFTA and GATS clearly permit governments to designate and maintain monopolies. Shared responsibility presents a more complex situation – how to do so without breaching rules respecting public-sector providers competing with private-sector counterparts.

A provincial government runs the risk of eroding the shield to NAFTA challenges afforded by Annex I grandfathering each time it amends its measures that implement its provincial health insurance plan. The challenge is to balance a changing, dynamic system with the benefit of the Annex I reservation. As part of the amending process, authorities should consider carefully the potential effect on the Annex I safe haven.

While it is easy to construct hypothetical worst-case scenarios under the trade-liberalizing agreements, a touch of realism is essential. Consider expropriation, which is the biggest single impediment to expanding the public component of the health-care system. The risk of expropriation claims is proportional to the extent to which private interests are engaged in the affected activity. For example, private insurers in Canada provide dental insurance. If all dental services were designated as insured health services covered exclusively by provincial plans, these insurers would be excluded, and NAFTA Chapter Eleven compensation claims would be likely. However, the situation with home-care services may be quite different. If private insurers are minimally involved in providing coverage for these services, or if such coverage that is provided is not profitable, the risk of claims is low. A risk analysis may disclose that the danger of a challenge or a claim vis-à-vis expansion of public health care under trade liberalization is both limited and manageable.

One dilemma for any expansion of the public component is whether or not to place a privative clause in the implementing legislation that forecloses or limits access to domestic courts. If such a clause is not included, the government may face claims from affected private parties in domestic courts. If one is included, the domestic risk is contained, but a NAFTA Chapter Eleven claim based on a denial of justice under Article 1105 is substantially more likely. Legislators must assessing possible claims and the relative chances under domestic law and NAFTA law of resisting or containing them.

Options

While presenting challenges, the trade-liberalizing agreements also leave ample options to governments as to organization of Canadian health care. Expansion of the public component may be problematic, but the agreements have virtually no impact on maintaining it at its current level.

The agreements also allow governments substantial freedom to regulate so long as they are not exclusionary or discriminatory. Most of the potential negative effect would arise from their excluding private interests from businesses previously open to them or from their discriminating against certain providers of services (for example, for-profit, U.S.-owned providers in favour of non-profit, Canadian-owned providers). The agreements leave governments wide latitude to regulate the terms of service delivery, including prices. As long as such regulations do not fall within the performance requirements prohibited by NAFTA Article 1106 (which are aimed at discriminatory treatment), governments retain a broad power to regulate. The agreements also do little to limit the ability of governments to regulate the prices of goods. While the intellectual-property agreements restrict use of less expensive generic drugs, governments are free to regulate the price of all drugs, including those subject to patents.

The Current Trade Negotiations: Challenges and Opportunities

The WTO Agreement, like GATT 1947 before it, is dynamic in that members periodically participate in major negotiating rounds, the objective of which is further to liberalize trade. As mentioned above, the Doha Round is currently under way. Can Canadian negotiators resist taking on new obligations that could erode the ability of the federal and provincial governments to maintain the health-care system? The most significant challenge will be the negotiation of further specific commitments under GATS. Canadian health-care businesses will seek to increase their ability to expand into markets in other member countries by requesting that the Canadian government increase GATS commitments by those member countries in the sectors in which these businesses wish to expand. There will be corresponding pressure on Canada to assume similar commitments. Canada's negotiators will have to balance the desire of certain Canadian businesses to secure market access in other countries with a need to keep the options open for Canadian governments in domestic health care.

One significant opportunity presented by the new WTO round arises from the heightened concern expressed at Doha with social issues and the ability of countries to address social problems. While the focus will be on the difficulties faced by developing countries, the issues should be the concern of all members. There should be opportunities to advocate new provisions in the WTO Agreement that assist members in, rather than impeding them from, reducing health-care costs.

Unlike the WTO Agreement, NAFTA is static. There has been one agreed interpretation under Chapter Eleven, and there have been some technical changes to certain trade-in-goods provisions. NAFTA Working Groups meet regularly on a variety of issues, but these usually involve technical matters arising from the application of existing NAFTA provisions. With a few minor exceptions, NAFTA does not contain any formal process for periodic negotiations for increased trade liberalization. However, the three NAFTA parties and thirty-one other Western Hemisphere countries are currently negotiating a Free Trade Agreement of the Americas (FTAA). Canadian negotiators will face similar pressures to assume obligations that curtail public involvement in the economy. However, there may also be opportunities in the FTAA negotiations. Negotiators from many countries will be very concerned about preserving and possibly enhancing the right of governments to address social issues. Also, there may be an opportunity to reconsider some of the more intrusive aspects of NAFTA's Chapter Eleven and to increase protection for the right of governments to regulate in the public interest without running the risk of facing compensation claims.

NOTES

1 In some provinces such as Alberta and Ontario, the legislation expressly prohibits private insurers from covering insured services under the Canada Health Act (Flood 1999, 29). However, even if there is no express prohibition, the fact that a provincial authority pays for insured services makes it unfeasible for private insurers to insure these services.
2 Canada is also party to bilateral free-trade agreements with Chile, Costa Rica, and Israel, as well as to bilateral foreign-investment-protection agreements (FIPAs) with a number of developing countries. As the economic interests in Canada of persons in these countries are negligible, the potential impact of these agreements on Canada's health-care system is minimal.
3 Annex 1B of the WTO Agreement.
4 See GATS Article I:3 and Article XXIV:12 of GATT 1994.
5 NAFTA's Chapter Fifteen also establishes obligations respecting state enterprises such as crown corporations. Canada's health-care system in its present form does not depend on the establishment and maintenance of such entities.
6 Annex 1C of the WTO Agreement.
7 Chapter Eleven does not apply to measures covered by Chapter Fourteen (Financial Services). While the definition of financial services in Article

1414 includes 'insurance,' Chapter Fourteen applies only to the cross-
border provision of financial services, which is not relevant to the activities
conducted by the public authorities in each province vis-à-vis health-
insurance plans. There is a corresponding exception in Article 1201(2)(a) for
Chapter Twelve.

8 *Pope & Talbot Inc. v. The Government of Canada* (Phase 2) [unreported (10
April 2001)]. http://www.naftalaw.org.

9 Secretariat File No. USA-MEX-98-2008-01. This case involved cross-border
services rather than investment, but Article 1202 is similar in its structure to
Articles 1102(1) and (2).

10 Article 1106(1)(c).

11 See the discussions of the potential shortcomings of the Annex II reservation in Schwartz 1997 and Appleton 2000, 2–7.

12 *Metalclad Corporation v. The United Mexican States* [unreported, ICSID Case
No. ARB(AF)/97/1 (30 Aug. 2000)]. http://www.naftalaw.org.

13 Investors have challenged the agreed interpretation in several cases. The
Pope & Talbot tribunal (damages phase) was highly critical of the agreed
interpretation but in the end did not challenge its binding character.

14 However, Sinclair and Grieshaber 2002, 21, assume that GATS Article I:3(c)
would be narrowly construed. This does not follow, because Article I:3(c)
defines scope and coverage and is not an exception.

15 CPC 8121.

16 Canada has also excluded certain services relating to health care from
broader service classifications. For example, it has assumed commitments
for wholesale trade services described in CPC 622 but has excluded from
the sector 62551 (pharmaceutical and medical goods) and 62252 (surgical
and orthopaedic instruments and devices).

17 Panel Report WT/DS114/R 7 March 2000.

18 The panel struck down a considerably less significant provision of Canada's patent legislation that permitted a generic manufacturer to produce
and stockpile a product during the six-month period before patent expiry.

19 Both the TRIPS Agreement and NAFTA Chapter Seventeen incorporate its
substantive provisions.

20 Annex 1A of the WTO Agreement.

21 Ibid.

22 Ibid.

23 Annex 4 of the WTO Agreement.

24 Annex 2 of the WTO Agreement.

25 See *United States – Import Prohibition of Certain Shrimp and Shrimp Products*,
Panel Report WT/DS58/R 15 May 1998, Appellate Body Report WT/

DS58/AB/R 12 Oct. 1998. The Appellate Body affirmed the right of the United States to enact the environmental measures in question, which prohibited the importation of shrimp harvested by a method that did not protect sea turtles. The Appellate Body took issue only with the less-than-even-handed application of the measures. This case has been incorrectly characterized as anti-environmental, which it clearly is not.

26 The sole exception is Article 1501, on competition laws.

27 In *Canada – Term of Patent Protection*, Panel Report WT/DS170/R 5 May 2000, Appellate Body Report WT/DS170/AB/R 18 Sept. 2000, the United States chose to challenge Canada's law on the term of patent protection under the DSU because TRIPS was favourable to its case. The corresponding provision in NAFTA Article Seventeen expressly permitted the term of protection provided by Canada.

28 Or of Articles 1502(3)(a) or 1503(2), which require that governmental authority delegated to a monopoly or state enterprise be exercised consistently with certain NAFTA provisions, including Chapter Eleven.

29 A tribunal cannot award punitive damages or order a party to change its law.

30 NAFTA Article 1120(1)(a) provides a third option – namely the International Centre for the Settlement of Investment Disputes (ISCID) Convention – but, as Canada is not yet a party to that convention, this option is not as yet available.

31 See DSU Article 22(4) and NAFTA Article 1029(1).

REFERENCES

Appleton, Barry. 2000. Opinion letter to Michael McBane, National Coordinator, Canadian Health Coalition re: NAFTA Investment Chapter Implications of Alberta Bill 11, 10 April.

Flood, Colleen M. 1999. 'The Structure and Dynamics of Canada's Health Care System.' In Jocelyn Downie and Timothy Caulfield, eds., *Canadian Health Law and Policy.* Toronto: Butterworths, 5–50.

Schwartz, Bryan. 1997. 'NAFTA Reservations in the Areas of Health Care.' *Health Law Journal* 5: 99–117.

Sinclair, Scott, and Jim Grieshaber-Otto. 2002. *Facing the Facts: A Guide to the GATS Debate.* Ottawa: Canadian Centre for Policy Alternatives.

12 The Effects of International Trade Agreements and Options for Upcoming Negotiations

RICHARD OUELLET

For half a century now, particularly since 1994, Canada has been a member of or party to a number of agreements on economic integration. These arrangements may be bilateral (for example, the Canada–Chile Free Trade Agreement), regional (the North American Free Trade Agreement [NAFTA]), or multilateral (the General Agreement on Tariffs and Trade [GATT] and the World Trade Organization [WTO]). Irrespective of their geographical scope, they all affect the role of Canadians' governments and many aspects of their lives.

As concrete expressions of the globalization phenomenon, these agreements affect the most significant areas of human activity, including the provision of health care. Many experts say unequivocally that the globalization of the economy poses a major challenge to national health-care policies. 'Globalization is one of the key challenges facing health policy makers and public health practitioners ... While there is a growing literature on the importance of globalization for health ... there is no consensus either on the pathways and mechanisms by which globalization affects the health of populations or on the appropriate policy responses. There is, however, an increasing tension between the rules, actors, markets that characterize the modern phase of globalization and the ability of countries to protect and promote health' (Woodward et al., 2001, 875).

There are essentially two sources for the growing tensions between health and freedom of trade. The first is the magnitude of the interests at stake. On the one hand, there are enormous business interests linked to health-care–related activities. Recent publications provide the clearest possible illustrations of the gains to be made, for example, from the provision of health services and the manufacture of drugs (Lexpert, March 2002, 64; *Business Week*, 28 May 2001, 40; Vellinga 2000, 130–9; WTO 1998a, 2–9). Yet, as one can imagine, there are social and health interests affecting Canadians' rights to accessible and quality health care. These rights are enshrined in domestic legislation, but they also reflect fundamental rights recognized in international instruments such as the Universal Declaration of Human Rights (article 25, para. 1) and the International Covenant on Economic, Social and Cultural Rights (article 12).

Second, recent economic agreements have opened to market forces a whole range of areas of activity that directly, indirectly, or potentially affect trade in health-related goods and services. Even today, however, it is hard to gauge accurately the potential impact of such agreements as NAFTA or the General Agreement on Trade in Services (GATS, of the WTO) in opening up markets for health care. Canadians legitimately want to know more about the long-term consequences of trade commitments entered into by their federal government, which are likely to change their health-care systems. This second source of tension is the subject of this study.

To gauge fully their effects, I examine first the legal scheme of Canada's major economic agreements. To that end I review their key provisions vis-à-vis health services in Canada. I note the somewhat ambivalent status assigned to health care in the commercial rules that now prevail. I also attempt to determine which agreements may materially affect Canadian health systems. Second, I consider potential approaches to health that Ottawa might adopt in ongoing multilateral trade negotiations and assess how best Canadian governments might reconcile trade and economic commitments with a responsive health system.

The purpose of this study is not to describe Canadian health-care systems or to assess citizens' expectations about them, but rather to explain how Canada has undertaken to 'liberalize' its health-care system, and how it may reconcile its international economic commitments with Canadians' desires vis-à-vis health care.

Effects of the Major Agreements

The general objective of this first section is to compile and review the provisions of international economic agreements that may affect the capacity of Canadian governments to adopt and maintain health-care measures. In addition to outlining arguments that could be used against Canada in a potential dispute, this inventory allows us to determine which agreements have the most significant bearing on Canadian health systems. The agreements examined here fall into three categories: multilateral, regional, and bilateral. Each category has displayed a particular approach with regard to health care. Some of these approaches form the basis for comments in the second section of the study.

Multilateral Agreements

Among Canada's multilateral trade agreements, it is essentially the WTO Agreements that currently affect health measures in Canada. I look in turn at GATT, GATS, and, collectively, the other relevant multilateral agreements.

The General Agreement on Tariffs and Trade (GATT)

Fundamental Principles. Immediately following the Second World War, the General Agreement on Tariffs and Trade (GATT) introduced new trade rules designed to liberalize international commercial transactions. A number of key principles put in place then have since become the foundation of most international trade agreements, especially the principle of non-discrimination and the prohibition of quantitative restrictions. I describe these last two fundamental principles, which entail the liberalization of trade in products. These principles have a particular significance as they are replicated in virtually all international economic agreements. I then consider major exceptions to these principles.

Principle of Non-Discrimination. The principle of non-discrimination hinges on two rules: most-favoured-nation treatment (article I of GATT) and national treatment (article III). Under article I, each member of the WTO must automatically extend to all others a treatment as favourable as that granted to any other country. Thus such treatment guarantees equal terms of market access to all trading partners. Linked with this rule is that on national treatment, which requires that each member grant to the products of all other members the treatment that it gives to its own products. This rule applies to all national measures of internal taxation and regulation. For example, all measures affecting the sale, purchase, transportation, or distribution of products must apply in the same way to both national products and like imported products.

Prohibition of Quantitative Restrictions. Quantitative restrictions generally take the form of quotas, licences, or other measures designed to limit the import of foreign products onto the national territory or the export of national products. Such restrictions therefore operate to disrupt if not to prevent trade in certain products. Article XI of GATT prohibits such restrictions.

There are, however, two types of exceptions to these basic principles, under article XX and under article III.

GATT Provisions. A number of provisions in GATT allow members of the WTO to take restrictive measures in relation to health products. This is the general exception that appears in article XX of GATT and in certain special regimes established by other GATT provisions.

The General Exception in Article XX(b). Article XX sets out some general exceptions for which the principles of the agreement will not apply, thereby recognizing the special nature of certain fundamental interests such as public morals, health, and the preservation of natural resources and national treasures. Thus, under certain conditions, measures 'necessary to protect human, animal or plant life or health' are compatible with GATT provisions.

The terms of implementation of article XX are restrictive, since they are subject to a number of cumulative conditions. First, the contentious measure must concern one of the interests appearing in one of the paragraphs of article XX – in this instance, the protection of health and human life. It is not sufficient that the measure be referred to in one of the paragraphs, it must also be necessary under the language of the preamble of article XX. This necessity criterion implies that the measure must not be excessive in relation to the contemplated purpose, that there exists a causal relationship between the measure and the intended objective, and that other means, less restrictive to the free movement of trade, do not exist. Furthermore, the preamble of article XX adds a major limitation, since the measure must not be used 'in a manner which would constitute a means of arbitrary or unjustifiable discrimination between countries where the same conditions prevail, or a disguised restriction on international trade.'

The scope of this exception has been amended over time. Quasi-judicial bodies of the WTO have not always given it the same purview. So this exception does have its own limits and risks.

Other GATT Provisions that Allow an Override of the Fundamental Principles. Article III: 8 (b) allows members that so desire to grant subsidies exclusively to domestic producers. Canada could therefore grant subsidies in such areas of activity as the manufacture of health equipment and drugs. Since 1995, article III: 8 (b) must be assessed in the light of the Subsidies and Countervailing Duties Agreement, which I examine below.

GATT legal regime therefore, requires that Canada comply with certain rules of equality of treatment between nations and between similar or competing products. It also allows for some special circumstances where Canada could derogate from these obligations, particularly in regard to health protection. GATT thus commits WTO members to general liberalization of trade in products while recognizing that health-related issues may enjoy a certain special status. I now look at how the GATS regime differs significantly from GATT's.

The General Agreement on Trade in Services (GATS)
As the Canadian minister of international trade has stated, health services available in Canada are excluded at this time from the application of GATS: "'I would like to stress that we will maintain and preserve the ability of all levels of government to regulate and set policy in areas of importance to Canadians," added Minister Pettigrew. '*We will not negotiate our health*, public education or social *services ...*" ' (add source).

It is true that each member of the WTO retains discretion to submit or not each services sector covered by the agreement to the major rules of GATS. As we see in greater detail below, Canada is fully entitled under GATS not to undertake to comply with its rules of market access and national treatment. It is up solely to Canada to decide the extent of its commitments to liberalize health services provided on its territory. Nevertheless, in examining the legal regime of GATS, I note that the provision of health services may, at least indirectly or potentially, already be affected by this accord. To gauge the GATS legal regime's ambivalence in regard to health services, I first analyse GATS's notion of service. I next consider the GATS provisions leading to gradual liberalization of health services. Finally, I examine the provisions allowing special status for the protection of health.

The Notion of Service. GATS does not provide an explicit definition of the notion of services. It defines only trade in services and, four modes of service. Article I, paragraph 2:

> trade in services is defined as the supply of a service:
> (a) from the territory of one Member into the territory of any other Member;
> (b) in the territory of one Member to the service consumer of any other Member;
> (c) by a service supplier of one Member, through commercial presence in the territory of any other Member;
> (d) by a service supplier of one Member, through presence of natural persons of a Member in the territory of any other Member.

Article I, paragraph 3(b), states that 'services' include '*any service in any sector* except services supplied in the exercise of governmental authority' (emphasis added). Article I, paragraph 3(c), provides that '"services supplied in the exercise of governmental authority" means any service which is supplied *neither on a commercial basis, nor in competition with one or more service suppliers*' (emphasis added). As some specialists note, this description encompasses all services, including health (Vellinga 2000, 138, 152; Pollock and Price 2000, 1996). As such, health services are thus covered by this WTO agreement.

However, in some situations and under some conditions, health services do not fall within the scope of GATS. Article I, paragraphs 3(b) and 3(c), exempts services supplied in the exercise of governmental authority. Thus, where only government provides health-care services on a non-commercial basis without competing with one or more service suppliers, health services are then excluded from the GATS. Moreover, if some services linked to health care supplied in the exercise of governmental authority are so provided on a commercial basis or in competition with private suppliers, the GATS provisions will cover the latter. In this regard, the WTO background note is explicit: 'The hospital sector in many countries, however, is made up of government- and privately-owned entities which both operate on a commercial basis, charging the patient or his insurance for the treatment provided. Supplementary subsidies may be granted for social, regional and similar policy purposes. It seems unrealistic in such cases to argue for continued application of Article 1:3 and/or maintain that no competitive relationship exists between the two groups of suppliers or services' (WTO 1998a, 11).

This statement has been relevant to Canada since the Alberta government opened the possibility private entities might provide some health services. Consequently, in the context of multilateral trade rules, its authorization of commercial provision of some health services could effectively exclude such services throughout Canada from the notion of 'public services.'

GATS does not clearly define services and public services. To establish clearly whether a service is likely to be covered by the GATS rules, we must first determine whether public authorities provide it non-commercially and non-competitively. But, as we can see in Canada, governments have a choice between opening and not opening the provision of health-care services to market forces. The application of the GATS general obligations and disciplines to health services depends not only on Canada's commitments or on exemptions under this agreement, but also on the possibility of its passing legislation allowing competition between public and private suppliers. In Canada, jurisdiction over health belongs to the provinces, and they may exclude health services provided on their territory from the notion of public services.

Liberalization of Health Services. As in the GATT framework, most-favoured-nation (MFN) treatment and national treatment underlie trade liberalization in GATS. Furthermore, the annex on financial services also relates to the insurance sector, especially with regard to health insurance.

Most-Favoured-Nation Treatment (Article II). One of the most important GATS obligations is most-favoured-nation (MFN) treatment, found in article II, paragraph 1: 'With respect to any measure covered by this Agreement, each Member shall accord immediately and unconditionally to services and service suppliers of any other Member treatment no less favourable than that it accords to like services and service suppliers of any other country.' However, paragraph 2 allows some temporary easing in the liberalization of certain services: 'A Member may maintain a measure inconsistent with paragraph 1 provided that such a measure is listed in, and meets the conditions of, the Annex on Article II Exemptions.' Thus paragraph 2 substantially diminishes the scope of paragraph 1, since it allows a member, under certain conditions, to circumvent the principle contained in paragraph 1.

To find out which health services are exempted, one must consult the schedule in the annex. At the close of the Uruguay Round of GATT, eight countries exempted their professional services and certain medical, health, and social services from MFN treatment: Bulgaria, Costa Rica, Cyprus, the Dominican Republic, Honduras, Panama, Turkey, and Venezuela (WTO, S/C/W/50, 18 Sept. 1998, 18, 28). Canada has made no such exemption for health services. Thus, to the degree that health care is subject to GATS – discussed more specifically below in connection with market access – Canada is bound to comply with paragraph 1.

Market Access and National Treatment (Articles XVI and XVII). During the negotiations on trade in services, the member countries hoped to proceed with a progressive liberalization of services (article XIX), so that market access and national treatment are not yet general obligations. In fact, the relevant provisions appear not in the general the GATS obligations, but only in the part listing each member's specific commitments, as recorded in the national schedules.

Article XVI states that 'each Member shall accord services and service suppliers of any other Member treatment no less favourable than that provided for under the terms, limitations and conditions agreed and specified in its Schedule.' Article XVII says, 'In the sectors inscribed in its Schedule, and subject to any conditions and qualifications set out therein, each Member shall accord to services and service suppliers of any other Member, in respect of all measures affecting the supply of services, treatment no less favourable than that it accords to its own like services and service suppliers.'

How the two rules are applied depends therefore on each member's specific commitments. The schedules detail areas of commitment, the degree of openness negotiated, and the exceptions to national treatment. Commitments are thereby consolidated – that is, the member may no longer reopen them or, if the member does, will have to bear the related costs by granting compensation to members adversely affected (article XXI of GATS). Thus members that have made specific commitments in the health-services sector will have to comply with those commitments.

A background note on health and social services the Council on Trade in Services of the WTO provides some clarification on members' commitments (WTO, S/C/W/50, 18 Sept. 1998, 15, 25). 'Schedules do not necessarily provide an accurate, let alone comprehensive, picture of actual trade and market conditions' (15). As well, 'Members generally found it easier to make commitments on health-related professional services (medical and veterinary services, etc.) than on "genuine" health and social services' (16). The note explains that in relation to modes of delivery 1, 2, and 3 (described above), 49 members have made commitments concerning medical and dental services, and 39 for hospital services; most of these members are developing countries. In relation to mode 4, of the 55 members that have committed themselves concerning medical, dental, and veterinarian services, two have not specified any limitation, while all the others substantially limited the scope of their commitments (18). Canada has made no commitment in this regard, since its schedule makes no reference to any such commitments (WTO, the GATS, Canada, SC/16, 15 April 1994).

A priori, since Canada has made no specific commitments on health-related services, it is under no obligations in such matters. However, GATS includes an annex on financial services that may affect health insurance.

The Annex on Financial Services. This annex covers measures that hinder or prevent the supply of financial services. Among services covered are those supplied in the exercise of governmental authority, which include '(b) ... (ii) *activities forming part of a statutory system of social security or public retirement plans*; and (iii) other activities conducted by a public entity for the account or with the guarantee or using the financial resources of the Government' (emphasis added).

At least one commentator argues that, in view of the definitions cited above, Canada's commitments with regard to financial services probably have some impact on health-insurance plans (Sanger, 2001, 75).

GATS Provisions Guaranteeing a Specific Status for Health. GATS includes some general exceptions, with one of them for health protection. This recent agreement also provides for gradual liberalization of services. Other provisions contain standards that remain tentative.

The General Exception (Article XIV). Article XIV of GATS – the corollary of article XX of GATT – lists some general exceptions: 'Subject to the requirement that such measures are not applied in a manner which would constitute a means of arbitrary or unjustifiable discrimination between countries where like conditions prevail, or a disguised restriction on trade in services, nothing in this Agreement shall be construed to prevent the adoption or enforcement by any Member of measures: ... (b) necessary to protect human, animal or plant life or health.'

No WTO Panel has yet had occasion to interpret this provision. Owing to similarities between this provision and GATT's article XX, it is conceivable that the same restrictive conditions apply. The protection of health is therefore recognized, but it has an exceptional status.

Progressive Liberalization (Article XIX). Article XIX, dealing with progressive liberalization, might actually allow members that so desire not to liberalize their health services. The first sentence in its paragraph 2 states: 'The process of liberalization shall take place with due respect for national policy objectives and the level of development of individual Members, both overall and in individual sectors.'

Health is an area included in a state's national policy objectives. Accordingly, it seems that a member could argue that total liberalization of health services would conflict with its national health policy.

Other WTO Agreements
Besides the GATT of 1994 and GATS, other WTO agreements – TRIPS and SPS – may have consequences for national measures directly or indirectly affecting health.

Agreement on Trade-Related Aspects of Intellectual Property Rights (TRIPs). A comprehensive analysis of the impact of the TRIPs Agreement requires expert knowledge of the national and international rules of intellectual property, which I do not possess. I limit myself here to a few general remarks about its substantial impact on health systems, particularly on drugs.

The TRIPs Agreement affects intellectual property rights associated with certain products such as drugs. These rights are intended to reserve the commercial use of a product for a limited period in order to cover research and development costs.

TRIPs and, more generally, the intellectual property regimes of the industrialized countries have been much criticized for exerting upward pressure on drug prices by substantially restricting the marketing opportunities for generic drugs. In developing countries, access to some drugs is also virtually ruled out by what many see as pharmaceutical companies' excessive protection of their patents. The Doha Conference in 2001 and the ensuing negotiations have begun to tackle this sensitive issue.

Agreement on the Application of Sanitary and Phytosanitary Measures (SPS Agreement). This WTO agreement essentially governs the measures that WTO members apply at their borders to protect the health and life of humans and animals and to preserve plant life within their territory. Obviously, it affects the provision of health care only indirectly, but its structure provides an example of the proper balancing of free trade with the right to health.

The SPS Agreement clearly establishes that each WTO member must determine its own level of SPS protection against parasites, illnesses, and pathogenic organisms. To adopt and apply the SPS measures of its choice, a member must prove scientifically that such measures are necessary for it to achieve its stated level of SPS protection. For example, if it determines the level by reference to the goal of minimizing negative effects on trade, and if the measure applied restricts trade no more than is necessary to obtain that level, it will be judged consistent with GATT, specifically with article XX(b), discussed above.

The rules under this agreement, consistent with members' intentions in health while not inconsistent with trade liberalization, should, I believe, be a source of inspiration for the future. What the agreement allows in terms of safety and wholesomeness of food should be replicable in health care. Each state should be able to determine the level of care that it seeks for its citizens, and any liberalization of trade in goods and services should be consistent with this guaranteed level of care. I reconsider this point in the paper's final recommendations.

Regional Agreements

The commitments made by the three contracting states in NAFTA reflect a regime that differs from that of the multilateral trade system. Although this instrument was negotiated concurrently with the WTO agreements – in the early 1990s, Canada, the United States, and Mexico chose not to establish general agreements with specific features and applications spelled out in sectoral agreements or through schedules containing piecemeal commitments. Rather, they created a single document that is divided into parts and chapters comprising general commitments to liberalize trade and detailed rules of application. Voluminous annexes contain reservations where each party indicates both those sectors of investment and trade in services to which the provisions of the agreement do not apply and those sectors where it reserves the right to maintain, adopt, and apply in future measures that are not consistent with the terms of the agreement. Thus, as we see below, it is fairly easy to determine, from reading the annexes, which aspects of Canada's health systems are likely to be covered by the commitments to liberalization contained in the agreement.

I describe, first, NAFTA provisions that could affect trade in health-related goods and, second, provisions on trade and investment in services that may affect the provision of health care. But we will pay particular attention to the reservations and exceptions which, at least until now, have kept NAFTA from having a direct and tangible application in the health services sector.

Trade in Goods under NAFTA

Like all international economic agreements, and like GATT, NAFTA contains many articles that apply the principle of non-discrimination between goods and that facilitate trade in those goods through the abolition of tariff and non-tariff barriers. Part II of NAFTA sets out the rules of national treatment, MFN treatment, market access, and export subsidies in terms similar to, if not identical with, GATT's. Part III, specifically the chapter on standards-related measures, is a close relative of the WTO's Agreement on Technical Barriers to Trade. Chapter 10 deals with government procurement and could affect trade in goods related to health care. Though circumscribed by many exceptions and rules dealing with the tendering entity, type of goods purchased, and contract price, it could in principle apply to the purchase by a Canadian public entity of health-related goods. Finally, chapter 17, which essentially forces the three parties to protect intellectual property rights, may relate to trade in drugs, just as does TRIPs. Some studies indicate that NAFTA-driven increases in patent protection of pharmaceuticals and elimination of compulsory licences have significantly raised prices drugs in Canada (Anderson et al. 1997; Lexchin 2001).

These provisions on trade in goods may all therefore influence trade in various health-related goods. However, they have not led to any significant change in Canada's health system, in its supply of health care, or in governments' capacity to provide the care that Canadians desire. NAFTA's possibly relevant provisions are primarily those that affect investment and services.

Investment and Trade in Services under NAFTA

Chapters 11 and 12 of NAFTA deal with investments and trade in services, but two annexes to NAFTA have prevented chapters 11 and 12 from having any real effect on health care.

Chapter 11 has three sections. Section A sets out the rules relating to the treatment that each NAFTA party must grant to investors and investments originating from the other two countries. Section B governs the dispute-settlement process between a NAFTA party and an investor from another party. Section C contains a series of definitions applicable to the terms and expressions commonly used in chapter 11.

Section A is relevant to our study, since it lays down (essentially in articles 1101–7) the parties' substantive obligations. It formulates rules without reference to the specific commercial activity targeted by the investment. For example, nothing in articles 1101–7 would seem to bar U.S. or Mexican investors or investments from entering Canada's health sector. Only article 1108, through exceptions and a reference to reservations found in annexes I to IV, intimates possible application of chapter 11 to Canadian health care. But articles 1101–8 make it clear that, for all intents and purposes, Canada has not undertaken to comply with chapter 11 in health care. Through reservations that it has recorded in various NAFTA annexes, Canada has retained the power to override the chapter's most important obligations, doing so most clearly and completely in annex II, at page II-C-a of the Canadian edition of NAFTA, relating to social services as a group. In addition to applying to pre-NAFTA measures in Canada, it covers the social-service measures that Canada will adopt and apply subsequently. Canada's reservation of its right to override the national treatment rule (article 1102) and the rule on senior management and boards of directors (article 1107) reads as follows:

Cross-Border Services and Investment
Canada reserves the right to adopt or maintain any measure with respect to the provision of public law enforcement and correctional services, and the following services to the extent that they are social services established or maintained for a public purpose: income security or insurance, social security or insurance, social welfare, public education, public training, health, and child care.

In legal terms, it is hard to define the resulting protection to the Canadian health system (Johnson 1998, 235). However, through this reservation and others, more general, pertaining to all sectors of economic activity, Canada has so far excluded health services from NAFTA's investment rules.

Chapter 12 of NAFTA, on cross-border trade in services, contains some general commitments to liberalize certain economic activities. In theory, nothing there prevents health services from being covered by NAFTA. Only paragraph 3(b) of article 1201 might put a damper on these general commitments, where it states that the parties cannot be prevented from providing certain social services. '3. Nothing in this Chapter shall be construed to: ... (b) prevent a Party from providing a service or performing a function such as law enforcement, correctional services, income security or insurance, social security or insurance, social welfare, public education, public training, health, and child care, in a manner that is not inconsistent with this Chapter.'

This paragraph is at the least obscure. Apparently the provisions of chapter 12 do not prevent NAFTA parties from providing services in a manner that is not inconsistent with the provisions of chapter 12! If this paragraph is suggesting that governments may continue to provide some social services, it is not clear what exactly these governments may do. The reservations to which article 1206 refers indicate the limits of Canada's commitments to liberalization of health services.

The reservations on application of chapter 12, particularly the one on page II-C-a, are the same as those that apply to chapter 11. The Canadian health system has thus been protected from the consequences of NAFTA's liberalization of services.

Chapter 16 of NAFTA relates to the temporary admission of business persons and has close links in its application to cross-border trade in services. It sets out a few guidelines as to the rules that a NAFTA party may apply when deciding to allow (or not) a national from another party to enter its territory to conduct business. The annexes to chapter 16 state quite precisely and comprehensively the classes of business persons involved. Annex 1603 – more precisely, appendix 1603.D.1 – provides for the temporary admission of physicians only for teaching or research activities. NAFTA says nothing about the admission, even temporary, of U.S. or Mexican physicians to Canada to practise medicine. This is therefore an additional obstacle to Canada's opening the market in health services to its NAFTA partners.

NAFTA has not yet appreciably affected Canadian governments' ability to maintain the health system and to provide health care as established in legislation. However, as we see in the second section of this study, the approach adopted in NAFTA – making general commitments and circumscribing them through reservations – is risky; it could in future fail to provide sufficient protection to the publicly funded health system.

Bilateral Agreements

Canada is a party to 25 bilateral economic agreements that are currently in force. To my knowledge, none of them materially affects health care in Canada. Twenty-two of them aim at protecting foreign investments; their complete texts are available on the web site of the Department of Foreign Affairs and International Trade. Canada conducts little or almost no trade with the vast majority of the countries with which it has signed these agreements. Strictly speaking, their acknowledged potential effects on Canada's health care are virtually nil. Moreover, the most recent – an agreement with Croatia to promote and protect investments, which came into force at the end of 2001 – includes, in an annex, exceptions to national treatment that cover social services, including health services. So there seems to be little to fear about the potential effects of such agreements.

The other three trade agreements involve Chile, Costa Rica, and Israel. Though much less complete and comprehensive than NAFTA, they resemble it in structure. All three are clearly oriented towards liberalization of trade in goods and reduction in tariffs. Only one (with Chile) contains separate provisions on cross-border trade in services; an annexed reservation is identical to the one found at page II-C-8 of NAFTA, reproduced above. Thus, on the bilateral level, Canada appears to have used the reservations approach in order to shield our health systems from the effects of international economic agreements.

Health Care and the Upcoming Trade Negotiations

The provisions in the major international instruments to which Canada adheres that could affect the Canadian health system indicate that the interface between health care and trade varies substantially among agreements. In NAFTA and in at least one bilateral agreement, Canada has undertaken in principle to liberalize trade in goods and services while including or annexing reservations and exceptions covering health care. As we saw above, a completely different regime has operated in the WTO. In Part III of GATS, which addresses market access and national treatment, there is no general commitment or reservation or exception – only piecemeal commitments by each member. Other WTO agreements explained briefly above do not contain any reservations, exceptions, or possibility for piecemeal undertakings. Rather, they, like the SPS Agreement, balance freedom of trade and protection of health.

So far, these approaches have not conflicted. Canada has not had to limit the meaning of its commitments or reservations about health care in one agreement in order to comply with its commitments in another. Its position on liberalization of health care thus seems consistent. But this consistency is only apparent and could be temporary. In any event, it is rather fragile.

The country is now engaged in major trade negotiations leading potentially to instruments that could all liberalize health care. As for multilateral negotiations, the Doha agenda contemplates renegotiation of GATS. Negotiations towards a Free Trade Area of the Americas (FTAA) proceed on the basis of NAFTA. Both cases may lead to increased liberalization of trade, particularly in services. It is conceivable therefore that new international agreements will differ from each another as much as do NAFTA and GATS — each with its own interpretation and features. Reservations and exceptions, so far the preferred approach at the regional level, and the piecemeal commitments of GATS may ultimately lead to contradictory and irreconcilable documents. General commitments (accompanied by reservations and exceptions) and some piecemeal commitments could make it extremely difficult to define Canada's commitments to liberalization.

Consequently, we would like to emphasize the risks related to the two approaches favoured in the NAFTA and the GATS and to stress the need for Canada and any other state keen to define the dimensions of health care that it hopes to open to adopt an overall approach so that citizens and governments can understand what is subject to international competition and what is protected.

This section complements the first section, which described all the agreements that can affect the health system. From the standpoint of international trade law, it presents two ways – reservations and exceptions, and piecemeal commitments – to ensure maintenance of a public system compatible with Canada's agreements. As I explain, whichever orientation Canadians and their governments choose, it is now urgent to present and defend internationally a clear and firm stand that has the same meaning in trade agreements. By way of conclusion, I venture some suggestions as to Canada's approach in current trade negotiations.

Risks of the Reservations and Exceptions Approach

This approach prevails in NAFTA and Canada's bilateral agreements on trade in services. Ultimately, it entails some risks. On the one hand, reservations and exceptions are always interpreted in a restrictive manner. Thus some services that Canada sees as covered might not seem so to trading partners or to a panel arbitrating a dispute between Canada and another party seeking access to Canada's health-care market for one of its nationals.

On the other hand, some reservations and exceptions are intended to circumvent the effect of general rules. However, in the FTAA talks, rules, not exceptions, are the main concern. The rules are aimed at liberalizing trade, not at protecting social services. The negotiated texts open up markets in accordance with agreed-on rules. If protection of health care appears not in the rules but solely in exceptions, protection of health care may become less important. Thus the balance sought by the Canadian government between opening foreign markets and protecting health care is secured by legal provisions that are unequal. A rule enshrines the goal of opening markets, but only an exception protects the health systems. Before deciding to value protection of the health system less than opening markets, shouldn't the federal government assess Canadians' priorities? What values should be enshrined in a broad rule, and what others, possibly in contradiction with freer trade, would warrant instead an exception?

Risks of the Piecemeal-Commitments Approach

The approach adopted by the WTO members in GATS – piecemeal commitments – would mean that only WTO members that have specifically undertaken to do so must provide access to their national market. A priori, if Canada has made no commitment with regard to health services, it need not admit private suppliers of such services. Therefore the risks do not lie in the wording of the commitments. A WTO member that remains silent about a service sector is not required to give access to its market in that sector. The risks, however, lie in the negotiation of commitments made by each WTO member. Because each member wants its nationals to be able to offer specific services to other members with attractive markets, give-and-take bidding ensues. For example, in return for access to markets in financial or professional services, some members will concede access to other services sectors such as transportation and audiovisual services. In the process, all services covered by GATS are likely to enter the negotiations. Political or economic pressures may then be exerted on a WTO member to open its market in specific services. Since, as we saw above, health services are potentially covered by GATS, the gradual liberalization of trade in services will eventually encompass health services. Here again, while this approach has protected health care until now, it is fraught with limitations and pitfalls.

Risks Related to the Absence of a Comprehensive Approach

The two agreements with the strongest potential impact on health – GATS and NAFTA – conflict with each other in at least one respect. In GATS, a WTO member's silence on access to a service sector allows it to protect that sector from foreign competition. But in NAFTA, a party must be explicit in its reservations if it wishes to exempt a service from application of the agreement. In two major rounds of trade negotiations – the WTO and the FTAA – Canada is using these contradictory approaches. Yet it must articulate a consistent global policy towards trade in health services. Pressed on all sides by various stakeholders, it has to defend a common policy and express its position through commitments (or lack thereof) in one forum and through reservations and exceptions in the other. Moreover, the ultimate goal – explicitly for the WTO – is liberalization of trade in services. If Canada wishes to argue that its health system is not negotiable, and if, above all, it seeks to ensure that international economic agreements have no bearing on national health policies, it should, in our view, spell out these principles explicitly in provisions and no longer express them simply through silence or through exceptions in annexes.

Concluding Remarks

Although Canada has used the latitude provided in the agreements to protect its health system, this latitude is quickly shrinking, in my view, and may no longer allow Canada to make international trade commitments that are consistent with the preferences of Canadians as to the effects, or lack of effect, that these agreements should have on their health systems. There are risks inherent in relying on exceptions or on piecemeal commitments, and they will surely increase with the FTAA and WTO talks. It is time for Canada to develop a single, clear position that it can express in the same terms, in all forums.

It should start to promote an international instrument that balances and opposes the principles of free trade with the principles of a public system of health care. The SPS Agreement, analysed above, might serve as a guide. Such an instrument should enable each state to establish, without risk of challenge, the desired level of public health services. It should also require that each state justify trade measures that would limit or prevent trade in health-related goods and services by demonstrating that they are necessary for achieving the chosen level of health care. That document would thereby reflect two values in democratic countries: free trade and the right to health. More important, a broad rule would state that liberalization of trade in health-related goods and services cannot undermine the right to health or a party's public health systems. While this balancing may seem hard to achieve, it seems to me essential to reconciling globalization with respect for the principles underlying the health-care system that countries such as Canada have put in place.

REFERENCES

Anderson, M., C. Auld, C. Bolton, A. Gregory, and J. McBride. 1997. 'The Economic Impact of Bill C-91 on the Cost of Pharmaceuticals in Canada.' Kingston, Ont.: Queen's Health Policy Research Unit, Queen's University.
Bettcher, D.W., D. Yach, and G.E. Guindon. 2000. 'Global Trade and Health: Key Linkages and Future Challenges,' Bulletin of the WHO 78, no. 4: 521–34. www.who.int/bulletin/tableofcontents/2000/vol.78no.4.html, April 2002.
Carey, John, 2001. 'Costly Drugs: An Even Bloodier Backlash Ahead.' Business Week, 28 May, 40.
Correa, Carlos, M. 2000. 'Implementing National Public Health Policies in the Framework of WTO Agreements.' Journal of World Trade 34, no. 5: 89–121.
Johnson, Jon R. 1998. International Trade Law. Concord, Ont.: Irwin Law.
Kinnon, C.M. 1998. 'World Trade: Bringing Health into the Picture.' World Health Forum 19: 397–405.
Lexchin, J. 2001. Globalization, Trade Deals and Drugs. Briefing Paper Series: Trade and Investment. Ottawa: Canadian Centre for Policy Alternatives, Nov. 2001.
Normand, François. 1998. 'L'AMI, prise trois.' Le Devoir, 26 Sept.

Pollock, M. Allyson, and David Price. 2000. 'Rewriting the Regulations: How the World Trade Organization Could Accelerate Privatisation in Health-Care Systems.' *Lancet* 356 (6 Dec.): 1995.

République française, Avis et rapports du Conseil économique et social. 2001. *Les négociations commerciales multilatérales: le cas des services*. Paris: Les Éditions des journaux officiels.

Sanger, Matthew. 2001. *Reckless Abandon: Canada, the GATS and the Future of Health Care*. Ottawa: Canadian Centre for Policy Alternatives.

Vellinga, Jake. 2000. 'International Trade, Health Systems and Services: A Health Policy Perspective.' *Trade Policy Research 2001*, 21 Jan. 137. www.dfait-maeci.gc.ca/eet/pdf/07-en.pdf Dec. 2001.

Woodward, David, Nick Drager, Robert Beaglehole, and Debra Lipson. 2001. 'Globalisation and Health: A Framework for Analysis and Action.' *Bulletin of the World Health Organization* 79, no. 9: 875–81.

World Health Organization. 2001. *Globalization, Patents and Drugs. An Annotated Bibliography*. 2nd ed. Geneva: Health Economics and Drugs, EDM Series no. 10.

World Health Organization and World Trade Organization. 2002. *WTO Agreements and Public Health*. Joint Study by WHO and the WTO Secretariat. Geneva: WTO Secretariat.

WTO. 1998a. Council for Trade in Services, Health and Social Services. *Background Note by the Secretariat*. S/C/W/50, 18 Sept.

– 1998b. *Communication of the United States*. S/C/W/56, 20 Oct.